RENAL DIET COOKBOOK FOR BEGINNERS

600+ Easy-to-Prepare & Tasty Recipes to Help You Manage Kidney Problems and Avoid Dialysis. Low-Sodium, Potassium, and Phosphorus Proposals to Living a Healthy Life

DR. LINDSAY BURTON

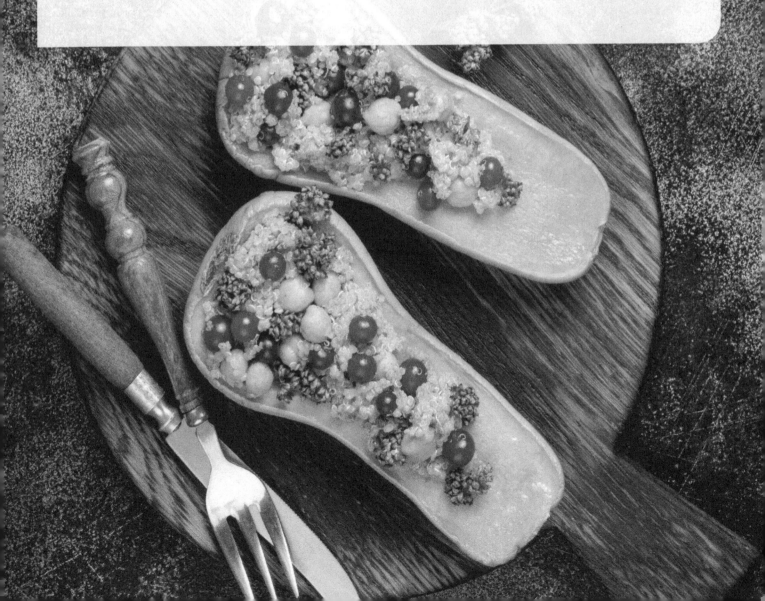

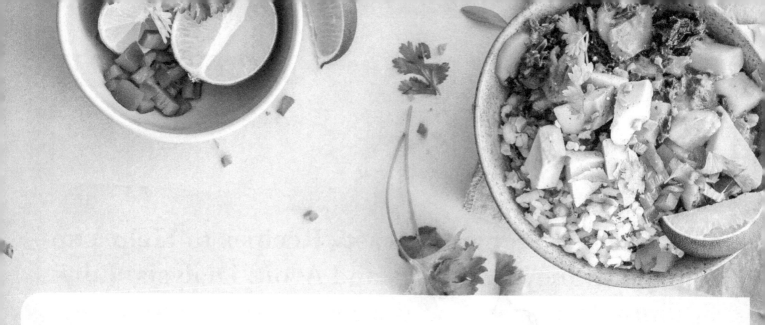

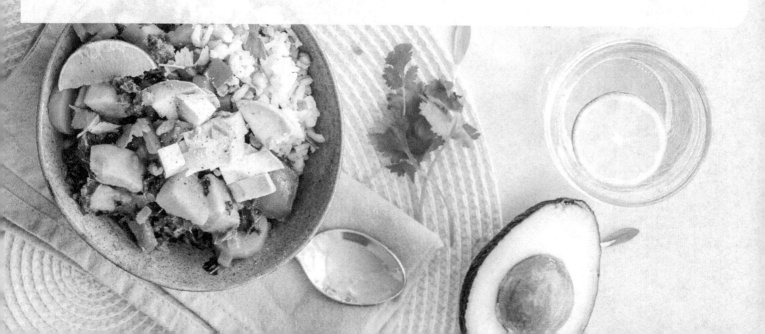

Table of Contents

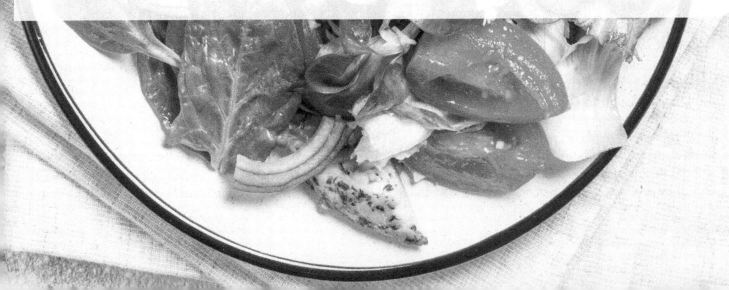

Introduction

A renal diet is actually a diet that is low in sodium, phosphorus, and potassium, which are three minerals that the system cannot metabolize properly and filter out (in excess levels) when renal function is compromised. To do that, you need to watch what you eat, carefully preparing or arranging your meals so that you receive the required nutrition, minus all the unnecessary components.

Whether you have kidney disease or related conditions, there are many benefits to adapting to the renal diet. It's a good way to eat and live, especially if you may be susceptible to kidney infections and other issues that impact this vital organ's function. This includes making changes early and paying close attention to your symptoms and any changes you notice, as these may indicate the progression in the kidney disease itself or a positive change in your kidneys' function. Keeping an eye on the slightest changes can make a significant difference in improving your health and taking charge of your well-being.

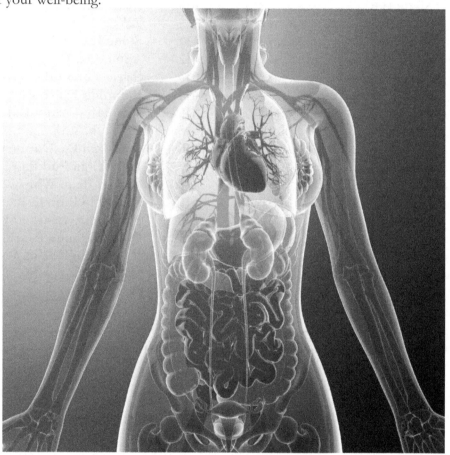

A proper renal diet is a non-medicinal solution to kidney problems. It is both preventive and restrictive to help treat kidney disease by controlling the consumption of kidney-damaging elements like sodium, potassium, and phosphorous. While these minerals are important for maintaining blood pressure, hydration, nerve impulses, and hormone regulation, too much can burden the kidneys, eventually damaging kidney cells called nephrons. The renal diet works to protect our kidneys.

Firstly, this specific diet calls for lower sodium consumption by restricting salts and products high in salt. It also proposes lower potassium consumption by restricting high-potassium salt substitutes and canned items. Similarly, it also limits phosphorus consumption in excessive amounts.

We have already gone through the list of the items suitable for low sodium, low phosphorus, and low potassium diet. The recipes shared in this book are created with these limits in mind.

Secondly, the diet prohibits all food that could indirectly affect kidney health related to high blood pressure, edema, heart problems, diabetes, etc. Here, high amounts of protein can contribute to kidney damage once they are digested since they produce toxic substances. This is why the renal diet recommends reducing protein consumption as much as possible.

Moreover, fruits, vegetables, juices, and water play an important role in the renal diet. Drinking more fluids creates an unclean environment inside the kidneys to provide instant relief to damaged or strained kidney cells. Exercise and physical activity also play their part in making this diet effective as they help improve your metabolism and break down the food you eat more.

An individualized renal diet works in various ways to support your remaining kidney function. This section reviews the renal diet guidelines, focusing on the nutrients that you may need to limit, as well as pointers to help you make smart choices for managing your CKD. The stage of your CKD, your individual lab values, and your other coexisting conditions are all important factors to consider. Before making dietary changes, always consult with your healthcare provider (HCP), who may provide you with more specific recommendations based on your unique health situation. Chronic kidney disease is a term used to describe how a person's kidneys gradually fail, resulting in the need for more and more dialysis treatments. In earlier times, when a person had kidney disease, they would be confined to a hospital bed. With the advent of dialysis machines and kidney transplantation, kidney disease can be managed at home.

Living with the renal disease doesn't mean that you have to give up eating food. You can still eat practically, but you'll need to change some of your habits and become more familiar with the renal diet. As with any diet or weight-loss strategies, it's essential to follow a routine to stray from your practice. Try one of these tips to stay on track: When it comes to chronic kidney disease, lifestyle changes, and kidney diet can help you survive kidney failure. The Renal Diet Cookbook for Beginners Renal Diet Cookbook for Beginners is full of advice to manage your condition. Kidney health is a significant part of overall health. Chronic kidney disease is no joke and can be fatal if it is not managed correctly. The Renal Diet Cookbook for Beginners gives you the knowledge needed to start working on your kidney disease. Some bad habits can influence your kidneys, but some good habits can help you lower blood pressure and increase blood flow to your kidneys. Below we have written down some tips that can help you with chronic renal disease and other topics related to kidney health.

The Renal Diet Cookbook for Beginners Renal Diet Cookbook is designed to give you the tips, ideas, and inspiration you need to manage and treat chronic kidney disease – also known as CKD.

Chronic kidney disease (CKD) is a severe condition that can cause kidney failure. There are two types of CKD: Chronic renal failure is caused by damaged kidneys and leads to kidney function loss. Congestive heart failure leads to an inability to get enough oxygen into the body, called hypoxia.

To control chronic kidney disease symptoms, it is necessary to know which foods are suitable for the kidneys and which kinds of food you should avoid. This article will give you tips about managing CKD, everyday habits that can lead to kidney problems, and more.

The Renal Diet Cookbook was created with dietitians and physicians' help to give you better control over your CKD. It gives you the understanding that you need to monitor your nutrition and adjust when necessary. A renal diet is a food that is recommended for people with chronic kidney disease. It works by lowering the amount of protein in your diet. The result is that you will need to use less dialysis treatment or kidney transplant for those people with chronic kidney disease.

If you are new to the system of renal diet, we will guide you through the process.

A renal diet is a particular type of eating plan that you need to follow if you have chronic kidney disease. It is not difficult to follow. It can be both uncomplicated and amusing!

Renal diet does not eliminate proteins; it simply cuts them back by 50% and adds fruits and vegetables. The goal of a renal diet is to prevent protein wasting by reducing the workload of your kidneys. This means that with a renal diet, fewer toxins are being produced in your body. This improves your overall health, increases energy levels, and reduces inflammation. It also helps you recover from illness faster, which will allow you to delay dialysis for more extended periods.

You will notice that your overall hunger will reduce while following a renal diet.

You can follow a renal diet to manage your chronic kidney disease without too much difficulty. You should be aware of various things, though: This book shows you how to incorporate a kidney diet into your lifestyle so that you can live a healthier life. It has recipes that are easy to follow with simple instructions. Each recipe will give you a complete breakdown of all the nutrients that it contains so that you can monitor your health while still eating delicious food! A renal diet is a diet that's specifically designed for people with kidney problems. A renal diet is low in potassium, phosphorus, protein, sodium, and fluid. People with kidney disease are at increased risk of developing cardiovascular disease, type 2 diabetes, high blood pressure, and osteoporosis.

A diabetic person must maintain his/her blood sugar by choosing the right food and beverages to prevent the worse condition of kidney disease. Only a kidney-friendly diet can help you in the protection of kidneys from more damage. By choosing a kidney-friendly diet, you can limit particular foods to avoid the build-up of minerals in your body.

Salt or sodium is one of the essential ingredients that the renal diet prohibits its use. This ingredient, although simple, can badly and powerfully affect your body and especially the kidneys. Any excess of sodium can't be easily filtered because of the failing condition of the kidneys. A massive build-up of sodium can cause catastrophic results on your body. Potassium and Phosphorus are also prohibited for kidney patients depending on the stage of kidney disease.

Kidney disease or "renal disease" and "kidney damage" is a health condition where the kidneys cannot function healthily and properly. Chronic kidney disease is a slow-moving disease and does not cause the patient many complaints in the initial stages. Chronic kidney disease includes a group of kidney diseases, in which case the renal function decreases for several years or decades. With the help of timely diagnosis and treatment, it can slow down and even stop kidney disease progression.

Anatomically, the kidneys are positioned in the abdomen, at the back, usually on both sides of the spine. The renal artery, which is a direct branch of the aorta, supplies blood to the kidneys. Renal veins empty the blood from kidneys to the vena cava, then the heart. The word "renal" originated from the Latin word for kidney.

There is a special connection between the health and function of our kidneys and the way we eat. How we eat and the foods we choose make a significant impact on how well we feel and our overall well-being. Making changes to your diet is often necessary to guard against medical conditions. While eating well can treat existing conditions, healthy food choices can also help prevent many other conditions from developing – including kidney disease.

Consider the related conditions that contribute to high blood pressure and type 2 diabetes. The dietary changes are often suggested to treat and, in some successful cases, reverse the damage of these conditions. Dietary changes for the treatment and prevention of disease often focus on limiting salt, sugar, and trans fats from our food choices, while increasing minerals, protein, and fiber, among other beneficial nutrients. The renal diet also focuses on eliminating, or at least limiting, the consumption of various ingredients to aid our kidneys to function better and to prevent further damage from occurring.

Other types of food may be harmful to kidneys infected with a disease, so you need to make sure you have a sound knowledge of the infection and how it affects the body.

You don't want kidney disease, but there are ways to boost your well-being by changing your diet. In reality, renal diets help you manage your health and reduce kidney disease.

You need to remember—changing your diet won't heal everybody, but it can help everyone. It doesn't mean a diet is a cure-all, so don't think of this article as medical advice; it's more of a guide.

Kidney disease is rarely thought about by people unless they have been diagnosed with it themselves. Yet, while many Americans go on their way, unaware an estimated thirty-seven million adults have been diagnosed with the condition. Not only that, but a person can feel fine and seem healthy and still be at a high risk of developing this disease if they don't take care of themselves, as millions of Americans are at risk. Thankfully, if a person is aware of the risk of kidney disease and the condition is detected early, it can help prevent the progression of the disease and potential kidney failure. Therefore, early diagnosis, treatment, and understanding of kidney disease and kidney health are vital.

People who can easily develope chronic kidney disease are those with a family history of kidney failure, diabetes, and high blood pressure. The elderly, Latinx people, Native people, Pacific Islanders, and black people are also at an increased risk of developing kidney disease.

If your doctor suspects you might have kidney disease or that you are at an increased risk of developing kidney problems, they will check your blood pressure, urine albumin, and serum creatinine. Increased markers on these three tests usually result in a kidney disease diagnosis, but your doctor who is familiar with your individual case will be able to know for sure and officially diagnose you. Keep in mind that nobody but your doctor can diagnose you with kidney disease, even if your test results indicate you might have one.

If you are worried that you or someone you care about may have developed kidney disease, then see your doctor right away. They will be able to run the necessary test to either confirm or deny whether you have the condition. Usually, both kidneys will be affected by the disease. As the kidneys become damaged, they will be unable to properly filter your blood, resulting in excess fluid and waste within your body. While there are often no symptoms present until the late stages of the disease, it is possible to experience side effects.

And, of course, you should be more careful of kidney disease if there is any history of it in your family. If you are concerned about an increased risk of developing the disease, ask your doctor about a plan to monitor your kidney health in the future to prevent any damage from going unchecked.

Track your phosphorous consumption——creamers, pasta, cereals, and rice are on the OK list.

Restrict liquid intake to 48 oz. Each day's recommended fluid level for renal diets is certain fluid in items like grapes, ice cream, oranges, etc.

Track your salt intake—you'll need to be a tag reader to make sure you keep your salt intake low——know what you're putting in your body and what it might contain.

Regulate your protein intake—maintain 5-7 ounces. Use egg replacements instead of regular eggs as a useful technique for low protein consumption.

If you choose to use a dietitian, they can point you precisely to what you should and shouldn't consume and why. Being aware of the effect food has on your body is essential and can help you feel good every day. Also, this design is not an alternative to clinical guidelines. Yet renal diets help most kidney disease sufferers to become and stay healthier.

As such, you have to watch the amount of sodium you consume per day. Try to limit your sodium consumption to 140 – 150 milligrams per serving for snacks and 400 – 500 mg per serving for meals. Generally, chronic kidney disease (CKD) patients are advised to keep their daily intake of sodium between 1500 to 2000 milligrams. However, you may need to consult a kidney dietitian to be sure of the right amount of sodium you are allowed to consume per day, depending on the condition of your kidneys and other variables

Human health hangs in a complete balance when all of its interconnected bodily mechanisms function properly in perfect sync. Without its major organs working normally, the body soon suffers permanent damage. Kidney malfunction is one such example, and it is not just the entire water balance that is disturbed by the kidney disease, but a number of other diseases also emerge due to this problem. Kidney diseases are progressive in nature, meaning that if left unchecked and uncontrolled, they can ultimately lead to permanent kidney damage. That is why it is essential to control and manage the disease and put a halt to its progress, which can be done through medicinal and natural means. While medicines can guarantee only thirty percent of the cure, a change of lifestyle and diet can prove to be miraculous with their seventy percent of guaranteed results. A kidney-friendly diet and lifestyle not only saves the kidneys from excess minerals but it also aids medicines to work actively. Treatment without a good diet, hence, proves to be useless. In this renal diet cookbook, we shall bring out the basic facts about kidney diseases, their symptoms, causes, and diagnosis. This preliminary introduction can help the readers understand the problem clearly; then, we shall discuss the role of renal diet and kidney-friendly lifestyle in curbing the diseases. And it's not just that. The book also contains a range of delicious renal diet recipes which will guarantee luscious flavors and good health. Despite their tiny size, the kidneys perform a number of functions, which are vital for the body to be able to function healthily.

These include:

- Filtering excess fluids and waste from the blood
- Creating the enzyme known as renin, which regulates blood pressure,
- Ensuring bone marrow creates red blood cells,
- They are controlling calcium and phosphorus levels through absorption and excretion.

Chapter 1. All about The Renal Diet

Renal Diet is a diet that aims to lower kidney stones or disease by eating an ultra-low sodium, low-phosphorus, low-sodium diet. Found on the internet and in some books, like Dr. Fuhrman's Eat to Live. It can help to dissolve kidney stones and dissolve plaque buildup within the kidneys caused by high levels of calcium in urine, which can often cause kidney disease or make it harder for us to recover from injury or illness. Renal Diet is vegan and promotes good health through proper nutrition like fruits and vegetables with lots of nutrients like antioxidants for healing wounds but not processed refined foods with artificial colors, flavors, preservatives etc. Dr. Fuhrman's site says "The first book to explain how to take control of heart disease and reverse the effects of high blood pressure and high cholesterol. This book has the most in-depth information on essential nutrients and how to obtain, store and use them for optimal health."

As we know we need a healthy diet in order to avoid disease, so we can eat any food we want, but your kidneys filter the excess salt in your body into urine which helps keep you alive. You need sodium in your body even though it is an excess that can be harmful when its within certain proportions in your blood when it becomes too much over time, when you drink excess water or when you eat too much salt. The Renal diet is a diet that takes this in mind and is aimed at people with kidney disease or high levels of calcium in their urine. When your body does not have enough sodium to create the salt you need, you become dehydrated and if not taken care of can die within 24 hours. In order to prevent this from happening, you need to watch the salt intake when on this diet which is why it's called a renal diet because people with renal disease must be careful about how much salt they consume.

How Does This Work?

There are a number of things that can cause an overabundance of calcium in the body. The main source is drinking too much water and peeing a flushed-out by-product called urine. It can also be found in the foods we eat. In order to prevent this, you need to avoid drinking excess water, including mouthwash or mouthwash containing fluoride rinse which have high levels of salt, and produce too much urine. Also, high amounts of sodium from processed foods can promote kidney disease so it's not worth consuming for your health either.

How To Use It?

The renal diet is a holistic way of making sure that your body is getting the best nutrients that it needs for health and to prevent diseases. This includes getting rid of excess salt from processed foods which you can get from things like pizzas, burgers, cookies, burgers, fries from fast-food places or anything with a high amount of sodium. You go through a transition phase where you'll slowly cut back on salt by consuming less and less processed foods and drink more water. Eventually this diet will make you healthier in the long run once all excess salt has been washed out your system and you won't have to worry about it anymore.

Renal Diet Tips:

If you're on a renal diet, basically what happens is that after a while of consuming less salt and drinking excess water, all this extra water will flush out the kidneys and clean them out. Your body will be uncomfortable during this time so you will start to drink less water so it makes it easier for your kidneys to filter more efficiently. During the transition phase of the diet, you won't feel good because your body has been overloaded with too much salt from processed foods and not enough water to wash it out. This can cause kidney stones another painful feeling. In order to avoid these things from happening, you need to make sure you're drinking enough water and limit your salt intake. So, what you would do is drink a lot of water until your body flushes out all the bad stuff that it doesn't need. You can use a website called medicinenet.com that has a lot of information on renal diets and how to get started. Below is some helpful information taken directly from their site:

This article is based on an interview with Dr. Fuhrman. Dr. Fuhrman is a board-certified family physician and chairman of the Nutritional Research Foundation.

Dr. Fuhrman has been working with patients with kidney disease for more than two decades, using diet to prevent and treat chronic illness. After performing an initial analysis of the patient's condition, he develops a treatment plan that includes a dietary change, exercise routine and supplements needed to obtain optimal nutrition.

Dr. Fuhrman's Renal Diet allows individuals with kidney disease to have a normal life, consuming all the nutrients they need while being able to adhere to a sodium-restricted diet that can help reduce or prevent blood pressure elevation.

Chapter 2. Shopping List

Vegetables:
- Arugula (raw)
- Alfalfa sprouts
- Bamboo shoots
- Asparagus
- Beans - pinto, wax, fava, green
- Bean sprouts
- Bitter melon (balsam pear)
- Broccoli
- Broad beans (boiled, fresh)
- Cactus
- Cabbage - red, swamp, Napa/ Suey Choy, skunk
- Carrots
- Calabash
- Celery
- Cauliflower
- Chayote
- Celeriac (cooked)
- Collard greens
- Chicory
- Cucumber
- Corn
- Okra
- Onions
- Pepitas
- Green Peas
- Peppers
- Radish
- Radicchio
- Seaweed
- Rapini (raw)
- Shallots
- Green lettuce (raw)
- Snow peas
- Dandelion greens (raw)
- Daikon
- Plant Leaves
- Drumstick
- Endive
- Eggplant
- Fennel bulb
- Escarole
- Fiddlehead greens
- Ferns
- Hearts of Palm
- Irish moss
- Hominy
- Jicama, raw
- Leeks
- Kale(raw)
- Mushrooms (raw white)
- Lettuce (raw)
- Mustard greens
- Squash
- Turnip
- Tomatillos (raw)
- Watercress
- Turnip greens
- Wax beans
- Water chestnuts (canned)
- Winter melon
- Wax gourd
- Zucchini (raw)

Fruits:
- Acerola Cherries
- Apple
- Blackberries
- Asian Pear
- Boysenberries
- Blueberries
- Cherries
- Casaba melon
- Clementine
- Chokeberries
- Crabapples
- Cloudberries
- Cranberries (fresh)
- Grapefruit
- Gooseberries
- Pomegranate
- Grapes
- Rambutan
- Quince
- Rhubarb
- Raspberries (fresh or frozen)
- Jujubes
- Golden Berry
- Kumquat
- Jackfruit
- Lingonberries
- Lemon
- Loganberries
- Lime
- Lychees
- Mango
- Mandarin orange
- Peach
- Pineapple
- Pear
- Plum
- Strawberries
- Rose-apple

- Tangerine
- Tangelo
- Watermelon

Fresh Meat, Seafood, and Poultry:
- Chicken
- Beef and Ground Beef
- Goat
- Duck
- Wild Game
- Pork
- Lamb
- Veal
- Turkey
- Fish

Milk, Eggs, and Dairy: Milk:
- Milk (½-1 cup/day)

Non-Dairy Milk:
- Almond Fresh (Original, Unsweetened, Vanilla)
- Almond Breeze (Original, Vanilla, Vanilla Unsweetened, Original Unsweetened)
- Silk True Almond Beverage (Unsweetened Original, Original, Vanilla, Unsweetened Vanilla)
- Good Karma Flax Delight (Vanilla, Original, Unsweetened)
- Rice Dream Rice Drink (Vanilla Classic, Non-Enriched Original Classic)
- Silk Soy Beverage (Original, Vanilla, Unsweetened)
- Natura Organic Fortified Rice Beverage (Original, Vanilla)
- PC Organics Fortified Rice Beverage

Other Dairy Products:
- Non-Hydrogenated Margarine (Salt-Free or Regular)
- Butter (Unsalted or Regular)
- Whipping Cream
- Sour Cream
- Whipped Cream

Chapter 3. A 7-Step Guide To A Plant-Based Renal Diet

This post covers some of the basics of how to go vegan and is a general guide for those who are interested and new to the diet. This is a more detailed post on some of the food you can eat on a plant-based renal diet, as well as key nutrients that may be lacking in this type of diet. Some dietary supplements will be mentioned, but this list does not cover all plants or their corresponding nutrient values.

General Principles of a Plant-Based Renal Diet.

1) Avoid all animal products. Basically any animal product should be avoided. This includes flesh, milk, eggs, cheese, ice cream or other dairy products; fish; poultry; and cooked foods that contain gelatin (such as jello or puddings), shellfish including shrimp and lobster; meat extracts like gravy mixes (spices) and basting sauces (e.g. ketchup); fish oils; gelatin desserts (e.g. marshmallows) or Jello; gelatin-based candies (e.g. jellies) or marshmallows; gelatin molds or jellied shellfish molds; pistachios, almonds, cashews, hazelnuts, sunflower seeds, sesame seeds and all other nuts that are processed with shells on them (e.g. oil roasted nuts) except for peanuts which are recommended.

2) It is important to understand the terminology used to quantify food. There are many different types of food that are used in the study of nutrition. For the plant-based diet, there are three terms that you need to learn about: plant, whole food, and nutrient density. A plant is any raw or cooked vegetable or fruit that has not been processed with an animal product or bone broth (e.g., fruits are considered fruits). A whole food is any plant that has not been refined, processed, or modified in any form. Processed foods are anything containing an animal-product (including meat, dairy, eggs), cooked with meat or bone broth products or products containing gelatin, has sugar added to it (no matter the source), or has any other forms of artificial modification.

3) All plant-based foods should be whole foods unless packaged/bottled by the manufacturer. Whole foods include tubers (e.g., potatoes, beets, carrots, yams), fruits, beans and legumes. All plant-based foods should be eaten in a 100% whole food form.

4) Focus on eating a variety of fruits and vegetables. Fruits and vegetables have a wide variety of nutritional values due to their fiber content. Vegetables have more fiber than fruits and fruit juices do not contain enough fiber to benefit the body in any way. Therefore, veggies are more beneficial than fruit.

5) A person on a plant-based diet for the person with diabetes should eat 2-3 cups of vegetables with each meal. A cup is approximately 150 grams or 5 ounces. Vegetables have the most benefits of all food groups, therefore consuming them regularly is important. The main things to aim for are steamed, or stir fried (if using oil), or roasted (if using oil), or cooked in some other healthy way with herbs/spices/minerals for flavor (e.g. fresh tomato sauce or a stir-fry, a soup or a stew) with no animal products added.

6) The best way to prepare vegetables is to steam them in a pressure cooker for 5 to 10 minutes. If steaming is not practical, roasting them in the oven (at 400 degrees F.) is another good option. However, roasting at high temperatures will cause the vegetable to lose some of its nutritional value. A better option would be to roast them for 30 mins at 225 degrees F.

7) A person on a plant-based diet for the person with diabetes should eat 1 ½ to 2 cups of fruit with each meal. A cup is approximately 145 grams or 5 ounces. Fruits are known to have more carbohydrates than vegetables, so they are not recommended for the evening meal. For this reason, they are recommended for eating in the morning and afternoon meals.

Chapter 4. Breakfast

1. Bowl of Oatmeal

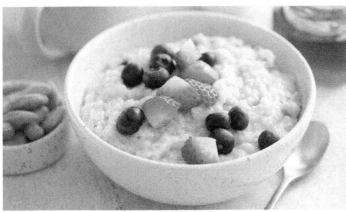

Preparation Time: 5 minutes
Cooking Time: 5 minutes
Servings: 2
Ingredients:
- ½ C. of quick oatmeal
- ½ to 2/3 C. of hot or cold water
- ½ C. of vegetable milk
- 1 tsp. of maqui berry powder or acai powder (optional)
- ½ C. of fresh grapes or berries
- ½ banana (or a whole banana, if you prefer)
- ¼ Walnuts

Directions:
1. Put together the oatmeal and water in a bowl. Let them soak for a few minutes.
2. Cut the banana and grapes or berries as you wish and add them to the oatmeal.
3. Pour vegetable milk over oatmeal and fruits.
4. Cover with nuts, seeds, powdered maqui berry, or acai powder.

Nutrition: Calories: 222 Fat: 4g Carbohydrates: 40g Protein: 9.9g

2. Oatmeal Seasoned with Vegetables

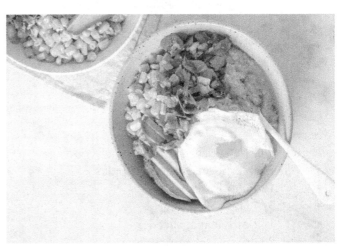

Preparation Time: 10 minutes
Cooking Time: 7 minutes
Servings: 2
Ingredients:
- 4 cups of water
- 2 cups of "cut" oatmeal (quick-cooking steel-cut oats)
- 1 teaspoon Italian spices
- 1/2 teaspoon Herbamare or sea salt
- 1 teaspoon garlic powder
- 1 teaspoon onion powder
- 1/2 cup nutritional yeast
- 1/4 teaspoon turmeric powder
- 1 1/2 cup kale or tender spinach
- 1/2 cup sliced mushrooms
- 1/4 cup grated carrots
- 1/2 cup small chopped peppers

Directions:
1. Boil the water in a saucepan.
2. Add the oatmeal and spices and lower the temperature.
3. Cook over low heat without lid for 5 to 7 minutes.
4. Add the vegetables.
5. Cover and set aside for 2 minutes.
6. Serve immediately.

Nutrition: Calories: 90 Fat: 3.3g Carbohydrates: 13g Protein: 2g

3. Fruit and Nut Oatmeal

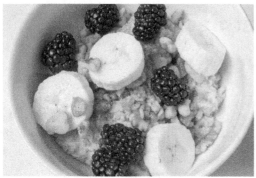

Preparation Time: 5 minutes
Cooking Time: 10 minutes
Servings: 3
Ingredients:
*   2 tablespoons chopped apples
*   1/4 cup fresh berries
*   3/4 cup rolled oats
*   1/2 of banana, sliced
*   2 tablespoons apricot
*   2 tablespoons cranberries
*   1/4 teaspoon ground cinnamon
*   1/4 teaspoon of sea salt
*   2 tablespoons chopped walnuts
*   2 tablespoons raisins
*   2 tablespoons maple syrup
*   1 1/2 cup water

Directions:
1.   Take a small saucepan, place it over high heat, add oats, pour in water, and bring it to a boil.
2.   Switch heat to medium-low level, simmer for 5 minutes until oats have cooked.
3.   Get the pan from heat then stir in salt and cinnamon.
4.   Distribute oats evenly among bowls, top with remaining ingredients, drizzle with maple syrup in the end, and then serve.
Nutrition: Calories: 250 Fat: 11g Carbohydrates: 34g Protein: 8g

4. Flaxseed Pancakes

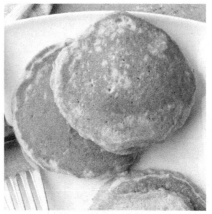

Preparation Time: 10 minutes
Cooking Time: 10 minutes
Servings: 6
Ingredients:
*   3 cups oatmeal
*   1/2 cup of millet flour
*   1/2 cup ground flax seeds
*   1 teaspoon of sea salt
*   1 1/2 teaspoon baking soda
*   2 teaspoons baking powder
*   4 cups vanilla almond milk
*   2 tablespoons rice vinegar
*   1 tablespoon maple honey or date paste
*   1 tablespoon pure vanilla extract
*   3 tablespoons unsweetened applesauce

Directions:
1.   Put and mix all dry ingredients in a bowl.
2.   In a different bowl, mix the liquid ingredients.
3.   Add the liquid ingredients over the dry ones and combine them well.
4.   Process the mixture well in a blender until smooth and lump-free.
5.   Heat a pan over medium-low heat.
6.   Using a spoon, pour the desired amount of mixture into the pan.
7.   Turn the pancake when bubbles appear on the top, and underneath it is firm for approximately 5 minutes.
Nutrition: Calories: 161.5 Fat: 7g Carbohydrates: 10g Protein: 16g

Nutrition: Calories: 83 Fat: 1.6g Carbohydrates: 15g Protein: 4g

5. Oatmeal Breakfast Muffins

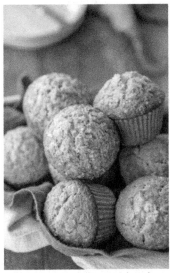

Preparation Time: 20 minutes
Cooking Time: 45 minutes
Servings: 6
Ingredients:
- 2 1/2 cups of flaked oatmeal
- 1/2 cup oatmeal
- 1 teaspoon baking powder
- 1/2 teaspoon baking soda
- 1/2 teaspoon salt
- 1 tablespoon cinnamon
- 1/2 teaspoon ground nutmeg
- 4 ripe bananas, crushed
- 1 grated apple
- 1/2 cup non-dairy milk
- 2 teaspoons vanilla extract
- 1/2 cup raisins
- 1/2 cup chopped walnuts (optional)

Directions:
1. Preheat the oven to 300-350 F (177 C).
2. In a large bowl, combine and beat the dry ingredients.
3. In a small bowl, combine bananas, apple, non-dairy milk, vanilla, and stir until well combined.
4. Put together the wet ingredients to the dry ones and combine them well.
5. Add raisins and nuts if you use them.
6. If you use a mold for 6 muffins, bake for 45 minutes. If you use a mold of 12 muffins, bake for 35 minutes.

6. Cherry and Poppy Seed Muffins

Preparation Time: 10 minutes
Cooking Time: 30 minutes
Servings: 12
Ingredients:
- 1 cup (120 g) raw buckwheat flour
- 1 1/4 cup oatmeal (155 g) oatmeal
- 2 tablespoons poppy seeds
- 2 teaspoons cinnamon
- 1/2 teaspoon cardamom
- 2 teaspoons baking powder
- 10 chopped figs
- A little more than 1 cup (260 ml) of vegetable milk, without sugar
- 2 ripe bananas
- 2 heaped tablespoons unsweetened applesauce
- 2 tablespoons peanut butter
- 1 pinch of sea salt (optional)
- 1/2 cup (50 g) dark chocolate (at least 70% cocoa), chopped
- 24 fresh or frozen cherries

Directions:
1. Preheat the oven to 355 F.
2. Cut the figs and soak them in vegetable milk for at least 30 minutes. If you want to dip it further, put it in the refrigerator.
3. While the figs are soaked, chop the chocolate, and place it aside. Prepare all other dry ingredients in a bowl. Put the figs and milk into the mixer.
4. Put all remaining wet ingredients and mix until smooth.
5. Pour the wet mixture over the dry ingredients and mix well. Make sure there are no lumps. Add chopped chocolate.
6. The mold is filled with 12 muffins (molded using silicon) with a lump and finally hits two cherries in each muffin.
7. Bake for 25-30 minutes. Allow it to cool a little before trying to remove it from the mold.

Nutrition: Calories: 114.5 Fat: 2g Carbohydrates: 22g Protein: 2.53

7. Brown Rice Breakfast Pudding with Dates

Preparation Time: 10 minutes
Cooking Time: 15 minutes
Servings: 2
Ingredients:
* 1 cup dates, pitted, chopped
* 3 cups cooked brown rice
* 1 apple, cored, chopped
* 1/4 teaspoon salt
* 1 cinnamon stick
* 1/4 cup raisins
* 1/4 teaspoon ground cloves
* 1/4 cup slivered almonds, toasted
* 2 cups almond milk, unsweetened

Directions:
1. Take a medium saucepan, place it over medium-low heat, add rice, stir in dates, cinnamon, and cloves, pour in milk, stir until mixed, and then cook for 12 minutes until thickened.
2. Then, remove the cinnamon stick from the pudding and remove the pan from heat.
3. Add apple and raisins into the pudding, season with salt, and stir until mixed.
4. Garnish pudding with almonds and then serve.

Nutrition: Calories: 118 Fat: 0.7g Carbohydrates: 21g Protein: 7.6g

8. Quinoa with Berries

Preparation Time: 5 minutes
Cooking Time: 15 minutes
Servings: 4
Ingredients:
* 2 cups almond milk
* 3/4 cups uncooked quinoa
* 1 tbsp. Almond butter
* 3 chopped walnuts
* 1 tbsp. Maple syrup
* 1 cup strawberries
* 1 oz. Sunflower seeds

Directions:
1. Warm nonstick pan over medium heat and pour milk into a saucepan.

2. Once the milk boils, add quinoa, and reduce heat to medium.
3. With cover, let it simmer for 15 minutes or until the milk has been absorbed.
4. Remove from the heat, add some milk, almond butter, walnuts, and maple syrup.
5. Mix well and place the quinoa in a bowl.
6. Top with strawberries and sunflower seeds.
7. Serve and enjoy!

Nutrition: Calories: 224 Fat: 2.5g Carbohydrates: 43g Protein: 4g

9. Breakfast Scramble

Preparation Time: 5 minutes
Cooking Time: 20 minutes
Servings: 2
Ingredients:
* 1 cup of fresh spinach
* 1/8 teaspoon of black pepper
* 1/2 a teaspoon of onion powder
* 1/2 teaspoon of garlic powder
* 1 tablespoon of vegetable broth
* 2 tablespoons of nutritional yeast
* 1/2 a diced bell pepper
* 4 ounces of sliced mushrooms
* 1 packet of extra firm tofu

Directions:
1. Prepare frying pan over medium temperature.
2. Drain off the tofu, place it in a bowl and mash it down with a fork.
3. Transfer the tofu into the frying pan and add pepper, garlic powder, onion powder, broth, nutritional yeast, bell pepper, and mushrooms.
4. Add cover on the frying pan and leave it to cook for 10 minutes. Stir the ingredients after 5 minutes.
5. Put spinach and cook for another 5 minutes, divide onto plates, and serve.

Nutrition: Calories: 121 Fat: 5g Carbohydrates: 10.6g Protein: 10g

10. Simple Granola Platter

Preparation Time: 5 minutes
Cooking Time: 25 minutes
Serving: 4
Ingredients:
* 1-ounce porridge oats

- 2 teaspoons of maple syrup
- Cooking spray as needed
- 4 medium bananas
- 5-ounce fresh fruit salad, such as strawberries, blueberries, and raspberries
- 1/4-ounce pumpkin seeds
- 1/4-ounce sunflower seeds
- 1/4-ounce dry Chia seeds
- 1/4-ounce desiccated coconut

Directions:
1. Preheat your oven to 300°F.
2. Take a baking tray with baking paper.
3. Prepare a large bowl, then put the oats, seeds, and maple syrup.
4. Arrange mix on a baking tray.
5. Put coconut oil on top and bake for 20 minutes, making sure to keep stirring it from time to time.
6. Sprinkle coconut after the first 15 minutes.
7. Remove from oven and let it cool.
8. Take a bowl and layer sliced bananas.
9. Lay out cooled granola mix on top and serve with a topping of berries. Enjoy!

Nutrition: Calories: 446 Fat: 29g Carbohydrates: 37g Protein: 13g

11. Delicious Apple and Cinnamon Oatmeal

Preparation Time: 5 minutes
Cooking Time: 10 minutes
Serving: 2
Ingredients:
- 1 1/4 cups apple cider
- 1 apple, peeled, cored, and chopped
- 2/3 cup rolled oats
- 1 teaspoon ground cinnamon
- 1 tablespoon pure maple syrup

Directions:
1. Take a medium-sized saucepan, bring apple cider to boil over medium-high heat
2. Stir in apples, oats, cinnamon
3. Bring cereal to a boil and lower heat, simmer for 3-4 minutes until thickened
4. Spoon between two bowls and serve with maple syrup. Enjoy!

Nutrition: Calories: 339 Fat: 14g Carbohydrates: 40g Protein: 8g

12. Vegan Pancakes

Preparation time: 5 minutes
Cooking time: 5 minutes
Servings: 2
Ingredients:
For the pancakes
- ½ cup chickpea flour
- ½ cup of water
For filling:
- 1 large zucchini
- 2 carrots
- 1 onion
- Garlic
- Salt
- Turmeric
- Pepper
- Coconut milk or other vegetable cream

Direction:
1. Place the chickpea flour and water in a deep bowl and beat to integrate well with an electric or wire whisk.
2. Heat over medium-low heat in a medium nonstick skillet to cook pancakes. Add a few drops of oil to prevent the dough from sticking. Once the pan is very hot, add a few tablespoons of the preparation to make the first pancake. Once the edges begin to peel off, turn it over to cook on the other side. Repeat the process two more times. Reserve the pancakes.
For the filling:
3. Chop the onion and cook it in a pan with oil until it becomes transparent. Meanwhile, peel and cut the carrot and zucchini into cubes of the desired size. Also chop the garlic. Pour the garlic, carrot and zucchini into the pan and cook for a few minutes until the vegetables are tender. Finally add turmeric, pepper and serve.

Nutrition: Calorie: 73.9 Protein: 3g Fat: 0.3g Carbohydrates: 15.8

13. Instant Oats

Preparation time: 5 minutes
Cooking time: 5 minutes
Servings: 2-4
Ingredients:
- ½ cup oatmeal
- ½ - 2/3 cup hot or cold water

- ½ cup of vegetable milk
- 1 teaspoon of maqui berry powder
- ½ cup fresh grapes or berries
- Half banana
- Walnuts
- Seeds

Direction:

1. Combine the oatmeal and water in a bowl, and let them soak for a few minutes.
2. Cut the banana and the grapes or berries as desired, and add them to the oats.
3. Pour the vegetable milk over the oats and fruits.
4. Top with nuts, seeds, powdered maqui berry, or acai powder. You can use walnut nuts and hemp seeds.

Nutrition: Calorie: 389 Protein: 16.9g Fat: 6.9g Carbohydrates: 66.3g

14. Zucchini Rolls Stuffed with Dried Tomato Paté

Preparation time: 10 minutes
Cooking time: 10 minutes
Servings: 2-4
Ingredients:

- 1 zucchini
- ½ cup cashews or cashews
- 8 dried tomatoes
- Fresh basil leaves
- A few drops of lemon
- 1 tablespoon of olive oil
- Salt and pepper to taste

Direction:

1. Wash the zucchini well. Using a mandolin or a knife, cut it into very thin sheets. Arrange them on a plate and add salt so that they soften a little so that they can be rolled up more easily.
2. To prepare the filling, place the dried tomatoes in a bowl, add boiling water to hydrate them and let them rest for about 10 minutes.
3. Place the cashews in the glass of the blender or food processor. Add salt, a few drops of lemon, a tablespoon of olive oil, fresh basil and the hydrated tomatoes. Process until all the ingredients are well integrated and obtain a homogeneous paste.

4. To finish, arrange a sheet of zucchini on a plate, spread it with a teaspoon of dried tomato paté and roll it up.

Nutrition: Calorie: 489 Protein: 13g Fat: 4g Carbohydrates: 96g

15. Vegetable Seasoned Oats

Preparation time: 10 minutes
Cooking time: 7-10 minutes
Servings: 4-6
Ingredients:

- 2 cups of "cut" oats
- ½ teaspoon sea salt
- 1 teaspoon Italian spices
- 1 tsp garlic powder
- 4 cups of water
- ½ cup nutritional yeast
- 1 teaspoon onion powder
- ¼ tsp turmeric powder
- ½ cup mushrooms
- ¼ cup grated carrots
- 1 ½ cup kale or tender spinach
- ½ cup small peppers

Direction:

1. Boil the water in a saucepan.
2. Add the oats and spices and lower the temperature.
3. Cook over low heat without lid for 5 to 7 minutes.
4. Add the vegetables.
5. Cover and set aside for 2 minutes.
6. Serve immediately.

Nutrition: Calorie: 90 Protein: 2.4g Fat: 3.3g Carbohydrates: 12.7g

16. Vegan Pea Burger

Preparation time: 20 minutes
Cooking time: 35 minutes
Servings: 12
Ingredients:

- 2 cups cooked peas
- 1 cup of oatmeal
- 1 cooked carrot
- ½ cup black olives
- Garlic

- Salt and spices to taste

Direction:

1. Put the oats in a mixer and process it into a thick flour (you can also use the whole flakes if you prefer)

2. On the other hand, pour the peas or peas, the carrot, the olives and the garlic in the glass of a food processor or minipimer. Crush well to a sticky mass.

3. Place the preparation in a bowl and add the desired salt and spices. Mix well.

4. Finally add the oats to give a more compact consistency to the dough. Integrate well.

5. Take portions of dough by hand and form hamburgers of the desired size.

6. Arrange them on a previously oiled baking sheet. Cook in a preheated oven at 180 °C for about 15 minutes on each side or until the surface of the patties is golden

Nutrition: Calorie: 167 Protein: 21.3g Fat: 4.1g Carbohydrates: 11g

17. Vegan Tart

Preparation time: 20 minutes
Cooking time: 20 minutes
Servings: 8
Ingredients:
For the mass:
- ½ lbs. whole wheat flour
- 4 tablespoons of oil
- 2 cups of water
- 1 pinch of salt

For the filling:
- 2 leeks
- 2 cups of mushrooms
- 2 small onions
- 1 clove garlic
- 6 cherry tomatoes
- Salt, pepper and spices to taste
- 6 tbsp of chickpea flour
- 18 tablespoons of water
- 1 teaspoon of vinegar

Direction:
For the mass:

1. In a bowl place the flour, oil, water and salt and mix well to form smooth dough.

2. Roll it out on a previously oiled cake pan or upholstered with vegetable paper. Pinch the dough with a fork.

3. Bake at 180°C for 10 minutes until slightly cooked.

For the filling:

4. In a frying pan, sauté the onions, leeks and garlic in olive oil. Add the mushrooms, salt, pepper and spices and sauté for a few more minutes.

5. Once it is well cooked, pour into a bowl and let it cool down a bit.

6. In another bowl place the chickpea flour, vinegar and water and form an egg-like cream.

7. Add this mixture to the vegetables and mix well.

8. Pour it over the previously cooked dough, decorate with cherry's cut in half and take to the oven for 10-15 more minutes until the edges of the dough are well cooked and the mixture of chickpea flour, vinegar and water has linked the ingredients.

Nutrition: Calorie: 278 Protein: 4.4g Fat: 16.7g Carbohydrates: 28.9g

18. Oatmeal with Chia Seeds

Preparation time: 2h
Cooking time: 0 minutes
Servings: 1
Ingredients:
- 1.7 oz oats
- ¼ cup milk of your choice
- 2 tbsp chia seeds

Direction:

1. Firstly, once you have your ingredients ready, in a bowl or glass add the oats, the chia seeds and finally the milk until it completely covers the container.

2. Mix the ingredients well.

3. Refrigerate for at least 2 hours so that the oats and chia absorb the milk and soften.

4. After 2 hours, add a little more milk so that it moistens more and the mixture does not dry out.

Nutrition: Calorie: 353.8 Protein: 15.6g Fat: 8g Carbohydrates: 55.3g

19. Apple & Cauliflower Porridge

Preparation time: 15 minutes
Cooking time: 25 minutes
Serving: 4
Ingredients:
- 2 cups apple, peeled, cored and shredded
- ½ cup cauliflower rice
- ½ cup coconut, shredded
- 1¾ cups unsweetened coconut milk
- 1 teaspoon vanilla extract
- ¾ cup fresh strawberries, hulled and sliced

Direction:
1. In a large pan, add all the ingredients except strawberries over medium heat and bring to gentle simmer, stirring frequently.
2. Reduce the heat to low and simmer for about 15-20 minutes.
3. Serve warm with the topping of strawberries.

Meal Prep Tip:
1. Remove from heat and set aside to cool.
2. After cooling, divide the porridge into 4 containers.
3. Refrigerate for 1-2 days.
4. Remove from refrigerator and reheat in microwave before serving. Top with strawberries and serve.

Nutrition: Calories: 266, Fats: 18.1g, Carbs: 22.4g, Fiber: 4.5g, Sugar: 16.6g, Proteins: 2.4g, Sodium: 40mg

20. Pumpkin Porridge

Preparation time: 15 minutes
Cooking time: 25 minutes
Serving: 4
Ingredients:
- 1 cup water
- Pinch of salt
- 1 cup almond flour
- 2 tablespoons maple syrup
- ½ cup pumpkin puree
- ½ teaspoon ground cinnamon
- Pinch of ground nutmeg
- ½ cup almonds, chopped

Direction:

1. In a pan add water and salt over medium-high heat and bring to a boil.
2. Slowly, add the almond flour, stirring continuously.
3. Reduce the heat to medium and cook for about 15-20 minutes or until all the liquid is absorbed, stirring continuously.
4. Add the remaining ingredients except the almonds and stir to combine well.
5. Remove from the heat and serve immediately with the topping of almonds.

Meal Prep Tip:
1. Remove from heat and set aside to cool.
2. After cooling, divide the porridge into 4 containers.
3. Refrigerate for 1-2 days.
4. Remove from refrigerator and reheat in microwave before serving. Top with strawberries and serve.

Nutrition: Calories: 274, Fats: 19.4g, Carbs: 18g, Fiber: 5.5g, Sugar: 7.5g, Proteins: 8.9g, Sodium: 53mg

21. Date & Walnut Oatmeal

Preparation time: 10 minutes
Cooking time: 0 minute
Serving: 2
Ingredients:
- ½ cup rolled oats
- ¼ cup walnuts, chopped
- 2 large dates, pitted and chopped
- ½ teaspoon ground cinnamon
- ¼ teaspoon ground nutmeg
- Pinch of sea salt
- 1 cup of water

Direction:
1. In a Mason jar, place all the ingredients except the water and cover with the lid.
2. Refrigerate overnight.
3. Just before serving, add the water and microwave for about 2 minutes.
4. You can serve this oatmeal with your favorite non-dairy milk.

Meal Prep Tip:
1. Place the oatmeal into a jar and refrigerate for 2-3 days.
2. Just before serving, reheat in the microwave.

Nutrition: Calories: 202, Fats: 10.7g, Carbs: 22.8g, Fiber: 4.2g, Sugar: 6.2g, Proteins: 6.7g, Sodium: 122mg

22. Fruity Oatmeal

Preparation time: 10 minutes
Cooking time: 20 minutes
Serving: 4
Ingredients:
• 4 cups water
• 1 cup dry steel cut oats
• 1 banana, peeled and mashed
• 1 cup fresh strawberries, hulled and sliced
• ½ cup mixed nuts, chopped
Direction:
1. In a large pan, add the water and oats over medium-high heat and bring to a boil.
2. Reduce the heat to low and simmer for about 20 minutes, stirring occasionally.
3. Remove from heat and set aside to cool slightly.
4. Stir in the mashed banana.
5. Top with strawberries and nuts and serve.
Meal Prep Tip:
1. Divide the oatmeal between 4 jars and refrigerate for 2-3 days.
2. Just before serving, reheat in the microwave.
Nutrition: Calories: 226, Fats: 11.7g, Carbs: 27.4g, Fiber: 4.6g, Sugar: 6.4g, Proteins: 6g, Sodium: 64mg

23. Simple Garlic and Kale

Preparation Time: 5 minutes
Cooking Time: 10 minutes
Serving: 4
Ingredients:
• 1 bunch kale
• 2 tablespoons olive oil
• 4 garlic cloves, minced
Directions:
1. Carefully tear the kale into bite-sized portions, making sure to remove the stem
2. Discard the stems
3. Prepare a large deep pot and place it over medium heat
4. Add olive oil and let the oil heat up
5. Add garlic and stir for 2 minutes
6. Add kale and cook for 5-10 minutes. Serve!

Nutrition: Calories: 121 Fat: 8g Carbohydrates: 5g Protein: 4g

24. Crispy Morning Tofu

Preparation Time: 5 minutes
Cooking Time: 20 – 30 minutes
Serving: 8
Ingredients:
• 1-pound extra-firm tofu, drained and sliced
• 2 tablespoons olive oil
• 1 cup almond meal
• 1 tablespoon yeast
• 1/2 teaspoon onion powder
• 1/2 teaspoon garlic powder
• 1/2 teaspoon oregano
• 1/4 teaspoon salt
Directions:
1. Add all ingredients except the tofu and olive oil in a shallow bowl. Mix well.
2. Prepare your oven to 400 degrees Fahrenheit
3. In a mixing bowl, put the almond meal and mix well
4. Glaze tofu with olive oil, dip into the mix, and coat well
5. Prepare a baking sheet with parchment paper
6. Transfer coated tofu to the baking sheet
7. Bake for 30 minutes, flip once until golden brown
8. Serve and enjoy!
Nutrition: Calories: 282 Fat: 20g Carbohydrates: 9g Protein: 12g

25. Morning Eggplant Soup

Preparation Time: 10 minutes
Cooking Time: 15 minutes
Serving: 8
Ingredients:
• 1 large eggplant, washed and cubed
• 1 tomato, seeded and chopped
• 1 small onion, diced
• 2 tablespoons parsley, chopped
• 2 tablespoons extra virgin olive oil
• 2 tablespoons distilled white vinegar
• 1/2 cup cashew cheese
Directions:
1. Preheat grill to medium to high

2. Prick the eggplant a few times using a fork/knife
3. Grill eggplants for 15 minutes until they are charred
4. Set aside and allow to cool
5. Take out the skin from the eggplant and dice the pulp
6. Transfer the pulp to a mixing bowl and add parsley, onion, tomato, olive oil, feta cheese, and vinegar
7. Mix well and chill for 1 hour.
Nutrition: Calories: 99 Fat: 7g Carbohydrates: 7g Protein: 3.4g

26. Simple Guacamole

Preparation Time: 15 minutes
Cooking Time: 0 minutes
Serving: 4
Ingredients:
• 3 large ripe avocados
• 1 large red onion, peeled and diced
• 4 tablespoons of freshly squeezed lime juice
• Sunflower seeds as needed
• Freshly ground black pepper as needed
• Cayenne pepper as needed
Directions:
1. Halve the avocados and discard the stone
2. Scoop the flesh from 3 avocado halves and transfer to a large bowl. Mash using a fork.
3. Put 2 tablespoons of lime juice and mix
4. Dice the remaining avocado flesh (remaining half) and transfer to another bowl
5. Add remaining juice and toss
6. Add the diced flesh with the mashed flesh and mix
7. Add chopped onions and toss
8. Season with sunflower seeds, pepper, and cayenne pepper
9. Serve and enjoy!
Nutrition: Calories: 172 Fat: 15g Carbohydrates: 11g Protein: 2g

27. Original Garlic Toast

Preparation Time: 5 minutes
Cooking Time: 5 minutes
Serving: 4
Ingredients:

• 1 teaspoon coconut oil
• Pinch of salt
• 1-2 teaspoons nutritional yeast
• 1 small garlic clove, pressed
• 1 slice wholegrain bread
Directions:
1. Take a small-sized bowl and add all ingredients except bread. Mix well
2. Toast your bread with seasoned oil or use a toaster. It should take about 5 minutes
3. Once done, spread garlic mix all over toast and serve
4. Enjoy!
Nutrition: Calories: 120 Fat: 6g Carbohydrates: 16g Protein: 7g

28. Cool Buffalo Cashew

Preparation Time: 5 minutes + 2 hours
Cooking Time: 55 minutes
Serving: 4
Ingredients:
• 2 cups raw cashews
• 3/4 cup red hot sauce
• 1/3 cup avocado oil
• 1/2 teaspoon garlic powder
• 1/4 teaspoon turmeric
Directions:
1. Take a bowl and mix wet ingredients in a bowl and stir in seasoning
2. Add cashews to the bowl and mix
3. Soak cashews in hot sauce mix for 2 hours
4. Preheat your oven to 325-degree Fahrenheit
5. Spread cashews onto the baking sheet
6. Bake for 35-55 minutes, turning after every 10-15 minutes
7. Let them cool and serve!
Nutrition: Calories: 120 Fat: 6g Carbohydrates: 20g Protein: 14g

29. Chia Mix

Preparation Time: 10 minutes
Cooking Time: 3 minutes
Serving: 1
Ingredients:
• 1 tablespoon chia seeds
• 2 cups strongly brewed coffee, chilled
• 1-ounce Macadamia nuts

- 1-2 packets Stevia, optional
- 1 tablespoon MCT oil

Directions:
1. Add all ingredients to a blender
2. Blend well on high until smooth and creamy
3. Enjoy your smoothie

Nutrition: Calories: 123 Fat: 8g Carbohydrates: 17g Protein: 5.2g

30. Curious Roasted Garlic Soup

Preparation Time: 10 minutes
Cooking Time: 1 hour
Serving: 10
Ingredients:
- 1 tablespoon olive oil
- 2 bulbs garlic, peeled
- 3 shallots, chopped
- 1 large head cauliflower, chopped
- 6 cups vegetable broth
- Salt and pepper to taste

Directions:
1. Ready your oven to 400 degrees Fahrenheit
2. Slice 1/4-inch top of the garlic bulb and place it in aluminum foil
3. Grease with olive oil and roast in the oven for 35 minutes
4. Get the flesh out of the roasted garlic
5. Put oil in a saucepan and add shallots. Sauté for 6 minutes.
6. Add garlic and remaining ingredients
7. Add lid to the pan and reduce the heat to low.
8. Let it cook for 15-20 minutes
9. Use a blender to puree the mixture
10. Season soup with salt and pepper. Serve and enjoy!

Nutrition: Calories: 142 Fat: 8g Carbohydrates: 3.4g Protein: 4g

31. Roasted Cashew and Almond Butter Delight

Preparation Time: 5 minutes
Cooking Time: 5 minutes
Serving: 1
Ingredients:

- 1 cup almonds, blanched
- 1/3 cup cashew nuts
- 2 tablespoons coconut oil
- 1/2 teaspoon cinnamon

Directions:
1. Prepare oven to 350 degrees Fahrenheit.
2. Bake almonds and cashews for 12 minutes. Let them cool
3. Place to a food processor together with the remaining ingredients
4. Add oil and keep blending until smooth
5. Serve and enjoy!

Nutrition: Calories: 205 Fat: 19g Carbohydrates: g Protein: 2.8g

32. Cashew Cheese and Walnut Crumbles

Preparation Time: 10 minutes
Cooking Time: 8 minutes
Serving: 10
Ingredients:
- 6 ounces' cashew cheese
- 2 tablespoons walnuts, chopped
- 1 tablespoon unsalted butter
- 1/2 tablespoon fresh thyme chopped

Directions:
1. Prepare oven to 350 degrees Fahrenheit
2. Get two rimmed baking sheets and line them with parchment
3. Add cheese, butter to a food processor and blend
4. Add walnuts to the mix and pulse
5. Take a tablespoon and scoop mix onto a baking sheet
6. Top with chopped thyme
7. Bake for 8 minutes, transfer to a cooling rack
8. Let it cool for 30 minutes
9. Serve and enjoy!

Nutrition: Calories: 80 Fat: 3g Carbohydrates: 7g Protein: 7g

33. Tasty Nut Packed Porridge

Preparation Time: 10 minutes
Cooking Time: 15 minutes

Serving: 4

Ingredients:

- 1 cup cashew nuts, raw and unsalted
- 1 cup pecans, halved
- 2 tablespoons Stevia
- 4 teaspoons coconut oil, melted
- 2 cups of water

Directions:

1. Prepare a food processor and add nuts. Process well to form a smooth paste.
2. Add water, oil, Stevia to the nut paste and transfer the mix to a saucepan.
3. Stir cook for 5 minutes on high heat.
4. Reduce heat to low and simmer for 10 minutes.
5. Serve warm and enjoy!

Nutrition: Calories: 260 Fat: 22g Carbohydrates: 12g Protein: 6g

34. Crazy Quinoa Protein Muffins

Preparation time: 15 minutes
Cooking time: 35 minutes
Serving: 6
Ingredients:

- ½ cup quinoa
- 2 tablespoons ground chia seeds
- ¼ cup almond flour
- 3 tablespoons vanilla protein powder
- ½ teaspoon salt (optional)
- ½ cup dates, chopped small
- 2 tablespoons coconut oil (optional)
- 3 tablespoons maple syrup (optional)
- 1 teaspoon vanilla extract
- ¼ cup unsweetened shredded coconut
- ½ cup raisins

Direction:

1. Rinse the quinoa and place in a small saucepan with a lid. Cover with ½ cup water and bring to a boil over medium-high heat. Cover and turn down to low. Let cook for 20 minutes and then remove from the heat. Take off the lid and let cool.
2. Preheat the oven to 450°F (235°C). Line six muffin cups with paper liners.
3. Mix the ground chia seeds with ¼ cup plus 2 tablespoons water and set aside.

4. Add the almond flour, protein powder, and salt (if desired) to a small bowl. Mix well. Add the dates and mix to coat. Set aside.
5. Put the coconut oil (if desired) in a medium bowl. If it is not liquid already, put in the microwave and heat for 10 to 20 seconds or until melted. Remove from microwave and add the maple syrup, if desired. Stir well. When cool, add the chia seed mixture, vanilla extract, coconut, almond flour mixture, cooked quinoa, and raisins. Mix well.
6. Divide the batter between the six muffin cups and bake 12 to 15 minutes, until a toothpick inserted in the center comes out clean.

Nutrition: Calories: 179 | fat: 6g | protein: 7g | carbs: 26g | fiber: 5g

35. Maple-Spice Buckwheat Crispiest Cereal

Preparation time: 15 minutes
Cooking time: 50 minutes
Serving: 5 cups
Ingredients:

- 1 cup raw buckwheat groats, soaked for at least 1 hour
- 1 cup sliced almonds
- 1 cup large-flake coconut
- ½ cup raw sunflower seeds
- 2 tablespoons chia seeds
- 3 tablespoons maple sugar or coconut sugar (optional)
- ¼ teaspoon fine sea salt (optional)
- 1½ teaspoons ground cinnamon
- ¼ teaspoon ground ginger
- ¼ teaspoon ground nutmeg
- 2 tablespoons liquid virgin coconut oil
- ¼ cup pure maple syrup (optional)
- 1 teaspoon pure vanilla extract

Direction:

1. Preheat the oven to 325°F (165°C). Line a large baking sheet with parchment paper and set aside.
2. Lay out a clean kitchen towel or a couple of lengths of doubled paper towels. In a fine-mesh strainer, rinse the buckwheat groats thoroughly. You're aiming to

remove as much of the slimy soaking liquid as possible. Scrape the rinsed buckwheat groats onto the clean kitchen towel and spread them out. Lightly pat the buckwheat groats dry and then transfer them to a large bowl.

3. To the large bowl, add the sliced almonds, coconut flakes, sunflower seeds, chia seeds, maple sugar, sea salt, if using, cinnamon, ginger, and nutmeg. Toss everything to coat.

4. In a small bowl, whisk together the coconut oil, maple syrup, if using, and vanilla, and then pour that over the buckwheat groats mixture. Stir with a rubber spatula to coat.

5. Scrape the wet cereal mixture onto the prepared baking sheet. Flatten and spread everything out with the back of your spatula as much as possible. Slide the baking sheet into the oven and bake for 50 minutes, stirring and flipping the crispiest a few times to ensure even browning. Once the cereal is evenly golden brown and lightly crispy, it's ready.

Nutrition: Calories: 195 | fat: 14g | protein: 4g | carbs: 16g | fiber: 3g

36. Breakfast Quinoa

Preparation time: 10 minutes
Cooking time: 25 minutes
Serving: 4
Ingredients:
- 2 cups plant-based milk
- 1 cup quinoa
- ½ cup frozen berries
- 1½ teaspoons cinnamon
- 1 banana, sliced

Optional Toppings:
- Walnuts or almonds
- Raw sunflower seeds
- Coconut shreds

Direction:
1. In a medium pot over medium-high heat, bring the milk to a boil.
2. Reduce the heat to low, add the quinoa, and cover.
3. Let the quinoa simmer for 15 minutes. Add the frozen berries and cinnamon, stir, cover, and simmer for 5 more minutes. Remove from the heat.
4. Fluff the quinoa by mixing it with a spoon.
5. Serve with the sliced banana and any optional toppings.

Nutrition: Calories: 269 | fat: 7g | protein: 11g | carbs: 33g | fiber: 5g

37. Zucchini Bread Oatmeal

Preparation time: 5 minutes
Cooking time: 20 minutes
Serving: 4
Ingredients:
- 2 cups rolled oats
- 1 medium zucchini, grated
- 4 cups water
- ½ cup unsweetened plant-based milk
- 1 tablespoon ground cinnamon
- ½ cup raisins
- 1 tablespoon maple syrup (optional)
- Pinch of salt (optional)
- 2 medium bananas, sliced
- 4 tablespoons chopped walnuts (optional)

Direction:
1. In a medium saucepan over medium-high, combine the oats, zucchini, and water and bring to a boil. Remove from the heat, add the plant-based milk, cinnamon, raisins, maple syrup, and salt (if using) and stir well.
2. Divide the oatmeal among 4 bowls and top each portion with ½ sliced banana and 1 tablespoon of walnuts (if using).

Nutrition: Calories: 301 | fat: 4g | protein: 9g | carbs: 62g | fiber: 8g

38. Toasty French Toast Bake

Preparation time: 10 minutes
Cooking time: 35 minutes
Serving: 6
Ingredients:
- Virgin coconut oil, for greasing the pan (optional)
- 1½ cups unsweetened almond milk or coconut milk
- ¼ cup plus 1 tablespoon pure maple syrup, divided (optional)

- 2 teaspoons orange zest
- 3 tablespoons fresh orange juice
- 2 teaspoons pure vanilla extract
- 1 teaspoon ground cinnamon
- 2 tablespoons arrowroot powder
- 12 to 14 slices of stale, whole-grain bread

Serve:
- Unsweetened coconut flakes
- Sliced fresh fruit or whole berries
- Pure maple syrup (optional)

Direction:

1.   Preheat the oven to 350°F (180°C). Lightly grease an 8-inch ovenproof dish with coconut oil, if using.

2. In a medium bowl, whisk together the almond milk, ¼ cup of maple syrup, orange zest, orange juice, vanilla, cinnamon, and arrowroot powder. Keep whisking until combined and there are no dry traces of arrowroot in the mix.

3. Arrange the bread slices in your dish. You can do two flat layers of bread or you can fan them out like a tian. You may have to cut your bread slices in half to accomplish this. Press the bread into the dish.

4. Pour about half the almond milk mixture over the bread. Push the bread down to absorb some of the liquid. Pour the remaining half of the almond milk mixture over the bread. Press down on the bread once more. Let the bread soak in the liquid for 10 minutes.

5. Slide the French toast bake into the oven, and bake until lightly browned on top and much of the liquid has been absorbed, about 30 minutes. Remove the bake from the oven and set the broiler to high

Nutrition: Calories: 335 | fat: 17g | protein: 8g | carbs: 39g | fiber: 6g

39. Choco Almond Mousse Pudding

Preparation time: 5 minutes
Cooking time: 0 minutes
Serving: 2
Ingredients:
- 2 cups soy milk
- 1 cup pomegranate seeds
- 2 peeled bananas
- 2 scoops soy protein isolate, chocolate flavor

- ¼ cup almond butter
- 1 cup water (optional)

Optional Toppings:
- Blueberries
- Shredded coconut

Direction:

1. Add all the ingredients to a blender and blend until smooth. Alternatively, blend the bananas, soy isolates and almond butter until smooth.

2. Add a heaped tablespoon of the almond butter mixture to 2 large glasses or Mason jars.

3. Add ¼ cup of soy milk and a tablespoon of pomegranate seeds to each glass or jar.

4. Store the pudding in an airtight container in the fridge, and consume within 2 days. Alternatively, store in the freezer for a maximum of 60 days and thaw at room temperature.

Nutrition: Calories: 596 | fat: 23g | protein: 43g | carbs: 55g | fiber: 12g

40. Banana and Oat Muffins

Preparation time: 10 minutes
Cooking time: 20 minutes
Serving: 12
Ingredients:
- 1 ripe banana, mashed
- ½ cup unsweetened applesauce
- ¾ cup coconut milk
- 1 teaspoon baking soda
- 1 tablespoon lemon juice
- ½ cup quick-cook rolled oats, uncooked
- ½ cup whole-wheat flour
- 2 tablespoons ground flaxseed
- 1 teaspoon ground cinnamon
- 1 teaspoon baking powder
- 1/3 cup chopped pecans, toasted
- 1/3 cup raisins, no sugar added

Direction:

1. Preheat the oven to 425°F (220°C) and line 12 muffin cups with paper liners.

2. In a medium bowl, mix the banana, applesauce, and coconut milk.

3. In a small bowl, combine the baking soda and lemon juice. Add to the banana mixture.

4. In a large bowl, mix the quick oats, whole-wheat flour, flaxseed, cinnamon, and baking powder.

5. Bake for 20 minutes or until a toothpick inserted in the center of a muffin comes out clean. Store the muffins in an airtight container or a zip-top bag in the refrigerator for up to 5 days.

Nutrition: Calories: 222 | fat: 12g | protein: 4g | carbs: 28g | fiber: 4g

41. Oatmeal Protein Mix

Preparation time: 5 minutes
Cooking time: 0 minutes
Serving: 3
Ingredients:
- 1 cup dry oatmeal
- 3 scoops of chocolate or vanilla flavor vegan protein powder
- ½ teaspoon cinnamon
- ½ teaspoon maple syrup (optional)
- ¼ cup almonds
- 1 cup almond milk
- 2 ice cubes
- 2 tablespoons peanut butter (optional)

Direction:
1. Add the required ingredients, including the optional peanut butter if desired, to a blender. Blend for 2 minutes. Transfer to a large cup or shaker and enjoy!

Nutrition: Calories: 298 | fat: 9g | protein: 29g | carbs: 25g | fiber: 4g

42. Savory Rosemary–Black Pepper Scones

Preparation time: 10 minutes
Cooking time: 20 minutes
Serving: 8 scones
Ingredients:
- 1 cup whole wheat flour
- ¾ cup old-fashioned rolled oats
- 2 tablespoons minced fresh rosemary
- ½ teaspoon baking powder
- ½ teaspoon freshly ground black pepper
- ½ teaspoon salt (optional)
- 3 tablespoons puréed white beans or tahini

- ¾ cup almond milk
- 1 tablespoon fresh lemon juice

Direction:
1. Preheat the oven to 475°F (245°C). Lightly grease a baking sheet or use parchment paper.

2. Mix the flour, oats, rosemary, baking powder, pepper, and salt (if desired) in a medium bowl. Add the puréed white beans and use a pastry cutter, two forks, or your fingers to mix until well combined. Add the almond milk and lemon juice and mix with a fork until it forms a shaggy ball of dough; do not overmix.

3. Split the dough into two balls. Spread one ball of dough into a circle on one end of the sheet. It should be 1 inch thick. Repeat on the other side. Use a knife to cut each circle into 4 wedges.

4. Bake for 20 minutes, or until a toothpick inserted in the middle comes out clean and the scones are golden brown. Serve warm. (Toast any leftovers before serving.)

Nutrition: Calories: 237 | fat: 9g | protein: 10g | carbs: 41g | fiber: 7g

43. Peanut Butter and Strawberry Jam Oatmeal

Preparation time: 5 minutes
Cooking time: 20 minutes
Serving: 4
- 2 cups rolled oats
- 4 cups water
- ½ cup unsweetened plant-based milk
- 1 tablespoon maple syrup (optional)
- Pinch of salt (optional)
- 4 tablespoons natural peanut butter, divided
- 4 tablespoons no-sugar-added strawberry jam, divided

Direction:
1. In a medium saucepan, combine the oats and water and bring to a boil over medium-high heat. Lower the heat to medium-low and simmer, stirring often, until the oats are soft and creamy, about 15 minutes. Remove from the heat. Add the plant-based milk, maple syrup, and salt (if using) and stir well.

2. Divide the oatmeal among 4 bowls, top each with 1 tablespoon of peanut butter and 1 tablespoon of jam, and serve immediately.

3. The oatmeal can be stored in an airtight container in the refrigerator for up to 4 days. To serve, reheat

the oatmeal in a medium saucepan over low heat with 2 tablespoons water to loosen it up, as oatmeal can get quite solid when chilled. Add the peanut butter and jam just before serving.

Nutrition: Calories: 284 | fat: 12g | protein: 11g | carbs: 35g| fiber: 6g

44. Warm Maple Protein Oatmeal

Preparation time: 5 minutes
Cooking time: 30 minutes
Serving: 2
Ingredients:
- 1 cup steel-cut oats
- 3 tablespoons raw shelled hempseed, divided
- 3 tablespoons maple syrup (optional)
- 2 teaspoons cinnamon
- 1 tablespoon slivered almonds
- 1 tablespoon currants

Direction:
1. Bring 4 cups of water to a boil in a large saucepan. Add the steel-cut oatmeal, 2 tablespoons hempseed, maple syrup (if desired), and cinnamon and bring back to a boil. Reduce heat to low and cook uncovered for 30 minutes, stirring occasionally.
2. Serve in bowls, garnished with almond slivers, currants, and the remaining hempseed.

Nutrition: Calories: 229 | fat: 6g | protein: 23g | carbs: 47g | fiber: 9g

45. Vanilla Breakfast Smoothie

Preparation time: 10 minutes
Cooking time: 0 minutes
Serving: 1
- 1 frozen banana, sliced
- 1 cup vanilla almond milk
- ¼ cup old-fashioned oats
- ¼ cup raisins
- 1 tablespoon flaxseed meal
- ¼ teaspoon cinnamon
- 3 tablespoons vanilla protein powder

Direction:

1. Add all the ingredients to a blender and blend until very smooth.

Nutrition: Calories: 399 | fat: 12g | protein: 26g | carbs: 48g | fiber: 12g

46. Almond and Protein Shake

Preparation time: 5 minutes
Cooking time: 0 minutes
Serving: 2
Ingredients:
- 1½ cups soy milk
- 3 tablespoons almonds
- 1 teaspoon maple syrup (optional)
- 1 tablespoon coconut oil (optional)
- 2 scoops of chocolate or vanilla flavor vegan protein powder
- 2 to 4 ice cubes
- 1 teaspoon cocoa powder (optional)

Direction:
1. Add all the required ingredients, and if desired, the optional cocoa powder, to a blender. Blend for 2 minutes. Transfer the shake to a large cup or shaker. Serve and enjoy!

Nutrition: Calories: 340 | fat: 17g | protein: 32g | carbs: 15g | fiber: 2g

47. Bulgur Porridge

Preparation time: 10 minutes
Cooking time: 15 minutes
Servings: 2
Ingredients:
- 2/3 cup unsweetened soy milk
- 1/3 cup bulgur, rinsed
- Pinch of salt
- 1 ripe banana, peeled and mashed
- 2 kiwis, peeled and sliced

Direction:
1. In a pan, add the soy milk, bulgur, and salt over medium-high heat and bring to a boil.
2. Adjust the heat to low and simmer for about 10 minutes.
3. Remove the pan of bulgur from heat and immediately, stir in the mashed banana.
4. Serve warm with the topping of kiwi slices.

Nutrition: Calories 223 Total Fat 2.3 g Saturated Fat 0.3 g Cholesterol 0 mg Sodium 126 mg Total Carbs 47.5 g Fiber 8.6 g Sugar 17.4 g Protein 7.1 g

48. Sunrise Smoothie Bowl

Preparation time: 10 minutes
Cooking time: 0 minutes
Serving: 2
Ingredients:
- 2 cups fresh spinach
- ½ cup water
- 1 orange, peeled and segmented
- 2 cups sliced peaches, preferably frozen
- 1 ripe banana, frozen
- 1 tablespoon fresh lemon juice
- ½ cup sliced strawberries
- ½ cup diced peaches
- 1 kiwifruit, diced
- ¼ cup raw cashews
- 4 fresh mint leaves, chopped

Direction:
1. In a blender, purée the spinach, water, and orange until smooth. Add the sliced peaches and the banana and pulse a few times, then purée until the mixture is thick and smooth. You will need to stop the blender occasionally to scrape down the sides. Add a little extra water if needed. The texture should be thick and creamy like frozen yogurt.
2. Divide between 2 bowls and top each with half of the strawberries, diced peaches, kiwi, cashews, and mint. Serve immediately.
Nutrition: Calories: 307 | fat: 9g | protein: 7g | carbs: 56g | fiber: 9g

49. Irish Breakfast Oats

Preparation time: 5 minutes
Cooking time: 40 minutes
Serving: 4
Ingredients:
- 4 cups water
- ¼ teaspoon sea salt (optional)
- 1 cup gluten-free steel-cut oats
- 1 tablespoon pure maple syrup (optional)
- 1 tablespoon almond butter
Suggested Toppings:
- 1 ripe banana, sliced
- ½ cup sliced almonds
- Dash of ground cinnamon

Direction:
1. In a 4-quart saucepan, bring the water and salt (if using) to a boil. Add the oats and stir well. Reduce the heat to low and cook for 30 to 40 minutes, or until cooked through. The oats will be chewy, but they should not have any crunch.
2. Stir in the maple syrup (if using) and almond butter, then spoon the oatmeal into 4 bowls. If using any suggested toppings, add them now.
Nutrition: Calories: 188 | fat: 9g | protein: 7g | carbs: 28g | fiber: 6g

50. Avocado-Chia Protein Shake

Preparation time: 10 minutes
Cooking time: 0 minutes
Serving: 2
Ingredients:
- ¼ cup dry chia seeds, soaked for at least 1 hour
- 1 cup coconut milk
- ½ avocado, pitted and peeled
- 1½ tablespoon peanut butter
- 2 scoops of chocolate flavor vegan protein powder
- 1 cup water
- 3 ice cubes (optional)
- 1 to 2 teaspoons cacao powder (optional)

Direction:
1. Add all the required, and if desired, optional ingredients to a blender. When using ice cubes, the water can be left out. Blend for 2 minutes. Transfer the shake to a large cup or shaker. Top with some additional cacao powder. Serve and enjoy!
Nutrition: Calories: 379 | fat: 21g | protein: 30g | carbs: 17g | fiber: 10g

51. Homemade Granola Clusters

Preparation time: 15 minutes

Cooking time: 1 minute
Serving: 2 cups
Ingredients:

- 1½ creamy or chunky cups peanut butter
- ¼ cup agave or maple syrup (optional)
- 1½ cups old-fashioned rolled oats
- ¾ cup flaxseed meal
- ½ cup raisins
- ¾ cup raw sunflower seeds

Optional Toppings:

- ¼ cup coconut shreds
- 1 teaspoon cinnamon
- Pinch of salt (optional)

Direction:
1. Add the peanut butter and maple syrup (if desired) to a medium, microwave-safe bowl. Microwave on high for 30-second intervals, stirring between intervals until the mixture is creamy and well combined.
2. Add the oats, flaxseed meal, raisins, and sunflower seeds, and stir together with a spoon until thoroughly combined.
3. Transfer the mixture to a baking sheet.
4. Place in the freezer for at least 25 minutes. Store in the refrigerator in an airtight container for up to 7 days.
Nutrition: Calories: 510 | fat: 29g | protein: 31g | carbs: 34g | fiber: 11g

52. Spiced Pumpkin Muffins

Preparation time: 15 minutes
Cooking time: 20 minutes
Serving: 12 muffins
Ingredients:

- 2 tablespoons ground flaxseed
- ¼ cup water
- 1¾ cups whole wheat flour
- 2 teaspoons baking powder
- 1½ teaspoons ground cinnamon
- ½ teaspoon baking soda
- ½ teaspoon ground ginger
- ¼ teaspoon ground nutmeg
- 1/8 teaspoon ground cloves
- 1 cup pumpkin purée
- ½ cup pure maple syrup (optional)
- ¼ cup unsweetened applesauce
- ¼ cup unsweetened nondairy milk
- 1½ teaspoons vanilla extract

Direction:
1. Preheat the oven to 350ºF (180ºC). Line a 12-cup metal muffin pan with parchment-paper liners or use a silicone muffin pan.
2. In a small bowl, whisk together the flaxseed and water. Set aside.
3. In a large bowl, whisk together the flour, baking powder, cinnamon, baking soda, ginger, nutmeg, and cloves to combine.
4. In a medium bowl, stir together the pumpkin purée, maple syrup (if using), applesauce, milk, and vanilla. Using a spatula, fold the wet ingredients into the dry ingredients.
5. Fold the soaked flaxseed into the batter until evenly combined, but do not overmix the batter or your muffins will become dense. Spoon about ¼ cup of batter per muffin into your prepared muffin pan.
6. Store in an airtight container at room temperature for up to 1 week or freeze for up to 3 months.
Nutrition: Calories: 115 | fat: 1g | protein: 3g | carbs: 25g | fiber: 3g

53. Muesli and Berries Bowl

Preparation time: 10 minutes
Cooking time: 0 minutes
Serving: about 5 cups
Ingredients:
Muesli:

- 1 cup rolled oats
- 1 cup spelt flakes, quinoa flakes, or more rolled oats
- 2 cups puffed cereal
- ¼ cup sunflower seeds
- ¼ cup almonds
- ¼ cup raisins
- ¼ cup dried cranberries
- ¼ cup chopped dried figs
- ¼ cup unsweetened shredded coconut
- ¼ cup nondairy chocolate chips
- 1 to 3 teaspoons ground cinnamon

Bowl:

- ½ cup nondairy milk or unsweetened applesauce
- ¾ cup muesli
- ½ cup berries

Direction:

1. Put the muesli ingredients in a container or bag and shake.
2. Combine the muesli and bowl ingredients in a bowl or to-go container.

Nutrition: Calories: 450 | fat: 11g | protein: 17g | carbs: 83g | fiber: 13g

54. Sweet Potato Pie Oatmeal

Preparation time: 10 minutes
Cooking time: 22 minutes
Serving: 2
Ingredients:

- 1 large sweet potato, peeled and diced
- 1 cup rolled oats
- 1 cup unsweetened almond milk
- ½ cup date molasses
- ½ teaspoon ground cinnamon
- ½ teaspoon ground ginger
- ¼ teaspoon orange zest
- ¼ teaspoon ground allspice
- Pinch salt (optional)

Direction:

1. Steam or boil the sweet potato until tender, about 10 minutes. Drain and mash it and add it to a small saucepan with the oats, almond milk, molasses, cinnamon, ginger, orange zest, allspice, and salt (if using). Cook the mixture over medium heat until the oats are tender, 10 to 12 minutes.

Nutrition: Calories: 400 | fat: 3g | protein: 13g | carbs: 84g | fiber: 9g

55. Baked Flaxseed-Battered French Toast

Preparation time: 10 minutes
Cooking time: 15 minutes
Serving: 4
Ingredients:

- ¼ cup ground flaxseeds
- 1½ cups unsweetened plant-based milk, divided
- Olive oil cooking spray
- 1 tablespoon ground cinnamon
- 1 teaspoon vanilla extract
- 3 tablespoons maple syrup, plus more for serving (optional)
- 8 slices whole-grain bread

Direction:

1. In a medium bowl, combine the flaxseeds and ½ cup of plant-based milk. Let the mixture stand for 10 minutes to give the flaxseeds time to absorb the liquid and thicken, which will give them a consistency.
2. Preheat the oven to 400°F (205°C). Spray a sheet pan with olive oil cooking spray.
3. Add the remaining 1 cup plant-based milk, the cinnamon, vanilla, and maple syrup (if using) to the flax mixture and mix until combined. Dip each slice of bread into the flax mixture, making sure to cover in the liquid completely. Let any excess drip back into the bowl and then put the slices on the sheet pan.
4. Bake for 10 minutes. Using a spatula, carefully flip the bread and bake for 5 minutes. Serve with maple syrup.

Nutrition: Calories: 272 | fat: 7g | protein: 11g | carbs: 42g | fiber: 7g

56. Sweet Potato Waffles

Preparation time: 15 minutes
Cooking time: 20 minutes
Serving: 2
Ingredients:

- 2 medium sweet potatoes, peeled, grated and squeezed finely
- ½ teaspoon dried rosemary, crushed
- Salt and ground black pepper, as required

Direction:

1. Preheat the waffle iron and lightly grease it.
2. In a large bowl, mix together all ingredients.
3. Place half of the sweet potato mixture in preheated waffle iron.
4. Cook for 8-10 minutes or until waffles become golden brown.
5. Repeat with the remaining mixture.
6. Serve warm.

Meal Prep Tip:

1.	Store these cooled waffles in a container by placing a piece of wax paper between each waffle.
2.	Refrigerate up to 5 days.
3.	Reheat in the microwave for about 1-2 minutes.
Nutrition:
Calories: 178, Fats: 0.3g, Carbs: 42g, Fiber: 6.3g, Sugar: 0.8g, Proteins: 2.3g, Sodium: 91mg

57. Sweet Potato & Apple Hash

Preparation time: 15 minutes
Cooking time: 20 minutes
Serving: 2
Ingredients:
•	1½ tablespoons olive oil, divided
•	1 large apple, cored and cubed into 1-inch size
•	1 small onion, chopped finely
•	1 teaspoon ground cinnamon
•	1 large sweet potato, peeled and cubed into 1-inch size
•	2 tablespoons fresh cilantro, chopped
Direction:
1.	In a nonstick skillet, heat ½ tablespoon of oil over medium heat and cook the apple, onion and cinnamon and cook for about 4-5 minutes.
2.	Transfer the apple mixture into the bowl with bacon.
3.	In the same skillet, heat the remaining oil over medium heat and cook the sweet potato for about 10 minutes, stirring occasionally.
4.	Add the apple and cook for about 3-4 minutes.
5.	Serve hot with the topping of cilantro.
Meal Prep Tip:
1.	Remove from the heat and set the hash aside to cool completely.
2.	After cooling, divide the hash into 2 containers.
3.	Refrigerate for 1-2 days.
4.	Remove from refrigerator and reheat in microwave before serving.
Nutrition: Calories: 237, Fats: 10.9g, Carbs: 36.2g, Fiber: 6.8g, Sugar: 18.3g, Proteins: 2.4g, Sodium: 32mg

58. Chickpeas Scramble

Preparation time: 15 minutes
Cooking time: 5 minutes
Serving: 4
Ingredients:
•	15 ounces cooked chickpeas
•	2 tablespoons fresh lemon juice
•	6 tablespoons hummus
•	2 tablespoons nutritional yeast
•	1 teaspoon garlic powder
•	½ teaspoon ground turmeric
•	Ground black pepper, as required
Direction:
1.	In a bowl, add the chickpeas and the lemon juice and with a fork, mash slightly.
2.	Add the hummus and remaining ingredients and again, mash until well combined.
3.	Heat a lightly greased nonstick skillet over medium-high heat and cook the chickpeas mixture for about 5 minutes or until golden brown, stirring occasionally.
4.	Remove from the heat and serve warm.
Meal Prep Tip:
1.	Remove from the heat and set the hash aside to cool completely.
2.	After cooling, divide the chickpeas scramble into 2 containers.
3.	Refrigerate for 3-4 days.
4.	Remove from refrigerator and reheat in microwave before serving.
Nutrition: Calories: 172, Fats: 3.3g, Carbs: 24.6g, Fiber: 7.1g, Sugar: 0.3g, Proteins: 10.3g, Sodium: 111mg

59. Tofu Scramble

Preparation time: 15 minutes
Cooking time: 10 minutes
Serving: 2
Ingredients:
•	2 tablespoons nutritional yeast
•	1 teaspoon Dijon mustard
•	½ teaspoon paprika
•	½ teaspoon ground turmeric

- ¼ teaspoon garlic powder
- Salt and ground black pepper, as required
- 1/3 cup unsweetened almond milk
- 1 tablespoon coconut oil
- 8 ounces' extra-firm tofu, drained, pressed and mashed slightly
- 1 tablespoon fresh chives, chopped

Direction:
1. In a bowl, add the nutritional yeast, Dijon mustard, spices, salt, black pepper and almond milk and beat until well combined.
2. In a frying pan, melt the coconut oil over medium heat and cook the tofu for about 4-5 minutes, stirring frequently.
3. Add the spice mixture and cook for about 4-5 minutes or until all the liquid is absorbed, stirring occasionally.
4. Remove from the heat and serve hot with the topping of chives.

Meal Prep Tip:
1. Remove from the heat and set the hash aside to cool completely.
2. After cooling, divide the chickpeas scramble into 2 containers.
3. Refrigerate for 3-4 days.
4. Remove from refrigerator and reheat in microwave before serving.

Nutrition: Calories: 211, Fats: 14.8g, Carbs: 8.3g, Fiber: 3.6g, Sugar: 0.8g, Proteins: 16.3g, Sodium: 152mg

60. Tomato Omelet

Preparation time: 15 minutes
Cooking time: 25 minutes
Serving: 4
Ingredients:
- 1 cup chickpea flour
- ¼ teaspoon ground turmeric
- ¼ teaspoon red chili powder
- Pinch of ground cumin
- Pinch of salt
- 1½-2 cups water
- 1 medium onion, chopped finely
- 2 medium tomatoes, chopped finely
- 1 jalapeño pepper, chopped finely
- 2 tablespoons fresh cilantro, chopped
- 2 tablespoons olive oil, divided

Direction:

1. In a large bowl, mix together flour and seasoning.
2. Slowly, add water and mix until well combined.
3. Fold in the onion, tomatoes, green chili and cilantro.
4. In a large nonstick frying pan, heat ½ tablespoon of oil over medium heat.
5. Add ½ of tomato mixture and tilt the pan to spread it.
6. Cook for about 5-7 minutes.
7. Place the remaining oil over the omelet and carefully flip the side.
8. Cook for about 4-5 minutes or until golden brown.
9. Repeat with remaining mixture.

Meal Prep Tip:
1. In a resealable plastic bag, place the cooled omelet slices and seal the bag.
2. Refrigerate for about 2-3 days.
3. Reheat in the microwave on High for about 1 minute before serving.

Nutrition: Calories: 267, Fats: 10.3g, Carbs: 35.7g, Fiber: 10.2g, Sugar: 8.3g, Proteins: 10.6g, Sodium: 67mg

61. Vegetable Quiche

Preparation time: 10 minutes
Cooking time: 45-50 minutes
Servings: 4-6
Ingredients:
- Red cabbage
- White cabbage
- Onion
- Carrot
- Zucchini
- 2-3 eggs
- Liquid cream
- Salt
- cheese
- Puff pastry
- Tomatoes

Direction:
1. Grate all the vegetables except the tomato and mix with the eggs and the cream. You add cream depending on the texture there should not be a liquid texture, rather solid, all compact.
2. Next, add the cheese and mix again.

3.   Use a corrugated mold with a removable base, but put baking paper to extract the quiche once done. Spread the dough in it and prick several times with a fork. Bake the base at 1800C for 15 minutes.

4.   Extract the base and fill with the mixture. Cover with a layer of cheese and tomatoes. Put a little oregano on top to give it more taste.

5.   Bake the set for 30-35 minutes at 1800C. Until the filling is curdled and the golden mass. It is served hot and ready!

Nutrition: Calorie: 257 Protein: 6g Fat: 17g Carbohydrates: 17g

62. Black Bean Flutes

Preparation time: 5 minutes
Cooking time: 5 minutes
Servings: 10
Ingredients:
- 2 ½ cups cooked beans
- ½ chopped onion
- 2/3 cup Black Bean Broth
- 2 Chiles without seeds and chopped
- 1 tablespoon oil
- 12 corn tortillas
- ½ cup cream
- 1 cup cheese grated
- ¼ julienne romaine lettuce
- 2 cups red sauce oil to taste
- Salt, Pepper to taste

Direction:
1.   Season the onion and add the chilies.
2.   Cook for 5 minutes.
3.   Add the beans, the broth and the epazote.
4.   Crush and pepper.
5.   Cook until thick and dry. Remove and let cool.
6.   Heat the tortillas and fill with the previous mixture.
7.   Roll up to form flutes.
8.   Fry until golden brown and drain on absorbent paper.
9.   Serve and add the cream, lettuce and cheese and serve with the red sauce.

Nutrition: Calorie: 301.9 Protein: 14gFat: 4.3g Carbohydrates: 55.4g

63. Soy Milk and Oatmeal Smoothie

Preparation time: 5 minutes
Cooking time: 0 minutes
Servings: 1
Ingredients:
- ½ cup quick oatmeal
- 1 cup soy milk
- ½ cup of ice
- Sweetener to taste

Direction:
1.   Add all the ingredients to the blender for 5 minutes. It should be smooth.

Nutrition: Calorie: 120 Protein: 3g Fat: 5g Carbohydrates: 16g

64. Vegan Omelette

Preparation time: 5 minutes
Cooking time: 5 minutes
Servings: 1
Ingredients:
- 6 ounces Mori-nu lite silken tofu
- Cherry tomatoes
- Basil
- Olive oil
- cheese
- Salt and pepper

Direction:
1.   On a frying pan heat a teaspoon of olive oil and add 6 ounces Mori-nu lite silken tofu.
2.   Now add the tomatoes, cheese, and basil.
3.   Form a kind of omelette and roll.

Nutrition: Calorie: 104.5 Protein: 11.3g Fat: 1.9g Carbohydrates: 10.2g

65. Oatmeal Pancakes

Preparation time: 30 minutes
Cooking time: 10-15 minutes
 Servings: 4-6
Ingredients:
- 1 cup oatmeal
- Water with ½ cup
- Pinch of salt

- ¾ cup grated coconut
- 1 shoreline baking powder
- 1 tbsp vinegar

optional:
- a banana (sweet) or grated carrot (salty)

Direction:
1. Blend the cup of oatmeal with ½ cup of filtered water.
2. Add the rest of the ingredients minus the coconut.
3. Add more water until you get consistent dough like pancakes.
4. Add the grated coconut, stir well and let stand ½ hour in the fridge.
5. Heat a frying pan, cook the pancakes round and round and enjoy the topping you want.

Nutrition: Calorie: 159 Protein: 4.9g Fat: 7.4g Carbohydrates: 18g

66. Chia Vegan Pancakes

Preparation time: 15 minutes
Cooking time: 10 minutes
Servings: 1
Ingredients:
- 40 g oatmeal (if you don't have flour, grind the oatmeal)
- 1 tbsp chia seeds
- 1 tbsp sesame

Direction:
1. Mix all the ingredients (except the oil) until creating a homogeneous paste (it should be a little liquid but not like water).
2. Let stand about 15 minutes minimum (so that the chia seeds are hydrated).
3. It can also be done at night and left to rest in the fridge overnight.
4. In a frying pan, add a little extra virgin olive oil or coconut oil and add a ladle of dough. we leave 23 minutes and turn.
5. Repeat until we finish with the dough.
6. Accompany fruit, nuts, grated coconut, cinnamon, natural soy yogurt, pure cocoa powder.

Nutrition: Calorie: 229.9 Protein: 10.2g Fat: 6.9g Carbohydrates: 32.5g

67. Oatmeal Porridge

Preparation time: 5 minutes
Cooking time: 5 minutes
Servings: 1
Ingredients:
- 1 cup of oatmeal
- 2 cups of almond milk
- 1 teaspoon of peanut butter
- 1 banana
- Cinnamon
- Agave syrup

Direction:
1. In a saucepan, boil the oatmeal with the milk and cinnamon until the oats soften and we have a slightly thick mixture.
2. Pour the mixture into a bowl and put banana, peanut butter and syrup on top.

Nutritional Information: Calorie: 214 Protein: 11g Fat: 5.8g Carbohydrates: 30g

68. Blueberry Buckwheat Pancakes

Preparation time: 10 minutes
Cooking time: 25 minutes
Servings: 4
Ingredients:
- ¼ cup chia seeds
- 1 tsp of green powder (optional)
- 2 tbsp fresh berries
- 1 tsp of cinnamon
- ½ to 1 ripe banana, mashed
- 1 tbsp coconut softened oil or nut butter

Direction:
1. Stir in the soaked chia seeds until gelatinous consistency forms.
2. Add a little more liquid if desired. Add the banana puree.
3. Combine until the mixture has a consistency like porridge. Add cinnamon, green powder (if desired), coconut oil or pecan butter, and berries.
4. Serve in a deep plate and enjoy. Top with coconut flakes for added crunch.

Nutrition: Calorie: 91.4 Protein: 3.7g Fat: 3.7g Carbohydrates: 11.9g

69. Oatmeal Soaks with Goji Berries

Preparation time: 10 minutes
Cooking time: 2-10 minutes
Servings: 1-2
Ingredients:

- ¼ cup chia seeds
- 1 tsp of green powder (optional)
- 2 tbsp fresh berries
- 1 tsp of cinnamon
- ½ to 1 ripe banana, mashed
- 1 tbsp coconut softened oil or nut butter

Direction:
1.   Stir in the soaked chia seeds until gelatinous consistency forms.
2.   Add a little more liquid if desired. Add the banana puree.
3.   Combine until the mixture has a consistency like porridge. Add cinnamon, green powder (if desired), coconut oil or pecan butter, and berries.
4.   Serve in a deep plate and enjoy. Top with coconut flakes for added crunch.
Nutrition: Calorie: 353 Protein: 13g Fat: 10.5g Carbohydrates:51g

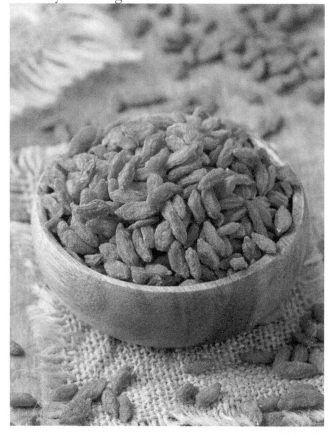

Chapter 5. Low-Potassium Recipes

70. Apple Oatmeal Crisp

Preparation Time: 5 minutes
Cooking Time: 5 minutes
Servings: 2
Ingredients:
- 5 Granny Smith apples
- 1 cup whole oatmeal
- 1/2 cup all-purpose flour
- 3/4 cup brown sugar
- 1/2 cup butter
- 1 teaspoon cinnamon

Directions:
1. Preheat the oven to 350 F.
2. Mix together oatmeal, brown sugar, flour, and cinnamon in a bowl.
3. With a pastry cutter to cut butter into oatmeal mixture until well blended.
4. Place sliced apples in a 9" x 9" baking pan and sprinkle oatmeal mixture over apples.
5. Bake for 30 to 35 minutes.

Nutrition:
Total Fat: 13 g
Cholesterol: 32 mg
Sodium: 95 mg
Total Carbohydrate: 42 g
Dietary Fiber: 2.4 g
Protein: 3 g
Potassium: 193 mg
Phosphorus: 74 mg

71. Apple Oatmeal Custard

Preparation Time: 5 minutes
Cooking Time: 5 minutes
Servings: 2
Ingredients:
- 1/3 cup quick-cooking oatmeal
- 1 large egg
- 1/2 cup almond milk
- 1/4 teaspoon cinnamon
- 1/2 medium apple, cored and finely chopped

Directions:
1. In a large mug, combine oats, egg, and almond milk. Stir well with a fork. Add cinnamon and apple. Stir again until fully mixed.
2. Cook in a microwave on high heat for 2 minutes. Fluff with a fork. If needed, cook for an additional 30 to 60 seconds.
3. Set in a little more milk or water if you prefer a thinner cereal.

Nutrition:
Total Fat: 8 g
Cholesterol: 186 mg
Sodium: 164 mg
Total Carbohydrate: 33 g
Dietary Fiber: 5.8 g
Protein: 11 g
Potassium: 362 mg
Phosphorus: 240 mg

72. Apple Cinnamon Rings

Preparation Time: 10 minutes
Cooking Time: 20 minutes
Servings: 6
Ingredients:
- 4 large apples cut in rings
- 1 cup flour
- 1/4 tsp. baking powder
- 1 tsp. stevia
- 1/4 tsp. cinnamon
- 1 large egg, beaten
- 1 cup milk
- Vegetable oil, for frying Cinnamon Topping:
- 1/3 cup of brown Swerve
- 2 tsps. cinnamon

Direction
1. Begin by mixing the flour with the baking powder, cinnamon and stevia in a bowl. Whisk the egg with the milk in a bowl. Stir in the dry flour mixture and mix well until it makes a smooth batter. Pour oil into a wok to deep fry the rings and heat it up to 375 degrees F. First, dip the apple in the flour batter and deep fry until golden brown. Transfer the apple rings on a tray lined with paper towel. Drizzle the cinnamon and Swerve topping over the slices. Serve fresh in the morning.

Nutrition

Calories 166
Total Fat 1.7g
Saturated Fat 0.5g
Cholesterol 33mg
Sodium 55mg
Carbohydrates 13.1g
Sugars 6.9g
Protein 4.7g
Phosphorus 241mg
Potassium 197mg

73. Kale and Garlic Platter

Preparation Time: 5 minutes
Cooking Time: 10 minutes
Serving: 4
Ingredients:
- 1 bunch kale
- 2 tablespoons olive oil
- 4 garlic cloves, minced

Directions:
1. Carefully tear the kale into bite-sized portions, making sure to remove the stem
2. Discard the stems
3. Set a large-sized pot and place it over medium heat
4. Add olive oil and let the oil heat up
5. Add garlic and stir for 2 minutes
6. Add kale and cook for 5-10 minutes
7. Serve!
Nutrition
Calories: 121
Fat: 8g
Carbohydrates: 5g
Protein: 4g

74. Cucumber Soup

Preparation Time: 14 minutes
Cooking Time: 15 minutes
Serving: 4
Ingredients:
- 2 tablespoons garlic, minced
- 4 cups English cucumbers, peeled and diced
- 1/2 cup onions, diced
- 1 tablespoon lemon juice
- 1 1/2 cups vegetable broth
- 1/2 teaspoon salt

- 1/4 teaspoon red pepper flakes
- 1/4 cup parsley, diced
- 1/2 cup Greek yogurt, plain

Directions:
1. Attach the listed ingredients to a blender and emulsify by blending them (except 1/2 cup of chopped cucumbers)
2. Blend until smooth
3. Divide the soup amongst 4 servings and top with extra cucumbers
4. Enjoy chilled!
Nutrition
Calories: 371
Fat: 36g
Carbohydrates: 8g
Protein: 4g

75. Eggplant Salad

Preparation Time: 10 minutes
Cooking Time: 30 minutes
Serving: 3
Ingredients:
- 2 eggplants, peeled and sliced
- 2 garlic cloves
- 2 green bell paper, sliced, seeds removed
- 1/2 cup fresh parsley
- 1/2 cup egg-free mayonnaise
- Salt and black pepper

Directions:
1. Preheat your oven to 480 F
2. Take a baking pan and add the eggplants and black pepper
3. Bake for about 30 minutes
4. Flip the vegetables after 20 minutes
5. Then, take a bowl and add baked vegetables and all the remaining ingredients
6. Mix well
7. Serve and enjoy!
Nutrition
Calories: 196
Fat: 108.g
Carbohydrates: 13.4g
Protein: 14.6g

76. Zucchini Pancakes

Preparation time: 10 minutes
Cooking time: 25 minutes
Serving: 4
Ingredients:
- 2 tablespoons ground flax seeds
- 1/3 cup water
- 1 teaspoon olive oil
- 3 large zucchinis, grated
- 1 jalapeño pepper, chopped finely
- Pinch of salt
- ¼ cup scallion, chopped finely

Direction:
1. In a bowl, mix together flax seeds and water and set aside.
2. In a large nonstick skillet, heat oil over medium heat and cook zucchini, salt and black pepper for about 2-3 minutes, stirring occasionally.
3. Transfer the zucchini into a large bowl and set aside to cool slightly.
4. Stir in flax seed mixture and scallion and mix well.
5. heat a greased griddle over medium heat
6. Place ¼ of the zucchini mixture into preheated griddle.
7. Cook for about 2-3 minutes.
8. Carefully flip the side and cook for 1-2 minutes more.
9. Repeat with the remaining mixture.
10. Serve warm.

Meal Prep Tip:
1. Set the crepes aside to cool completely before storing.
2. Store these cooled pancakes into an airtight container by placing a piece of wax paper between each pancake.
3. Refrigerate up to 4 days.
4. Reheat in the microwave for about 1½-2 minutes.

Nutrition: Calories: 70, Fats: 2.7g, Carbs: 9.8g, Fiber: 3.9g, Sugar: 4.5g, Proteins: 3.7g, Sodium: 66mg

77. Blueberry Waffles

Preparation time: 10 minutes
Cooking time: 24 minutes
Serving: 6
Ingredients:
- 2 cups almond flour
- 2 cups oat flour
- 2 tablespoons cornstarch
- 2 tablespoons baking powder
- 1 teaspoon ground cinnamon
- ½ teaspoon salt
- 4 tablespoons maple syrup
- 3 cups unsweetened almond milk
- 1 teaspoon pure vanilla extract
- 1 cup fresh blueberries

Direction:
1. In a large bowl, mix together the flours, cornstarch, baking powder, cinnamon and salt.
2. Add the almond milk and vanilla and mix until just combined.
3. Gently, fold in the blueberries.
4. Preheat the waffle iron and then grease it.
5. Place desired amount of the mixture into the preheated waffle iron and cook for about 5-6 minutes or until golden brown.
6. Repeat with the remaining mixture.
7. Serve warm.

Meal Prep Tip:
1. Store these cooled waffles in a container by placing a piece of wax paper between each waffle.
2. Refrigerate up to 5 days.
3. Reheat in the microwave for about 1-2 minutes.

Nutrition: Calories: 431, Fats: 21.6g, Carbs: 47.6g, Fiber: 8.4g, Sugar: 10.4g, Proteins: 12.7g, Sodium: 303mg

78. Gentle Apple Porridge

Preparation Time: 10 minutes
Cooking Time: 5 minutes
Serving: 2
Ingredients:
- 1 large apple, peeled, cored, and grated
- 1 cup unsweetened almond milk
- 1 1/2 tablespoon of sunflower seeds

- 1/8 cup of fresh blueberries
- 1/4 teaspoon of vanilla bean extract

Directions:
1. Prepare a large pan then add sunflower seeds, vanilla extract, almond milk, apples, and stir
2. Place it over medium heat.
3. Cook for 5 minutes, keep stirring the mixture
4. Transfer to a serving bowl
5. Serve and enjoy!

Nutrition: Calories: 123 Fat: 1.3g Carbohydrates: 23g Protein: 4g

79. Pasta with Lemon, Asparagus and Cauliflower

Preparation time: 5 minutes
Cooking time: 20 minutes
Servings: 2-4
Ingredients:
- 2 tbsp olive oil, divided
- 3 cups of various colored cauliflower sprigs
- 2 cups of water, divided
- ¼ cup 2% milk
- 1 package of Lemon & Asparagus with Cavatappi spaghetti
- 1 cup cannellini beans, canned, washed
- ¼ cup low-fat ricotta cheese
- ¼ cup chopped and toasted walnuts

Direction:
1. Heat 1 tablespoon of olive oil in a large nonstick skillet over medium-high heat and cook the cauliflower, stirring occasionally, until golden, about 5 minutes. Add ½ cup water to the skillet and cook 5 minutes or until cauliflower is tender. Remove the cauliflower and set aside.
2. Pour the remaining 1 ½ cups of water, milk, and the remaining tablespoon of olive oil in the same pan. Bring to a boil. Stir the package of spaghetti and bring to a boil, then lower heat to medium-high and simmer for 8 minutes, covered and stirring frequently.
3. Add the cauliflower and beans. Add ricotta to center. Garnish with walnuts and, if desired, with fresh parsley or chopped basil. Now it was delicious, try it!

Nutrition: Calorie: 489 Protein: 13g Fat: 4g Carbohydrates: 96g

80. French Toast with Applesauce

Preparation Time: 5 minutes
Cooking Time: 15 minutes
Servings: 6
Ingredients:
- ¼ cup unsweetened applesauce
- ½ cup milk
- 1 teaspoons ground cinnamon
- 2 eggs
- 2 tablespoons white sugar
- 6 slices whole wheat bread

Directions:
1. Mix well applesauce, sugar, cinnamon, milk, and eggs in a mixing bowl.
2. Dip the bread into applesauce mixture until wet; take note that you should do this one slice at a time.
3. On medium fire, heat a nonstick skillet greased with cooking spray.
4. Add soaked bread one at a time and cook for 2-3 minutes per side or until lightly browned.
5. Serve and enjoy.

Nutrition: Calories: 57 Carbs: 6g Protein: 4g Fats: 4g Phosphorus: 69mg Potassium: 88mg Sodium: 43mg

81. Bagels Made Healthy

Preparation Time: 5 minutes
Cooking Time: 25 minutes
Servings: 8
Ingredients:
- 2 teaspoons yeast
- 1 ½ tablespoon olive oil
- 1 ¼ cups bread flour
- 2 cups whole wheat flour
- 1 tablespoon vinegar
- 2 tablespoons honey
- 1 ½ cups warm water

Directions:
1. In a bread machine, mix all the ingredients, and then process on dough cycle.
2. Once done or end of the cycle, create 8 pieces shaped like a flattened ball.

3.　Using your thumb, you must create a hole at the center of each, and then create a donut shape.

4.　Place the donut-shaped dough on a greased baking sheet, then covers and let it rise about ½ hour.

5.　Prepare about 2 inches of water to boil in a large pan.

6.　In boiling water, drop one at a time the bagels and boil for 1 minute, then turn them once.

7.　Remove them and return them to a baking sheet and bake at 350oF (175oC) for about 20 to 25 minutes until golden brown.

Nutrition: Calories: 221 Carbs: 42g Protein: 7g Fats: 3g Phosphorus: 130mg Potassium: 166mg Sodium: 47mg

82. Cornbread with Southern Twist

Preparation Time: 15 minutes
Cooking Time: 60 minutes
Servings: 8
Ingredients:
- 2 tablespoons shortening
- 1 ¼ cups skim milk
- ¼ cup egg substitute
- 4 tablespoons sodium-free baking powder
- ½ cup flour
- 1 ½ cups cornmeal

Directions:
1.　Prepare an 8x8-inch baking dish or a black iron skillet, and then add shortening.

2.　Put the baking dish or skillet inside the oven at 425 °F; once the shortening has melted, that means the pan is hot already.

3.　In a bowl, add milk and egg, and then mix well.

4.　Take out the skillet, and add the melted shortening into the batter and stir well.

5.　Pour mixture into skillet after mixing all the ingredients.

6.　Cook the cornbread for 15-20 minutes until it is golden brown.

Nutrition: Calories: 166 Carbs: 35g Protein: 5g Fats: 1g Phosphorus: 79mg Potassium: 122mg Sodium: 34mg

83. Sweet Pancakes

Preparation Time: 10 minutes
Cooking Time: 5 minutes
Servings: 5
Ingredients:
- All-purpose flour – 1 cup
- Granulated sugar – 1 tablespoon
- Baking powder – 2 teaspoons.
- Egg whites – 2
- Almond milk - 1 cup
- Olive oil - 2 tablespoons.
- Maple extract – 1 tablespoon

Directions:
1.　Combine the flour, sugar and baking powder in a bowl.

2.　Make a well in the center and place to one side.

3.　Mx the egg whites, milk, oil, and maple extract, do this in another bowl.

4.　Add the egg mixture to the well and gently mix until a batter is formed.

5.　Heat skillet over medium heat.

6.　Cook 2 minutes on each side or until the pancake is golden only add 1/5 of the batter to the pan.

7.　Repeat with the remaining batter and serve.

Nutrition: Calories: 178 Potassium: 126mg Sodium: 297mg Protein: 6g

84. Rutabaga Latkes

Preparation Time: 15 minutes
Cooking Time: 7 minutes
Servings: 4
Ingredients:
- 1 teaspoon hemp seeds
- 1 teaspoon ground black pepper
- 7 oz rutabaga, grated
- ½ teaspoon ground paprika
- 2 tablespoons coconut flour
- 1 egg, beaten
- 1 teaspoon olive oil

Directions:
1.　Mix up together hemp seeds, ground black pepper, ground paprika, and coconut flour.

2.　Then add grated rutabaga and beaten egg.

3.　With the help of the fork combine all the ingredients into the smooth mixture.

4.　Preheat the skillet for 2-3 minutes over high heat.

5. Then reduce the heat till medium and add olive oil.

6. With the help of the fork, place the small amount of rutabaga mixture in the skillet. Flatten it gently in the shape of latkes.

7. Cook the latkes for 3 minutes from each side.

8. After this, transfer them to the plate and repeat the same steps with the remaining rutabaga mixture.

Nutrition: 64 Calories 3g Fiber 2.8g Protein 223mg Potassium 57mg Sodium

85. Cabbage Apple Stir-Fry

Preparation Time: 15 minutes
Cooking Time: 10 minutes
Servings: 4
Ingredients:
• 2 tablespoons extra-virgin olive oil
• 3 cups chopped red cabbage
• 2 tablespoons water
• 1 Granny Smith apple
• 3 scallions, both parts
• 1 tablespoon freshly squeezed lemon juice
• 1 teaspoon caraway seeds
• Pinch of salt

Directions:
1. In a big skillet or frying pan, heat the olive oil over medium-high temperature.

2. Add the cabbage and stir-fry for 2 minutes. Add the water, cover, and cook for 2 minutes.

3. Uncover and stir in the apple and scallions and sprinkle with the lemon juice, caraway seeds, and salt. Stir-fry for 4 to 6 minutes longer, or until the cabbage is crisp-tender. Serve.

Nutrition: 106 Calories 5.3g Fiber 2g Protein 214mg Potassium 55mg Sodium

86. Mushroom Tacos

Preparation Time: 10 minutes
Cooking Time: 15 minutes
Servings: 6
Ingredients:
• 6 leaves of collard greens
• 2 cups mushrooms, chopped
• 1 white onion, diced
• 1 tablespoon taco seasoning
• 1 tablespoon coconut oil
• ½ teaspoon salt
• ¼ cup fresh parsley
• 1 tablespoon mayonnaise

Directions:
1. Put the coconut oil in the skillet and melt it.

2. Add chopped mushrooms and diced onion. Mix the ingredients.

3. Close the lid and cook them for 10 minutes.

4. After this, sprinkle the vegetables with Taco seasoning, salt, and add fresh parsley.

5. Mix the mixture and cook for 5 minutes more.

6. Then add mayonnaise and stir well.

7. Chill the mushroom mixture a little.

8. Fill the collard green leaves with the mushroom mixture and fold up them.

Nutrition: 52 Calories 1.2g Fiber 1.4g Protein 251mg Potassium 81mg Sodium

Chapter 6. Low-Sodium Recipes

87. Frankenstein Avocado Toast

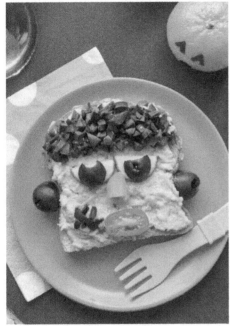

Preparation Time: 10 minutes
Cooking Time: 5 minutes
Servings: 2
Ingredients:
- 4 slices of whole wheat bread
- 1 avocado, cut in half, and seeded
- 1 tablespoon lemon juice
- 1/2 teaspoon garlic powder
- A pinch of sea salt

Decorative ingredients
- 1 nori leaf or a dark lettuce leaf
- 1/4 Black beans
- 1 small Sliced red pepper
- Mexicrema dressing

Directions:
1. Place bread in a toaster or a toaster oven.
2. While the bread is toasted, place the avocado in a bowl.
3. Add the lemon juice, garlic powder and salt, and pestle with a fork or potato masher.
4. Trim the nori leaf or dark lettuce to form the hair.
5. Decorate the toast forming the hair with the nori or the lettuce.

6. Put black beans as the eyes. The mouth with the sliced pepper, and the frame of the face with the dressing.
Nutrition: Calories: 230 Fat: 14g Carbohydrates: 22g Protein: 8g

88. Showy Avocado Toast

Preparation Time: 10 minutes
Cooking Time: 3 minutes
Servings: 2
Ingredients:
- 2 slices of bread
- 1 avocado, sliced
- 1/2 lemon juice
- 2 tablespoons pumpkin seeds
- 1 pinch red pepper flakes
- 1 pinch smoked paprika
- 1 pinch of sesame seeds
- 1 pinch of salt
- 1 pinch of black pepper

Directions:
1. Toast the bread.
2. Place the avocado slices on the toast.
3. Sprinkle the lemon juice over the avocado.
4. Sprinkle pumpkin seeds, red pepper flakes, sesame seeds, salt, and black pepper on top to taste.
Nutrition: Calories: 189 Fat: 11g Carbohydrates: 20g Protein: 3.8g

89. Beginnings with Sweet Potato

Preparation Time: 5 minutes
Cooking Time: 10 minutes
Servings: 2
Ingredients:
- 2 yams or baked sweet potatoes
- 2 peeled and sliced bananas
- 1 apple, without the heart and chopped
- 1/2 teaspoon ground cinnamon

Directions:
1. Peel and cut the yams or baked sweet potatoes.
2. Combine with bananas and apples.
3. Mix the cinnamon.

4. Briefly heat in a microwave oven. Serve hot.
Nutrition: Calories: 112 Fat: 0g Carbohydrates: 26g
Protein: 2g

90. Lovely Baby Potatoes

Preparation Time: 10 minutes
Cooking Time: 35 minutes
Serving: 4
Ingredients:
• 2 pounds' new yellow potatoes, scrubbed and cut into wedges
• 2 tablespoons extra virgin olive oil
• 2 teaspoons fresh rosemary, chopped
• 1/2 teaspoon ground black pepper and sunflower seeds
• 1 teaspoon garlic powder
Directions:
1. Prepare your oven to 400 degrees Fahrenheit
2. Arrange baking sheet with aluminum foil and set aside
3. Take a large bowl and add potatoes, olive oil, garlic, rosemary, sea sunflower seeds, and pepper
4. Prepare potatoes in a single layer on a baking sheet and bake for 35 minutes
5. Serve and enjoy!
Nutrition: Calories: 225 Fat: 7g Carbohydrates: 37g
Protein: 5g

91. Vegan Bread

Preparation time: 25 minutes
Cooking time: 45 minutes
Servings: 2-4
Ingredients:
• ½ lbs. coral lentils
• ¼ lbs. of millet
• 1 tablespoon of vinegar or lemon
• 1 teaspoon salt
• Water
• Spices to taste (turmeric, ginger, pepper, etc.)

Direction:
1. Place the lentils and millet in a bowl. Cover them with water and let stand 12 hours. After that time, rinse the grains, discarding the soaking water.
2. Crush the lentils and millet with a minimizer or food processor to form a sticky dough. Add the

vinegar or the lemon, the salt and the chosen spices and mix.
3. Let the dough rest in a bowl covered with plastic wrap or with a kitchen cloth at room temperature for two days. After that time, the dough begins to rise and you will feel an acidic smell due to the fermentation of the grains. Place the dough in a previously oiled bread pan or upholstered with vegetable paper.
4. Take in a preheated oven at 180 ° about 30-40 minutes or until a toothpick is inserted and it comes out dry.
Nutrition: Calorie: 80 Protein: 1g Fat: 2g
Carbohydrates: 14g

92. Pasta with Indian Lentils

Preparation Time: 5 minutes
Cooking Time: 0 minutes
Servings: 6
Ingredients:
• ¼-½ cup fresh cilantro (chopped)
• 3 cups water
• 2 small dry red peppers (whole)
• 1 teaspoons turmeric
• 1 teaspoons ground cumin
• 2-3 cloves garlic (minced)
• 1 can diced tomatoes (w/juice)
• 1 large onion (chopped)
• ½ cup dry lentils (rinsed)
• ½ cup orzo or tiny pasta
Directions:
1. Combine all the ingredients in the skillet except for the cilantro, and then boil on medium-high heat.
2. Ensure to cover and slightly reduce heat to medium-low and simmer until pasta is tender for about 35 minutes.
3. Afterwards, take out the chili peppers, then add cilantro and top it with low-fat sour cream.
Nutrition: Calories: 175 Carbs: 40g Protein: 3g Fats: 2g Phosphorus: 139mg Potassium: 513mg Sodium: 61mg

93. Apple Pumpkin Muffins

Preparation Time: 15 minutes

Cooking Time: 20 minutes
Servings: 12
Ingredients:
- 1 cup all-purpose flour
- 1 cup wheat bran
- 2 teaspoons Phosphorus Powder
- 1 cup pumpkin purée
- ¼ cup honey
- ¼ cup olive oil
- 1 egg
- 1 teaspoon vanilla extract
- ½ cup cored diced apple

Directions:
1. Preheat the oven to 400°F.
2. Line 12 muffin cups with paper liners.
3. Stir together the flour, wheat bran, and baking powder, mix this in a medium bowl.
4. In a small bowl, whisk together the pumpkin, honey, olive oil, egg, and vanilla.
5. Stir the pumpkin mixture into the flour mixture until just combined.
6. Stir in the diced apple.
7. Spoon the batter in the muffin cups.
8. Bake for about 20 minutes, or until a toothpick inserted in the center of a muffin comes out clean.
Nutrition: Calories: 125 Total Fat: 5g Saturated Fat: 1g Cholesterol: 18mg Sodium: 8mg Carbohydrates: 20g Fiber: 3g

94. Spiced French Toast

Preparation Time: 15 minutes
Cooking Time: 12 minutes
Servings: 4
Ingredients:
- 4 eggs
- ½ cup Homemade Rice Milk (here, or use unsweetened store-bought) or almond milk
- ¼ cup freshly squeezed orange juice
- 1 teaspoons ground cinnamon
- ½ teaspoons ground ginger
- Pinch ground cloves
- 1 tablespoon unsalted butter, divided
- 8 slices white bread

Directions:
1. Whisk eggs, rice milk, orange juice, cinnamon, ginger, and cloves until well blended in a large bowl.

2. Melt half the butter in a large skillet. It should be in medium-high heat only.
3. Dredge four of the bread slices in the egg mixture until well soaked, and place them in the skillet.
4. Cook the toast until golden brown on both sides, turning once, about 6 minutes' total.
5. Repeat with the remaining butter and bread.
6. Serve 2 pieces of hot French toast to each person.
Nutrition: Calories: 236 Total fats: 11g Saturated fat: 4g Cholesterol: 220mg Sodium: 84mg Carbohydrates: 27g

95. Mexican Scrambled Eggs in Tortilla

Preparation Time: 5 minutes
Cooking Time: 2 minutes
Servings: 2
Ingredients:
- 2 medium corn tortillas
- 4 egg whites
- 1 teaspoons cumin
- 3 teaspoons green chilies, diced
- ½ teaspoons hot pepper sauce
- 2 tablespoons salsa
- ½ teaspoons salt

Directions:
1. Spray some cooking spray on a medium skillet and heat for a few seconds.
2. Whisk the eggs with the green chilies, hot sauce, and comminute
3. Add the eggs into the pan, and whisk with a spatula to scramble. Add the salt.
4. Cook until fluffy and done (1-2 minutes) over low heat.
5. Open the tortillas and spread 1 tablespoon salsa on each.
6. Distribute the egg mixture onto the tortillas and wrap gently to make a burrito.
7. Serve warm.

96. Raspberry Overnight Porridge

Preparation Time: overnight

Cooking Time: 0 minute

Servings: 12

Ingredients:

- 1/3 cup rolled oats
- ½ cup almond milk
- 1 tablespoon honey
- 5-6 raspberries, fresh or canned and unsweetened
- 1/3 cup rolled oats
- ½ cup almond milk
- 1 tablespoon honey
- 5-6 raspberries, fresh or canned and unsweetened

Directions:

1. Combine the oats, almond milk, and honey in a mason jar and place into the fridge for overnight.
2. Serve the next morning with the raspberries on top.

Nutrition: calories: 143.6 kcal carbohydrate: 34.62 g protein: 3.44 g sodium: 77.88 mg potassium: 153.25 mg phosphorus: 99.3 mg dietary fiber: 7.56 g fat: 3.91 g

97. Buckwheat and Grapefruit Porridge

Preparation Time: 5 minutes

Cooking Time: 20 minutes

Servings: 2

Ingredients:

- Buckwheat – ½ cup
- Grapefruit – ¼, chopped
- Honey – 1 tablespoon
- Almond milk – 1 ½ cups
- Water – 2 cups

Directions:

1. Boil water on the stove. Add the buckwheat and place the lid on the pan.
2. Simmer for 7 to 10 minutes, in a low heat. Check to ensure water does not dry out.
3. Remove and set aside for 5 minutes, do this when most of the water is absorbed.
4. Drain excess water from the pan and stir in almond milk, heating through for 5 minutes.
5. Add the honey and grapefruit.
6. Serve.

Nutrition: Calories: 231 Fat: 4g Carb: 43g Phosphorus: 165mg Potassium: 370mg Sodium: 135mg

98. Egg and Veggie Muffins

Preparation Time: 15 minutes

Cooking Time: 20 minutes

Servings: 4

Ingredients:

- Cooking spray
- Eggs – 4
- Unsweetened rice milk – 2 tablespoons
- Sweet onion – ½, chopped
- Red bell pepper – ½, chopped
- Pinch red pepper flakes
- Pinch ground black pepper

Directions:

1. Preheat the oven to 350f.
2. Spray 4 muffin pans with cooking spray. Set aside.
3. Whisk together the milk, eggs, onion, red pepper, parsley, red pepper flakes, and black pepper until mixed.
4. Pour the egg mixture into prepared muffin pans.
5. Bake until the muffins are puffed and golden, about 18 to 20 minutes.
6. Serve

Nutrition: Calories: 84 Fat: 5g Carb: 3g Phosphorus: 110mg Potassium: 117mg Sodium: 75mg Protein: 7g

99. Cherry berry bulgur bowl

Preparation Time: 15 minutes

Cooking Time: 15 minutes

Servings: 4

Ingredients:

- 1 cup medium-grind bulgur
- 2 cups water
- Pinch salt
- 1 cup halved and pitted cherries or 1 cup canned cherries, drained
- ½ cup raspberries
- ½ cup blackberries
- 1 tablespoon cherry jam
- 2 cups plain whole-milk yogurt

Directions:

1.   Mix the bulgur, water, and salt in a medium saucepan. Do this in a medium heat. Bring to a boil.
2.   Reduce the heat to low and simmer, partially covered, for 12 to 15 minutes or until the bulgur is almost tender. Cover, and let stand for 5 minutes to finish cooking do this after removing the pan from the heat.
3.   While the bulgur is cooking, combine the raspberries and blackberries in a medium bowl. Stir the cherry jam into the fruit.
4.   When the bulgur is tender, divide among four bowls. Top each bowl with ½ cup of yogurt and an equal amount of the berry mixture and serve.
Nutrition: Calories: 242 Total Fat: 6g Saturated Fat: 3g Sodium: 85mg Phosphorus: 237mg Potassium: 438mg Carbohydrates: 44g Fiber: 7g Protein: 9g Sugar: 13g

100.   Couscous Salad

Preparation Time: 5 minutes
Cooking Time: 5 minutes
Servings: 5 servings
Ingredients:
- 3 cups of water
- 1/2 tsp. cinnamon tea
- 1/2 tsp. cumin tea
- 1 tsp. honey soup
- 2 tbsp. lemon juice
- 3 cups quick-cooking couscous
- 2 tbsp. tea of olive oil
- 1 green onion,
- Finely chopped 1 small carrot, finely diced
- 1/2 red pepper,
- Finely diced fresh coriander

Directions:
1.   Stir in the water with the cinnamon, cumin, honey, and lemon juice and bring to a boil. Put the couscous in it, cover it, and remove it from the heat.
2.   To swell the couscous, stir with a fork. Add the vegetables, fresh herbs, and olive oil. It is possible to serve the salad warm or cold.
Nutrition: Energy: 190 g, Protein: 6 g, Carbohydrates: 38 g, fibbers: 2 g, Total Fat: 1 g, Sodium: 4 mg, Phosphorus: 82 mg, Potassium: 116 mg

101.   Stuffed
Mushrooms with Cabbage

Preparation Time: 20 minutes
Cooking Time: 25 minutes
Serving: 6
Ingredients:
- 6 portobello mushrooms
- 3 tablespoons extra-virgin olive oil
- 1 onion, chopped
- 1 teaspoon minced peeled fresh ginger
- 2 cups shredded red cabbage
- 1/8 teaspoon salt
- 1/8 teaspoon freshly ground black pepper
- 3 tablespoons water
- 1 cup shredded Monterey Jack cheese

Direction
1.   Rinse the mushrooms briefly and pat dry. Remove the stems and discard. Scoop out the dark gills on the underside of the mushroom cap. Set aside.
2.   In a medium skillet, heat the olive oil over medium heat and cook the onion and ginger for 2 to 3 minutes, stirring, until fragrant.
3.   Add the cabbage, salt, and pepper and sauté for 3 minutes, stirring frequently.
4.   Add the water, cover, and steam the cabbage for 3 to 4 minutes, or until it is tender.
5.   Pull out vegetables from the skillet and place in a medium bowl; let cool for 10 minutes, then stir in the cheese.
6.   Preheat the oven to 400°F.
7.   Place the caps on a baking sheet and divide the filling among the mushrooms. Bake for 15 to 17 minutes, or until the mushrooms are tender and the filling is light golden brown. Serve.
Nutrition 163 Calories 179mg Sodium 173mg Phosphorus 360mg Potassium 7g Protein

102.   Carrot and
Parsnips French Fries

Preparation Time: 15 minutes
Cooking Time: 20 minutes
Servings: 2
Ingredients:
- 6 large carrots
- 6 large parsnips
- 2 tablespoons extra virgin olive oil
- ½ teaspoon of sea salt

Directions:
1.   Chop the carrots and parsnips into 2-inch slices and then cut each into thin sticks.

2.	Toss together the carrots and parsnip sticks with extra virgin olive oil and salt in a bowl and spread into a baking sheet lined with parchment paper.

3.	Bake the sticks at 425° for about 20 minutes or until browned.

Nutrition: Calories: 179 Fat: 4g Carbs: 14g Protein: 11g Sodium: 27.3mg Potassium: 625mg Phosphorus: 116mg

Sesame-Garlic Edamame

Preparation Time: 10 minutes

Cooking Time: 10 minutes

Servings: 4

Ingredients:

•	1 (14-ounce) package frozen edamame in their shells

•	1 tablespoon canola or sunflower oil

•	1 tablespoon toasted sesame oil

•	3 garlic cloves, minced

•	½ teaspoon kosher salt

•	¼ teaspoon red pepper flakes (or more)

Directions:

1.	Bring a large pot of water to a boil over high heat. Add the edamame, and cook just long enough to warm them up for 2 to 3 minutes.

2.	Meanwhile, heat the canola oil, sesame oil, garlic, salt, and red pepper flakes in a large skillet over medium heat for 1 to 2 minutes, then remove the pan from the heat.

3.	Drain the edamame and add them to the skillet, tossing to combine.

Nutrition: Calories: 173; Total Fat: 12g; Saturated Fat: 1g; Cholesterol: 0mg; Sodium: 246mg; Carbohydrates: 8g; Fiber: 5g; Added Sugars: 0g; Protein: 11g; Potassium: 487mg; Vitamin K: 34mcg Phosphorus 324mg

# 103.	Mixed Vegetable Barley

Preparation Time: 15 minutes

Cooking Time: 35 minutes

Servings: 6

Ingredients:

•	1 tablespoon olive oil

•	1 medium sweet onion, chopped

•	2 teaspoons minced garlic

•	2 cups fresh cauliflower florets

•	1 red bell pepper, diced

•	1 carrot, sliced

•	½ cup barley

•	½ cup white rice

•	2 cups water

•	1 tablespoon minced fresh parsley

Directions:

1.	In a large skillet over medium-high heat, heat the olive oil.

2.	Add the onion and garlic, and sauté until softened, about 3 minutes. Stir in the cauliflower, bell pepper, and carrot, and sauté for 5 minutes.

3.	Stir in the barley, rice, and water and bring to a boil.

4.	Reduce the heat to low, cover, and simmer until the liquid is absorbed and the barley and rice are tender, about 25 minutes. Serve topped with the parsley.

Nutrition (For Serving): Calories: 156, Total fat: 3g, Saturated fat: 0g, Cholesterol: 0mg, Sodium: 16mg, Carbohydrates: 30g, Fiber: 4g, Phosphorus: 83mg, Potassium: 220mg, Protein: 4g

Chapter 7. Low-Phosphorus Recipes

104.　　Almond Butter Toast with Sweet Potatoes and Blueberries

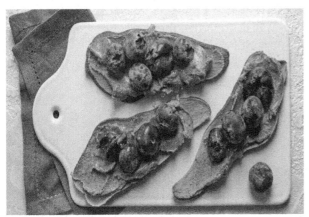

Preparation Time: 5 minutes
Cooking Time: 20 minutes
Servings: 2
Ingredients:
- 1 sweet potato, sliced half a centimeter thick
- 1/4 cup almond butter
- 1/2 cup blueberries

Directions:
1. Preheat the oven to 350-360 F (177 C).
2. Place the sweet potato slices on baking paper.
3. Bake until soft, approximately 20 minutes
4. Serve hot, coat with peanut butter and cranberries.

Nutrition: Calories: 264 Fat: 18g Carbohydrates: 19g Protein: 7g

105.　　American Blueberry Pancakes

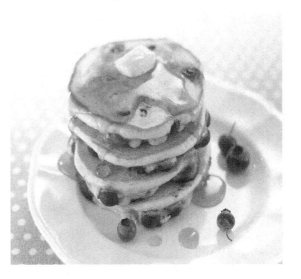

Preparation Time: 5 minutes
Cooking Time: 10 minutes
Servings: 6
Ingredients:
- 1 ½ cups all-purpose flour, sifted
- 1 cup buttermilk
- 3 tablespoons sugar
- 2 tablespoons unsalted butter, melted
- 2 teaspoons baking powder
- 2 eggs, beaten
- 1 cup canned blueberries, rinsed

Directions:
1. Combine the baking powder, flour, and sugar in a bowl.
2. Make a hole in the center and slowly add the rest of the ingredients.
3. Begin to stir gently from the sides to the center with a spatula until you get a smooth and creamy batter.
4. With cooking spray, spray the pan and place over medium heat.
5. Take one measuring cup and fill 1/3rd of its capacity with the batter to make each pancake.
6. Use a spoon to pour the pancake batter and let cook until golden brown. Flip once to cook the other side.
7. Serve warm with optional agave syrup.

Nutrition: Calories: 251.69 kcal Carbohydrate: 41.68 g Protein: 7.2 g Sodium: 186.68 mg Potassium: 142.87 mg Phosphorus: 255.39 mg Dietary Fiber: 1.9 g

106.   Cheesy Scrambled Eggs with Fresh Herbs

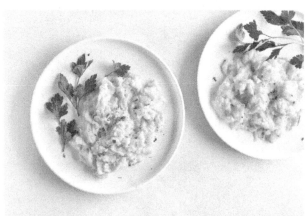

Preparation Time: 15 minutes
Cooking Time: 10 minutes
Servings: 4
Ingredients:
• 	Eggs – 3
• 	Egg whites – 2
• 	Cream cheese – ½ cup
• 	Unsweetened rice milk – ¼ cup
• 	Chopped scallion – 1 tablespoon green part only
• 	Chopped fresh tarragon – 1 tablespoon
• 	Unsalted butter – 2 tablespoons.
• 	Ground black pepper to taste
Directions:
1. 	In a container, mix the eggs, egg whites, cream cheese, rice milk, scallions, and tarragon until mixed and smooth.
2. 	Melt the butter in a skillet.
3. 	Pour in the egg mix and cook, stirring, for 5 minutes or until the eggs are thick and curds creamy.
4. 	Season with pepper and serve.
Nutrition: Calories: 221 Fat: 19g Carb: 3g Phosphorus: 119mg Potassium: 140mg Sodium: 193mg Protein: 8g

107.   Vegetable Omelet

Preparation Time: 15 minutes
Cooking Time: 10 minutes

Servings: 3
Ingredients:
• 	Egg whites – 4
• 	Egg – 1
• 	Chopped fresh parsley – 2 tablespoons.
• 	Water – 2 tablespoons.
• 	Olive oil spray
• 	Chopped and boiled red bell pepper – ½ cup
• 	Chopped scallion – ¼ cup, both green and white parts
• 	Ground black pepper
Directions:
1. 	Whisk together the egg, egg whites, parsley, and water until well blended. Set aside.
2. 	Spray a skillet with olive oil spray and place over medium heat.
3. 	Sauté the peppers and scallion for 3 minutes or until softened.
4. 	Over the vegetables, you can now pour the egg and cook, swirling the skillet, for 2 minutes or until the edges start to set. Cook until set.
5. 	Season with black pepper and serve.
Nutrition: Calories: 77 Fat: 3g Carb: 2g Phosphorus: 67mg Potassium: 194mg Sodium: 229mg Protein: 12g

108.   Squash and Turmeric Soup

Preparation Time: 10 minutes
Cooking Time: 30 minutes
Servings: 4
Ingredients:
• 	4 cups low-sodium vegetable broth
• 	2 medium zucchini squashes, peeled and diced
• 	2 medium yellow crookneck squashes, peeled and diced
• 	1 small onion, diced
• 	1/2 cup frozen green peas
• 	2 tbsp olive oil
• 	1/2 cup plain nonfat Greek yogurt
• 	2 tsp turmeric
Directions:
1. 	Warm the broth in a saucepan on medium heat.
2. 	Toss in onion, squash, and zucchini.
3. 	Let it simmer for approximately 25 minutes then add oil and green peas.

4.   Cook for another 5 minutes then allow it to cool.
5.   Puree the soup using a handheld blender then add Greek yogurt and turmeric.
6.   Refrigerate it overnight and serve fresh.
Nutrition: Calories 100. Protein 4 g. Carbohydrates 10 g. Fat 5 g. Cholesterol 1 mg. Sodium 279 mg. Potassium 504 mg. Phosphorus 138 mg. Calcium 60 mg. Fiber 2.8 g.

109.   Wild Rice Asparagus Soup

Preparation Time: 10 minutes
Cooking Time: 30 minutes
Servings: 4
Ingredients:
- 3/4 cup wild rice
- 2 cups asparagus, chopped
- 1 cup carrots, diced
- 1/2 cup onion, diced
- 3 garlic cloves, minced
- 1/4 cup unsalted butter
- 1/2 tsp thyme
- 1/2 tsp fresh ground pepper
- 1/4 tsp nutmeg
- 1 bay leaf
- 1/2 cup all-purpose flour
- 4 cups low-sodium vegetable broth
- 1/2 cup extra dry vermouth
- 4 cups unsweetened almond milk, unenriched

Directions:
1.   Cook the wild rice as per the cooking instructions on the box or bag and drain.
2.   Melt the butter in a Dutch oven and sauté garlic and onion.
3.   Once soft, add spices, herbs, and carrots.
4.   Cook on medium heat right until veggies are tender then add flour and stir cook for 10 minutes on low heat.
5.   Add 4 cups of broth and vermouth and blend using a handheld blender.
6.   Add asparagus to the soup.
7.   Stir in almond milk and cook for 20 minutes.
8.   Add the wild rice and serve warm.
Nutrition: Calories 295. Protein 21 g. Carbohydrates 28 g. Fat 11 g. Cholesterol 45 mg. Sodium 385 mg. Potassium 527 mg. Phosphorus 252 mg. Calcium 183 mg. Fiber 3.3

110.   Grated Carrot Salad with Lemon-Dijon Vinaigrette

Preparation Time: 15 minutes
Cooking Time: 10 minutes
Servings: 8
Ingredients:
- 9 small carrots (14 cm), peeled
- 2 tbsp. 1/2 teaspoon Dijon mustard
- 1 C. lemon juice
- 2 tbsp. extra virgin olive oil
- 1-2 tsp. honey (to taste)
- ¼ tsp. Salt
- ¼ tsp. freshly ground pepper (to taste)
- 2 tbsp. chopped parsley
- 1 green onion, thinly sliced

Directions:
1.   Grate the carrots in a food processor.
2.   Mix Dijon mustard, lemon juice, honey, olive oil, salt, and pepper in a salad bowl. Add the carrots, fresh parsley, and green onions. Stir to coat well. Cover and refrigerate until ready to be served.
Nutrition: Energy: 61 g, Proteins: 1 g, Carbohydrates: 7 g, fibbers: 1 g, Total Fat: 4 g, Sodium: 88 mg, Phosphorus: 22 mg, Potassium: 197 mg

111.   Cucumber Salad, Pulled Through Slowly

Preparation Time: 5 minutes
Cooking Time: 5 minutes
Servings: 4
Ingredients:
- 1 cucumber
- 1 tbsp. salt
- 100 ml of water
- 100 ml white wine vinegar
- 2 tbsp. cane sugar
- 5 peppercorns, crushed
- 1/2 teaspoon cinnamon
- 1/2 teaspoon of allspice
- 1 teaspoon chili powder
- 1 teaspoon ginger powder

Directions:

1. Wash the cucumber, cut it into thin slices, put them in a bowl, sprinkle with salt, and stir, shake well so that the salt gets everywhere. Then let it steep for half an hour.

2. Meanwhile, in a saucepan, mix water, vinegar, sugar, pepper, cinnamon, allspice, chili, ginger, and bring to a boil once, then let cool again with the lid closed.

3. Rinse the lettuce slices and pour off the water. If necessary, dry in a towel. Add the pot's dressing to the salad slices and let everything sit in the fridge for a day.

Nutrition: Energy: 49kcal, Protein: 1g, Carbohydrates: 5g, Potassium: 234mg, Sodium: 500mg, Calcium: 34mg, Phosphate: 21mg Phosphorus:142 mg

112. Cinnamon Apple Fries

Preparation Time: 5 minutes
Cooking Time: 15 minutes
Servings: 1
Ingredients:
- 1 apple, sliced thinly
- ¼ cup Dash of cinnamon
- 1 tbsp. Stevia

Directions:
1. Coat apple slices with cinnamon and stevia.
2. Bake for 15 minutes or until tender and crispy at 325 degrees F.

Nutrition: Calories: 146 Fat: 0.7 g Carbs: 36.4 g Protein: 1.6 g Sodium: 10 mg Potassium: 100mg Phosphorus: 0mg

113. Pear & Brie Salad

Preparation Time: 5 minutes
Cooking Time: 0 minutes
Servings: 4
Ingredients:
- 1 tablespoon olive oil
- 1 cup arugula
- ½ lemon
- ½ cup canned pears
- ¼ cucumber
- ¼ cup chopped brie

Direction:

1. Peel and dice the cucumber.
2. Dice the pear.
3. Wash the arugula.
4. Combine salad in a serving bowl and crumble the brie over the top.
5. Whisk the olive oil and lemon juice together.
6. Drizzle over the salad.
7. Season with a bit of black pepper to taste and serve immediately.

Nutrition: Calories 54, Protein 1 g, Carbs 12 g, Fat 7 g, Sodium 57mg, Potassium 115 mg, Phosphorus 67 mg

114. Caesar Salad

Preparation Time: 5 minutes
Cooking Time: 5 minutes
Servings: 4
Ingredients:
- 1 head romaine lettuce
- ¼ cup mayonnaise
- 1 tablespoon lemon juice
- 4 anchovy fillets
- 1 teaspoon Worcestershire sauce
- Black pepper
- 5 garlic cloves
- 4 tablespoons. Parmesan cheese
- 1 teaspoon mustard

Direction:
1. In a bowl mix all ingredients and mix well
2. Serve with dressing

Nutrition: Calories 44, Fat 2.1 g, Sodium 83 mg, Potassium 216 mg, Carbs 4.3 g, Protein 3.2 g, Phosphorus 45.6mg Calcium 19mg, Potassium 27mg Sodium: 121 mg

115. Roasted Chili-Vinegar Peanuts

Preparation Time: 5 minutes
Cooking Time: 10 minutes
Servings: 4
Ingredients:
- 1 tablespoon coconut oil
- 2 cups raw peanuts, unsalted
- 2 teaspoon sea salt
- 2 tablespoon apple cider vinegar
- 1 teaspoon chili powder

- 1 teaspoon fresh lime zest

Directions:

1. Preheat oven to 350°F.
2. In a large bowl, toss together coconut oil, peanuts, and salt until well coated.
3. Transfer to a rimmed baking sheet and roast in the oven for about 15 minutes or until fragrant.
4. Transfer the roasted peanuts to a bowl and add vinegar, chili powder, and lime zest.
5. Toss to coat well and serve.

Nutrition: Calories: 447 Fat: 39.5g Carbs: 12.3 g Protein: 18.9 g Sodium: 160 mg Potassium: 200mg Phosphorus: 0mg

116. Roasted Asparagus

Preparation Time: 5 minutes
Cooking Time: 10 minutes
Servings: 4
Ingredients:

- 1 tbsp. extra virgin olive oil
- 1-pound fresh asparagus
- 1 medium lemon, zested
- 1/2 tsp. freshly grated nutmeg
- 1/2 tsp. kosher salt
- ½ tsp. black pepper

Directions:

1. Preheat your oven to 500 degrees F.
2. Put asparagus on an aluminum foil and add extra virgin olive oil.
3. Prepare asparagus in a single layer and fold the edges of the foil.
4. Cook in the oven for 5 minutes. Continue roasting until browned.
5. Add the roasted asparagus with nutmeg, salt, zest, and pepper before serving.

Nutrition: Calories: 55 Fat: 3.8 g Carbs: 4.7 g Protein: 2.5 g Sodium: 98mg Potassium: 172mg Phosphorus: 35mg

117. Herbal Cream Cheese Tartines

Preparation Time: 15 minutes
Cooking Time: 15 minutes
Servings: 2
Ingredients:

- 1 clove garlic, halved

- 1 cup cream cheese spread
- ¼ cup chopped herbs such as chives, dill, parsley, tarragon, or thyme
- 2 tbsp. minced French shallot or onion
- ½ tsp. black pepper
- 2 tbsp. tablespoons water

Directions:

1. Combine the cream cheese, herbs, shallot, pepper, and water in a medium-sized bowl with a hand blender.
2. Serve the cream cheese with the rusks.

Nutrition: Calories: 476 Fat: 9g Carbs: 75g Protein: 23g Sodium: 885mg Potassium: 312mg Phosphorus: 165mg

118. Rosemary and White Bean Dip

Preparation Time: 10 minutes
Cooking Time: 10 minutes
Servings: 10 (¼ cup per serving)
Ingredients:

- 1 (15-ounce) can cannellini beans, rinsed and drained
- 2 tablespoons extra-virgin olive oil
- 1 garlic clove, peeled
- 1 teaspoon finely chopped fresh rosemary
- Pinch cayenne pepper
- Freshly ground black pepper
- 1 (7.5-ounce) jar marinated artichoke hearts, drained

Directions:

1. Blend the beans, oil, garlic, rosemary, cayenne pepper, and black pepper in a food processor until smooth.
2. Add the artichoke hearts, and pulse until roughly chopped but not puréed.

Nutrition: Calories: 75; Total Fat: 5g; Saturated Fat: 1g; Cholesterol: 0mg; Sodium: 139mg; Carbohydrates: 6g; Fiber: 3g; Added Sugars: 0g; Protein: 2g; Potassium: 75mg; Phosphorus 43mg Vitamin K: 1mcg

119. Salad with strawberries and goat cheese

Preparation time: 15 minutes
Cooking time: 0 minute
Servings: 2
Ingredients
- Baby lettuce, to taste
- 1-pint strawberries
- Balsamic vinegar
- Extra virgin olive oil
- 1/4 teaspoon black pepper
- 8-ounce soft goat cheese

Directions
1. Prepare the lettuce by washing and drying it, and then cut the strawberries.
2. Cut the soft goat cheese into 8 pieces.
3. Put together the balsamic vinegar and the extra virgin olive oil in a large cup with a whisk.
4. Mix the strawberries pressing them and putting them in a bowl, add the dressing and mix, then divide the lettuce into four dishes and cut the other strawberries, arranging them on the salad.
5. Put cheese slices on top and add pepper. Serve and enjoy!
Nutrition:

Calories: 300
Protein: 13 G
Sodium: 285 Mg
Potassium: 400 Mg
Phosphorus: 193 Mg

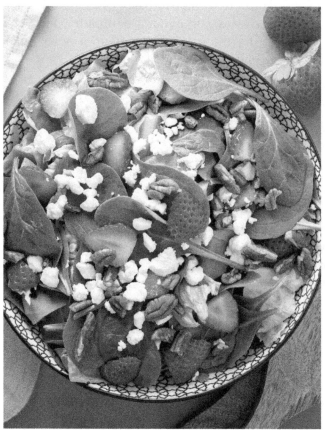

Chapter 8.   Snacks/Light bites/Entrée

120.   Popcorn Tofu Nuggets

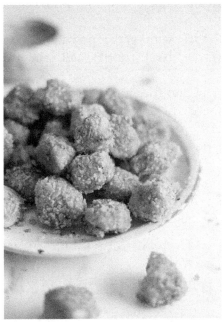

Preparation Time: 10 minutes
Cooking Time: 12 minutes
Serving: 2
Ingredients:
Popcorn Tofu
- 14 ounces' tofu, drained and pressed
- ½ cup quinoa flour
- ½ cup cornmeal
- 3 tablespoons nutritional yeast
- 2 tablespoons Bouillon Vegetarian
- 1 tablespoon Dijon mustard
- 2 teaspoon garlic powder
- 2 teaspoon onion powder
- ½ teaspoon salt
- ½ teaspoon pepper
- ¾ cup almond milk
- 1.5 cup panko breadcrumbs
Directions:
1.   At 350 degrees F, preheat your air fryer.
2.   Mix flour with milk, pepper, salt, onion, garlic, mustard and bouillon in a bowl until smooth.
3.   Dip the tofu in the batter and coat the panko breadcrumbs.
4.   Place the coated tofu in the air fryer basket, then air fry for 12 minutes.

5.   Flip the tofu nuggets once cooked halfway through.
6.   Serve.
Nutrition: Calories 392; Fat 8.7g; Cholesterol 0mg; Carbohydrate 59.3g; Sugars 5.1g; Protein 21.1g

121.   Vegan Onion Rings

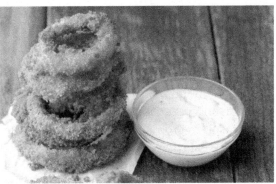

Preparation Time: 10 minutes
Cooking Time: 15 minutes
Serving: 4
Ingredients:
- 3 yellow onions
Wet mix:
- 1/2 cup flour
- 2/3 cup almond milk
- 1/2 teaspoon paprika
- 1/4 teaspoon turmeric
- 1/2 teaspoon salt
Dry mix:
- 1 cup panko breadcrumbs
- 1/2 teaspoon paprika
- 1/4 teaspoon turmeric
- 1/4 teaspoon salt
Directions:
1.   At 400 degrees F, preheat your Air fryer.
2.   Mix flour with milk, paprika, turmeric, and salt in a bowl until smooth.
3.   Toss breadcrumbs with salt, turmeric and paprika in a bowl.
4.   Cut the onions into ½ inch thick slices and separate them into rings.
5.   Dip each ring in the flour batter and coat with the panko crumbs.
6.   Place the onion rings in the air fryer basket and air fry for 15 minutes.
7.   Flip the onion rings once cooked halfway through, then resume cooking.

8.   Serve and enjoy.

Nutrition: Calories 139; Fat 1.4g; Cholesterol 0mg; Carbohydrate 27.1g; Sugars 4.2g; Protein 4.2g

122.   Kale and Potato Nuggets

Preparation Time: 10 minutes
Cooking Time: 19 minutes
Serving: 4
Ingredients:
- 2 cups chopped potatoes
- 1 teaspoon olive oil
- 1 clove garlic minced
- 4 cups chopped kale
- 1/8 cup almond milk
- 1/4 teaspoon sea salt
- 1/8 teaspoon ground black pepper
- Vegetable oil spray as needed

Directions:
1.   Add potatoes to a saucepan filled with boiling water and cook for 30 minutes until soft.
2.   Sauté garlic with oil in a skillet for 30 seconds until golden brown.
3.   Stir in kale and cook for 3 minutes, then transfer it to a bowl.
4.   Drain the cooked potatoes and allow them to cool.
5.   Mash the cooked potatoes in a bowl with a potato masher.
6.   Stir in kale, black pepper, milk, and salt, then mix well.
7.   At 390 degrees F, preheat your Air fry.
8.   Make 1-inch balls out of this potato mixture and place them in the air fryer basket.
9.   Spray the potato nuggets with vegetable oil and air fry them for 15 minutes.
10.   Flip the balls once cooked halfway through.
11.   Serve.

Nutrition: Calories 113; Fat 3g; Cholesterol 0mg; Carbohydrate 19.5g; Sugars 1.1g; Protein 3.5g

123.   Air Fryer Fries

Preparation Time: 10 minutes
Cooking Time: 30 minutes
Serving: 4
Ingredients:

- 3 medium red potatoes
- 1 teaspoon garlic powder
- 1 teaspoon onion powder
- ¼ teaspoon chilli powder
- ¼ teaspoon paprika
- ¼ teaspoon basil
- salt to taste

Directions:
1.   At 400 degrees F, preheat your air fryer.
2.   Peel, rinse and cut the potatoes into 1-inch matchsticks.
3.   Toss the fries with garlic powder, onion powder, chilli powder, basil, paprika and salt in a bowl.
4.   Spread the potato fries in the air fryer basket.
5.   Air fry these fries for 30 minutes in the preheated air fryer.
6.   Toss the fries after 15 minutes, then resume cooking.
7.   Serve warm.

Nutrition: Calories 117; Fat 0.3g; Cholesterol 0mg; Carbohydrate 26.6g; Sugars 2g; Protein 3.2g

124.   Za'atar Spiced Kale Chips

Preparation Time: 10 minutes
Cooking Time: 15 minutes
Serving: 2
Ingredients:
- 1 large bunch kale, washed and torn
- 1 tablespoon olive oil
- 2 tablespoons za'atar seasoning
- 1 teaspoon sea salt

Directions:
1.   Toss kale with olive oil and rub the leaves well.
2.   Mix the leaves with salt and za'atar seasoning, then spread in the air fryer basket.
3.   At 350 degrees F, preheat your air fryer.
4.   Spread the kale leaves in the air fryer basket, and air fry them for 15 minutes.
5.   Toss the kale leaves once cooked halfway through.
6.   Serve.

Nutrition: Calories 97; Fat 8g; Cholesterol 0mg; Carbohydrate 5.5g; Sugars 0g; Protein 2g

125.   Fried Ravioli

Preparation Time: 10 minutes
Cooking Time: 8 minutes
Serving: 4
Ingredients:
- ½ cup panko breadcrumbs
- 2 teaspoon nutritional yeast flakes
- 1 teaspoon dried basil
- 1 teaspoon dried oregano
- 1 teaspoon garlic powder
- Pinch salt and black pepper
- ¼ cup aquafaba liquid
- 8 ounces thawed vegan ravioli
- Spritz cooking spray

Directions:
1.   At 390 degrees F, preheat your air fryer.
2.   Mix panko crumbs with salt, black pepper, garlic powder, oregano, basil and yeast on a plate.
3.   Add aquafaba to a bowl and dip the ravioli in this liquid.
4.   Coat the ravioli with the panko crumbs mixture.
5.   Place the coated ravioli in the air fryer basket.
6.   Spray the ravioli with cooking spray and air fry for 8 minutes.
7.   Flip the ravioli once cooked halfway through.
8.   Serve warm.

Nutrition: Calories 120; Fat 1g; Cholesterol 0mg; Carbohydrate 23g; Sugars 1.5g; Protein 4.7g

126.   Nacho Kale Chips

Preparation Time: 10 minutes
Cooking time: 14 hours
Servings: 10
Ingredients:
- 2 bunches of curly kale
- 2 cups cashews, soaked, drained
- 1/2 cup chopped red bell pepper
- 1 teaspoon garlic powder
- 1 teaspoon salt
- 2 tablespoons red chili powder
- 1/2 teaspoon smoked paprika
- 1/2 cup nutritional yeast
- 1 teaspoon cayenne
- 3 tablespoons lemon juice
- 3/4 cup water

Direction:

1. Put all the shopping list: except the kale in a food processor and blend for 2 minutes until smooth.
2. Place the kale in a large bowl, pour the blended mixture, mix until coated and dehydrate for 14 hours at 120 degrees F until crisp.
3. If the dehydrator is not available, spread the kale between two baking sheets and bake for 90 minutes at 225 degrees F until crisp, turning halfway.
4. When finished, let the chips cool for 15 minutes and then serve.

Nutrition: Calories: 191 Cal Fat: 12 g Carbs: 16 g Protein: 9 g Fiber: 2 g

127.   Zucchini Fritters

Preparation Time: 10 minutes
Cooking time: 6 minutes
Servings: 12
Ingredients:
- 1/2 cup quinoa flour
- 3 1/2 cups shredded zucchini
- 1/2 cup chopped scallions
- 1/3 teaspoon ground black pepper
- 1 teaspoon salt
- 2 tablespoons coconut oil
- 2 flax eggs

Direction:
1. Squeeze the moisture from the zucchini by wrapping them in cheesecloth and then transfer them to a bowl.
2. Add the remaining shopping list: except the oil, mix until well blended and then form twelve meatballs.
3. Take a pan, put it on medium-high heat, add the oil and, when hot, add the patties and cook for 3 minutes on each side until golden.
4. Serve the meatballs with your favorite vegan sauce.

Nutrition: Calories: 37 Cal Fat: 1 g Carbs: 4 g Protein: 2 g Fiber: 1 g

128.   Tomato and Avocado Salsa

Preparation Time: 10 minutes
Cooking time: 0 minutes
Servings: 6
Ingredients:
- 3 cups chopped tomatoes
- 1 cup avocado, peeled, pitted and chopped

- 1 tablespoon black olives, pitted and sliced
- 1 red onion, chopped
- 2 teaspoons capers
- 3 garlic cloves, minced
- 2 teaspoons balsamic vinegar
- 1 tablespoon chopped basil
- A pinch of salt and black pepper

Direction:

1. In a bowl, mix the tomatoes with the avocado, the olives and the other shopping list: and toss.

2. Serve as an appetizer.

Nutrition: calories 201, fat 4.9, fiber 3.2, carbs 8, protein 6

129. Pea Dip

Preparation Time: 10 minutes
Cooking time: 0 minutes
Servings: 8
Ingredients:
- 2 cups canned black-eyed peas, drained and rinsed
- ½ teaspoon chili powder
- ½ cup coconut cream
- A pinch of salt and black pepper
- ½ teaspoon garlic powder
- 1 teaspoon Italian seasoning
- ½ teaspoon chili sauce
- 1 teaspoon hot paprika

Direction:

1. In a blender, mix the peas with the chili powder, cream and other grocery list: whisk and serve as a party sauce.

Nutrition: calories 127, fat 5, fiber 7, carbs 18, protein 8

130. Avocado Salsa

Preparation Time: 10 minutes
Cooking time: 0 minutes
Servings: 4
Ingredients:
- ½ cup leeks, chopped
- ½ cup spring onions, chopped
- 1 cup avocado, peeled, pitted and cubed
- 1 cup cherry tomatoes, chopped
- 1 tablespoon balsamic vinegar
- 1 tablespoon olive oil
- 1 teaspoon ground sage

- 1 teaspoon rosemary, dried
- A pinch of salt and black pepper

Direction:

1. In a bowl, mix the leeks with the spring onions, avocado and the other shopping list: mix, divide into smaller bowls and serve

Nutrition: calories 202, fat 5.2, fiber 4.3, carbs 8, protein 7

131. Quinoa Broccoli Tots

Preparation Time: 10 minutes
Cooking time: 20 minutes
Servings: 16
Ingredients:
- 2 tablespoons quinoa flour
- 2 cups steamed and chopped broccoli florets
- 1/2 cup nutritional yeast
- 1 teaspoon garlic powder
- 1 teaspoon miso paste
- 2 flax eggs
- 2 tablespoons hummus

Direction:

1. Put the whole shopping list: in a bowl, mix until well blended, then form the mixture into sixteen balls.

2. Arrange the balls on a baking sheet lined with parchment paper, drizzle with oil and bake at 400 ° F for 20 minutes until golden, turning halfway.

3. When cooked, leave to cool for 10 minutes and serve immediately.

Nutrition: Calories: 19 Cal Fat: 0 g Carbs: 2 g Protein: 1 g Fiber: 0.5 g

132. Thai Snack Mix

Preparation Time: 15 minutes
Cooking time: 90 minutes
Servings: 4
Ingredients:
- 5 cups mixed nuts
- 1 cup chopped dried pineapple
- 1 cup pumpkin seed
- 1 teaspoon onion powder
- 1 teaspoon garlic powder
- 2 teaspoons paprika
- 1/2 teaspoon ground black pepper

- 1 teaspoon of sea salt
- 1/4 cup coconut sugar
- 1/2 teaspoon red chili powder
- 1 tablespoon red pepper flakes
- 1/2 tablespoon red curry powder
- 2 tablespoons soy sauce
- 2 tablespoons coconut oil

Direction:

1. Turn on the slow cooker, add all the shopping list: in it except the dried pineapple and chili flakes, stir until combined and cook for 90 minutes on high heat, stirring every 30 minutes.

2. When cooked, spread the walnut mixture on a baking sheet lined with parchment paper and let it cool.

3. Then spread the dried pineapple on top, sprinkle with red pepper flakes and serve.

Nutrition: Calories: 230 Cal Fat: 17.5 g Carbs: 11.5 g Protein: 6.5 g Fiber: 2 g

133.   Red Salsa

Preparation Time: 10 minutes
Cooking time: 0 minute
Servings: 8
Ingredients:
- 30 ounces diced fire-roasted tomatoes
- 4 tablespoons diced green chilies
- 1 medium jalapeño pepper, deseeded
- 1/2 cup chopped green onion
- 1 cup chopped cilantro
- 1 teaspoon minced garlic
- ½ teaspoon of sea salt
- 1 teaspoon ground cumin
- ¼ teaspoon stevia
- 3 tablespoons lime juice

Direction:

1. Put the whole shopping list: in a food processor and work for 2 minutes until smooth.

2. Pour the sauce into a bowl, taste to adjust the seasoning and then serve.

Nutrition: Calories: 71 Cal Fat: 0.2 g Carbs: 19 g Protein: 2 g Fiber: 4.1 g

134.   Zucchini Chips

Preparation Time: 10 minutes
Cooking time: 120 minutes
Servings: 4

Ingredients:
- 1 large zucchini, thinly sliced
- 1 teaspoon salt
- 2 tablespoons olive oil

Direction:

1. Pat dry the zucchini slices and then spread them in an even layer on a baking sheet lined with parchment paper.

2. Whisk together the salt and oil, brush this mixture over the courgetti slices on both sides and bake for 2 hours or more until brown and crisp.

3. When cooked, let the chips cool for 10 minutes and then serve immediately.

Nutrition: Calories: 54 Cal Fat: 5 g Carbs: 1 g Protein: 0 g Fiber: 0.3 g

135.   Broccoli Spread

Preparation Time: 10 minutes
Cooking time: 15 minutes
Servings: 4
Ingredients:
- 4 cups broccoli florets
- 1 tablespoon olive oil
- 2 spring onions, chopped
- 1 cup coconut cream
- ½ cup cashews
- A pinch of salt and black pepper
- 1 teaspoon smoked paprika
- ½ teaspoon chili powder
- ½ teaspoon ground jalapeno
- ½ cup chopped chives

Direction:

1.   Heat a pan with the oil over medium heat, add the spring onions, paprika, jalapeño and chili powder and cook for 5 minutes.

2.   Add the rest of the shopping list: cook everything for another 10 minutes, blend with an immersion blender, divide into bowls and serve.

Nutrition: calories 210, fat 5.4, fiber 6.6, carbs 6, protein 7

136.   Tomato Hummus

Preparation Time: 5 minutes
Cooking time: 0 minute
Servings: 4
Ingredients:
- 1/4 cup sun-dried tomatoes, without oil

- 1 ½ cups cooked chickpeas
- 1 teaspoon minced garlic
- 1/2 teaspoon salt
- 2 tablespoons sesame oil
- 1 tablespoon lemon juice
- 1 tablespoon olive oil
- 1/4 cup of water

Direction:

1. Put the whole shopping list: in a food processor and work for 2 minutes until smooth.
2. Pour the hummus into a bowl, drizzle with more oil and serve immediately.

Nutrition: Calories: 122.7 Cal Fat: 4.1 g Carbs: 17.8 g Protein: 5.1 g Fiber: 3.5 g

137.   Chard Dip

Preparation Time: 10 minutes
Cooking time: 10 minutes
Servings: 4
Ingredients:
- 2 garlic cloves, minced
- 2 cups Swiss chard leaves
- ½ cup coconut cream
- 1 teaspoon turmeric powder
- 1 teaspoon curry powder
- ¼ cup sesame paste
- A pinch of salt and black pepper
- 2 teaspoons olive oil
- Juice of 1 lime
- 1 tablespoon chopped chives

Direction:

1. In a pan, mix the chard with the cream, turmeric and the other Shopping List: mix and cook over medium heat for 10 minutes.
2. Blend with a hand blender, divide into bowls and serve as a party sauce.

Nutrition: calories 142, fat 6, fiber 3, carbs 7, protein 4

138.   Nacho with Cheese Sauce

Preparation Time: 5 minutes
Cooking time: 10 minutes
Servings: 4
Ingredients:
- 3 tablespoons flour
- 1/4 teaspoon garlic salt
- 1/4 teaspoon salt
- 1/2 teaspoon cumin
- 1/4 teaspoon paprika
- 1 teaspoon red chili powder
- 1/8 teaspoon cayenne powder
- 1 cup vegan cashew yogurt
- 1 1/4 cups vegetable broth

Direction:

1. Take a saucepan, put it on medium heat, pour in the vegetable broth and bring it to a boil.
2. Then whisk together the flour and yogurt, add to the boiling broth, add all the spices, bring the heat to medium-low and cook for 5 minutes until thickened.
3. Serve immediately.

Nutrition: Calories: 282 Cal Fat: 1 g Carbs: 63 g Protein: 3 g Fiber: 12 g

139.   Vegan Pulled Pork

Preparation Time: 15 minutes
Cooking Time: 8 minutes
Serving: 2
Ingredients:
- 1 cup warm water
- 1 teaspoon vegetarian Bouillon
- 1 cup soy curls
- ¼ cup BBQ sauce
- 1 teaspoon canola oil

Directions:

1.   Mix water with bouillon in a large bowl.
2.   Soak soy curls in this water for 10 minutes, then drain.
3.   At 400 degrees F, preheat your air fryer.
4.   Pull the curls to shred them into finer strips.
5.   Spread the soy curls in the air fryer basket and air fry for 3 minutes.
6.   Mix the soy curls with ¼ cup of BBQ sauce in a bowl.

7.	Return these curls to the air fryer basket and air fry for 5 minutes.
8.	Serve warm.
Nutrition: Calories 117; Fat 4.7g; Cholesterol 0mg; Carbohydrate 13.8g; Sugars 8.6g; Protein 5g

# 140.	Apple and Honey Toast

Preparation Time: 5 minutes
Cooking time: 0 minute
Servings: 4
Ingredients:
- ½ of a small apple, cored, sliced
- 1 slice of whole-grain bread, toasted
- 1 tablespoon honey
- 2 tablespoons hummus
- 1/8 teaspoon cinnamon

Direction:
1.	Spread hummus on one side of the toast, top with apple slices and then drizzle with honey.
2.	Sprinkle cinnamon on it and then serve straight away.
Nutrition: Calories: 212 Cal Fat: 7 g Carbs: 35 g Protein: 4 g Fiber: 5.5 g

# 141.	Zucchini Muffins

Preparation Time: 10 minutes
Cooking time: 30 minutes
Servings: 12
Ingredients:
- 2 cups almond flour
- 2 teaspoons baking powder
- 2 tablespoons coconut sugar
- A pinch of black pepper
- 2 tablespoons flaxseed meal mixed with 3 tablespoons water
- ¾ cup almond milk
- 1 cup zucchinis, grated
- ½ cup tofu, shredded

Direction:
1.	In a bowl combine the flour with the baking powder, the flax seeds and the other shopping list: mix well, divide into a lined muffin pan, place in the oven and bake at 400 ° C for 30 minutes.
2.	Serve as a snack.

Nutrition: calories 149, fat 4, fiber 2, carbs 14, protein 5

# 142.	Chili Walnuts

Preparation Time: 10 minutes
Cooking time: 10 minutes
Servings: 4
Ingredients:
- ½ teaspoon chili flakes
- ½ teaspoon curry powder
- ½ teaspoon hot paprika
- A pinch of cayenne pepper
- 14 ounces' walnuts
- 2 teaspoons avocado oil

Direction:
1.	Spread the walnuts on a lined baking sheet, add the chili pepper and the other shopping list: mix, place in the oven and bake at 400 degrees for 10 minutes.
2.	Divide the mixture into bowls and serve as a snack.
Nutrition: calories 204, fat 3.2, fiber 5, carbs 7.4, protein 7

# 143.	Spicy Roasted Chickpeas

Preparation Time: 10 minutes
Cooking time: 20 minutes
Servings: 6
Ingredients:
- 30 ounces cooked chickpeas
- ½ teaspoon salt
- 2 teaspoons mustard powder
- ½ teaspoon cayenne pepper
- 2 tablespoons olive oil

Direction:
1. Put the whole Shopping List: in a bowl and mix until well covered, then distribute the chickpeas in an even layer on an oiled pan.
2. Cook the chickpeas for 20 minutes at 400 degrees F until golden brown and crisp and then serve immediately.
Nutrition: Calories: 187.1 Cal Fat: 7.4 g Carbs: 24.2 g Protein: 7.3 g Fiber: 6.3 g

144. Carrot Chips

Preparation Time: 10 minutes
Cooking time: 20 minutes
Servings: 6
Ingredients:
- 1-pound carrots, peeled and thinly sliced
- 1 teaspoon sweet paprika
- 1 teaspoon coriander, ground
- 2 tablespoons olive oil
- 1 tablespoon chili powder
- A pinch of cayenne pepper

Direction:
1. Spread the carrot chips on a lined baking sheet, add the paprika and the other shopping list: mix, put in the oven and bake at 350 degrees for 20 minutes.
2. Divide them into bowls and serve as a snack.
Nutrition: calories 219, fat 6.1, fiber 4, carbs 12, protein 5

145. Tomatillo Salsa

Preparation Time: 5 minutes
Cooking Time: 20 minutes
Serving: 2 cups
Ingredients:
- 5 medium tomatillos, chopped
- 3 cloves of garlic, peeled, chopped
- 3 Roma tomatoes, chopped
- 1 jalapeno, chopped
- ½ of a medium red onion, peeled, chopped
- 1 anaheim chili
- 2 teaspoons salt
- 1 teaspoon ground cumin
- 1 lime, juiced
- ¼ cup cilantro leaves
- ¾ cup of water

Directions:
1. Take a medium pot, place it over medium heat, pour in water, and then add onion, tomatoes, tomatillo, jalapeno, and Anaheim chili.
2. Sauté the vegetables for 15 minutes, remove the pot from heat, add cilantro and lime juice and then stir in salt.
3. Remove pot from heat and then pulse by using an immersion blender until smooth.
4. Serve the salsa with chips.

Nutrition: Calories: 317.4 Cal; Fat: 0 g; Protein: 16 g; Carbs: 64 g; Fiber: 16 g;

146. Spinach Dip

Preparation Time: 10 minutes
Cooking time: 0 minutes
Servings: 4
Ingredients:
- 1 tablespoon olive oil
- 10 ounces' spinach
- 1 teaspoon sweet paprika
- 1 teaspoon oregano, dried
- 1 teaspoon salt
- 1 teaspoon black pepper
- 3 tablespoons coconut cream

Direction:
1. In your blender, combine the spinach with the oil, paprika and the other shopping list, blend and serve.
Nutrition: calories 200, fat 3, fiber 5, carbs 14, protein 7.7

147. Rosemary Beet Chips

Preparation Time: 10 minutes
Cooking time: 20 minutes
Servings: 3
Ingredients:
- 3 large beets, scrubbed, thinly sliced
- 1/8 teaspoon ground black pepper
- ¼ teaspoon of sea salt
- 3 sprigs of rosemary, leaves chopped
- 4 tablespoons olive oil

Direction:
1. Spread the beetroot slices in a single layer between two large baking sheets, brush the slices with oil, then season with spices and rosemary, mix until well coated and cook for 20 minutes at 375 degrees F until crisp., turning halfway.
2. When finished, let the chips cool for 10 minutes and then serve.
Nutrition: Calories: 79 Cal Fat: 4.7 g Carbs: 8.6 g Protein: 1.5 g Fiber: 2.5 g

148.   Strawberry Salsa

Preparation Time: 10 minutes
Cooking time: 0 minutes
Servings: 4
Ingredients:
- 2 cups strawberries, halved
- ½ cup sunflower seeds
- ½ cup mango, peeled and cubed
- 1 teaspoon coconut sugar
- 12 apricots, dried and quartered

Direction:
1.   In a bowl, mix the strawberries with the seeds and the other shopping list: mix, divide into bowls and serve.
Nutrition: calories 137, fat 2, fiber 5, carbs 3.2, protein 3.3

149.   Artichoke Dip

Preparation Time: 10 minutes
Cooking time: 15 minutes
Servings: 4
Ingredients:
- 12 ounces canned artichoke hearts, no-salt-added, drained and chopped
- 1 cup coconut cream
- 1 cup tofu, shredded
- 1 teaspoon salt
- 1 teaspoon turmeric powder
- A pinch of black pepper

Direction:
1.   In a baking dish, mix the artichokes with the cream and the other Shopping List: sauté, place in the oven and bake at 400 degrees for 15 minutes.
2.   Divide into bowls and serve as a party sauce.
Nutrition: calories 200, fat 7.7, fiber 6, carbs 14, protein 8.2

150.   Rosemary Popcorn

Preparation Time: 10 minutes
Cooking time: 10 minutes
Servings: 4
Ingredients:
- 1/2 cup popcorn kernels
- 1/2 teaspoon sea salt
- 1 tablespoon and 1/2 teaspoon minced rosemary
- 3 tablespoons unsalted vegan butter
- 1/4 cup olive oil
- 1/3 teaspoon ground black pepper

Direction:
1.   Take a saucepan, put it on medium-low heat, add the oil and when it has melted, add four grains and wait for them to sizzle.
2.   Then add the remaining kernel, stir until coated, add 1 tablespoon of chopped rosemary, close the pot with the lid and shake the kernels until they are completely popped.
3.   Once all the kernels have popped, transfer them to a bowl, cook the remaining rosemary in the melted butter, then pour this mixture over the popcorn and stir until well coated.
4.   Season the popcorn with salt and black pepper, mix until smooth and serve.
Nutrition: Calories: 160 Cal Fat: 6 g Carbs: 28 g Protein: 3 g Fiber: 4 g

151.   Turmeric Snacks

Preparation Time: 35 minutes
Cooking time: 0 minute
Servings: 10
Ingredients:
- 1 cup Medjool dates, pitted, chopped
- 1/2 cup walnuts
- 1 teaspoon ground turmeric
- 1 tablespoon cocoa powder, unsweetened
- 1/2 teaspoon ground cinnamon
- 1/2 cup shredded coconut, unsweetened

Direction:
1.   Put the whole shopping list: in a food processor and blend for 2 minutes until the mixture is smooth.
2.   Pour the mixture into a bowl and then shape it into ten balls, 1 tablespoon of mixture per ball and then refrigerate for 30 minutes.
3.   Serve immediately.
Nutrition: Calories: 109 Cal Fat: 2 g Carbs: 13 g Protein: 1 g Fiber: 0 g

152. Hummus Quesadillas

Preparation Time: 5 minutes
Cooking time: 15 minutes
Servings: 1
Ingredients:
- 1 tortilla, whole wheat
- 1/4 cup diced roasted red peppers
- 1 cup baby spinach
- 1/3 teaspoon minced garlic
- ¼ teaspoon salt
- ¼ teaspoon ground black pepper
- 1/4 teaspoon olive oil
- 1/4 cup hummus
- Oil as needed

Direction:
1. Place a large skillet over medium heat, add the oil and, when hot, add the red peppers and garlic, season with salt and black pepper and cook for 3 minutes until sautéed.
2. Then add the spinach, cook for 1 minute, remove the pan from the heat and transfer the mixture to a bowl.
3. Prepare the quesadilla and for this, spread the hummus on half of the tortilla, then spread the spinach mixture on it, cover the filling with the other half of the tortilla and cook in a pan for 3 minutes on each side until golden brown.
4. When finished, cut the quesadilla into wedges and serve.

Nutrition: Calories: 187 Cal Fat: 9 g Carbs: 16.3 g Protein: 10.4 g Fiber: 0 g

153. Pico de Gallo

Preparation Time: 5 minutes
Cooking Time: 0 minutes
Serving: 3 cups
Ingredients:
- ½ of a medium red onion, peeled, chopped
- 2 cups diced tomato
- ½ cup chopped cilantro
- 1 jalapeno pepper, minced
- 1/8 teaspoon salt
- ¼ teaspoon ground black pepper
- ½ of a lime, juiced
- 1 teaspoon olive oil

Directions:
1. Take a large bowl, place all the ingredients in it and then stir until well mixed.
2. Serve the Pico de Gallo with chips.
Nutrition: Calories: 790 Cal; Fat: 6.4 g; Protein: 25.6 g; Carbs: 195.2 g; Fiber: 35.2 g;

154. Beet Balls

Preparation Time: 10 minutes
Cooking Time: 0 minutes
Serving: 18 balls
Ingredients:
- ½ cup oats
- 1 medium beet, cooked
- ½ cup almond flour
- 1/3 cup shredded coconut and more for coating
- ¾ cup Medjool dates, pitted
- 1 tablespoon cocoa powder
- ½ cup peanuts
- ¼ cup chocolate chips, unsweetened

Directions:
1. Place cooked beets in a blender and then pulse until chopped into very small pieces.
2. Add remaining ingredients and then pulse until the dough comes together.
3. Shape the dough into eighteen balls, coat them in some more coconut and then serve.
Nutrition: Calories: 114.2 Cal; Fat: 2.4 g; Protein: 5 g; Carbs: 19.6 g; Fiber: 4.9 g;

155. Cheesy Crackers

Preparation Time: 10 minutes
Cooking Time: 20 minutes
Serving: 3
Ingredients:
- 1 ¾ cup almond meal
- 3 tablespoons nutritional yeast
- ½ teaspoon of sea salt
- 2 tablespoons lemon juice
- 1 tablespoon melted coconut oil
- 1 tablespoon ground flaxseed
- 2 ½ tablespoons water

Directions:
1. Switch on the oven, then set it to 350 degrees F and let it preheat.

2. Meanwhile, take a medium bowl, place flaxseed in it, stir in water, and then let the mixture rest for 5 minutes until thickened.

3. Place almond meal in a medium bowl, add salt and yeast and then stir until mixed.

4. Add lemon juice and oil into the flaxseed mixture and then whisk until mixed.

5. Pour the flaxseed mixture into the almond meal mixture and then stir until dough comes together.

6. Place a piece of a wax paper on a clean working space, place the dough on it, cover with another piece of wax paper, and then roll dough into a 1/8-inch-thick crust.

7. Cut the dough into a square shape, sprinkle salt over the top and then bake for 15 to 20 minutes until done.

8. Serve straight away.

Nutrition: Calories: 30 Cal; Fat: 1 g; Protein: 1 g; Carbs: 5 g; Fiber: 0 g;

156. Nacho Cheese

Preparation Time: 10 minutes
Cooking Time: 15 minutes
Serving: 1 ½ cups
Ingredients:
- 1 cup chopped carrots
- ½ teaspoon onion powder
- 2 cups peeled and chopped potatoes
- ½ teaspoon garlic powder
- 1 teaspoon salt
- ½ cup nutritional yeast
- 1 tablespoon lemon juice
- ¼ cup of salsa
- ½ cup of water

Directions:
1. Take a medium pot, place carrots and potato in it, cover with water and then place the pot over medium-high heat.
2. Boil the vegetables for 10 minutes, drain them, and then transfer into a blender.
3. Add remaining ingredients and then pulse until smooth.
4. Tip the cheese into a bowl and then serve with vegetable slices.

Nutrition: Calories: 611.7 Cal; Fat: 17.2 g; Protein: 32.1 g; Carbs: 62.1 g; Fiber: 12.1 g;

157. Masala Popcorn

Preparation Time: 5 minutes
Cooking time: 15 minutes
Servings: 4
Ingredients:
- 3 cups popped popcorn
- 2 hot chili peppers, sliced
- 1 teaspoon ground cumin
- 6 curry leaves
- 1 teaspoon ground coriander
- 1/3 teaspoon salt
- 1/8 teaspoon chaat masala
- 1/4 teaspoon turmeric powder
- ¼ teaspoon red pepper flakes
- 1/4 teaspoon garam masala
- 1/3 cup olive oil

Direction:
1. Take a large pot, put it on medium heat, add half of the oil and when it is hot adding the chili and curry leaves and cook for 3 minutes until golden brown.
2. When done, transfer the curry leaves and pepper to a paper towel-lined dish and set aside until needed.
3. Add the remaining oil to the pot, add the remaining shopping list: except for the popcorn, stir until blended and cook for 1 minute until fragrant.
4. Then pour in the popcorn, remove the pan from the heat, mix well until coated, then sprinkle with bay leaves and red pepper.
5. Stir until combined and serve immediately.

Nutrition: Calories: 150 Cal Fat: 9 g Carbs: 15 g Protein: 2 g Fiber: 4 g

158. Buffalo Cauliflower

Preparation Time: 10 minutes
Cooking Time: 18 minutes
Serving: 4
Ingredients:
- 2 cups cauliflower florets
- 1 cup panko breadcrumbs

Buffalo Coating:
- ¼ cup melted vegan butter
- ¼ cup vegan Buffalo sauce

Directions:
1. At 350 degrees F, preheat your air fryer.
2. Melt the vegan butter in a bowl by heating it in the microwave for 30 seconds.
3. Stir in buffalo sauce and mix well.

4.   Dip the cauliflower florets in the buffalo sauce mixture and then coat them with breadcrumbs.

5.   Spread the coated florets in the air fryer basket.

6.   Air fry the buffalo cauliflower florets for 17 minutes.

7.   Flip the florets once cooked halfway through.

8.   Serve warm.

Nutrition: Calories 190; Fat 2.2g; Cholesterol 0mg; Carbohydrate 37.7g; Sugars 3.5g; Protein 6.4g

159.   Slow Cooker Versatile Seitan Balls

Preparation time: 15 minutes
Cooking time: 6 hours
Serving: 34 balls
Ingredients:

- 1½ cups vital wheat gluten
- ½ cup chickpea flour
- 1 tablespoon mushroom powder
- ½ teaspoon dried oregano
- ½ teaspoon onion powder
- ¼ teaspoon garlic powder
- ¼ teaspoon nutmeg
- ¼ teaspoon ground ginger
- ¼ teaspoon ground cloves
- ¼ teaspoon ground sage
- ½ teaspoon salt (optional)
- ½ cup tomato sauce, divided
- 1 teaspoon liquid smoke
- 1½ cups vegetable broth, divided

Direction:

1. Mix the gluten, flour, mushroom powder, oregano, onion and garlic powders, nutmeg, ginger, cloves, sage, and salt (if desired) in a large bowl.

2. In a small bowl, add ¼ cup tomato sauce, ¼ cup water, liquid smoke, and ½ cup vegetable broth. Mix well.

3. Make a well in the center of the dry ingredients and pour in the tomato sauce mixture. Mix well and start to knead. Knead for 1 minute or until the dough becomes mildly elastic. You will see the dough slightly pull back as you are kneading and it will be a bit sticky. Pour remaining ¼ cup tomato sauce, 1 cup vegetable broth, and 3 cups water into the slow cooker. Stir.

4. Tear off small chunks of the dough, squeeze into a round shape, and drop into the liquid in the slow cooker. There will be forty-four balls. You can also make seventeen larger balls and cut them after cooking and cooling. Or make two logs and cut into desired shapes. Cover and cook on low for 4 to 6 hours. They will grow in size as they cook. Check at 4 hours and see if you like the texture. They will become firmer as they sit in the refrigerator.

5. Remove from the pot and let cool. Store in the refrigerator for up to 5 days or freeze for up to 4 months.

Nutrition: Calories: 161 | fat: 1g | protein: 30g | carbs: 10g | fiber: 2g

160.   Rainbow Veggie Protein Pinwheels

Preparation time: 20 minutes
Cooking time: 0 minutes
Serving: 6
Ingredients:

- ¼ cup hummus
- ¼ cup tempeh, crumbled in a food processor
- 2 large spinach tortillas
- ¼ cup thinly sliced red bell pepper
- ¼ cup thinly sliced yellow bell pepper
- 1 thinly sliced carrot
- ¼ cup thinly sliced purple cabbage

Direction:

1. Mix together the hummus and tempeh.

2. Lay out tortillas. Spread hummus mixture in a thin layer over the whole surface of each tortilla stopping 1 inch from the edges. Lay a thin strip of each of the four vegetables, next to each other, over the hummus mixture.

3. Roll each tortilla tightly and cut crosswise into pinwheels. You can use toothpicks if needed, but the hummus helps them stick together at the edges.

Nutrition: Calories: 66 | fat: 2g | protein: 9g | carbs: 8g | fiber: 4g

161.   Classic Italian Mushrooms

Preparation time: 10 minutes
Cooking time: 2 hours
Serving: 4 to 6
Ingredients:
• 2 pounds (907 g) white button mushrooms, stemmed
• 1 medium onion, sliced into half-moons
• 3 to 5 tablespoons store-bought low-sodium vegetable broth
• 3 teaspoons Italian seasoning
• Ground black pepper
• Salt (optional)

Direction:
1. Cut any extra-large mushrooms in half. Place the mushrooms in the slow cooker. Add the garlic and onion.
2. Pour in the broth and sprinkle with the Italian seasoning. Season with black pepper and salt (if using). Stir to combine. Cover and cook on Low for 2 hours, or until the mushrooms are cooked through.
Nutrition: Calories: 68 | fat: 1g | protein: 8g | carbs: 12g | fiber: 3g

162.   15-Minute French Fries

Preparation time: 10 minutes
Cooking time: 1 hour
Serving: 6
Ingredients:
• 2 pounds (907 g) medium white potatoes
• 1 to 2 tablespoons no-salt seasoning

Direction:
1. Preheat the oven to 400ºF (205ºC). Line a baking sheet with parchment paper.
2. Wash and scrub the potatoes, then place them on the baking sheet and bake for 45 minutes, or until easily pierced with a fork.
3. Remove the potatoes from the oven, and allow to cool in the refrigerator for about 30 minutes, or until you're ready to make a batch of fries.
4. Preheat the oven to 425ºF (220ºC). Line a baking sheet with parchment paper.

5. Slice the cooled potatoes into the shape of wedges or fries, then toss them in a large bowl with the no-salt seasoning.
6. Spread the coated fries out in an even layer on the baking sheet. Bake for about 7 minutes, then remove from the oven, flip the fries over, and redistribute them in an even layer. Bake for another 8 minutes, or until the fries are crisp and golden brown, and serve.
Nutrition: Calories: 104 | fat: 0g | protein: 3g | carbs: 24g | fiber: 4g

163.   White Bean Caponata

Preparation time: 10 minutes
Cooking time: 0 minutes
Serving: 4 to 6
Ingredients:
• ¼ cup dry-packed, oil-free sun-dried tomatoes
• 1 (15-ounce / 425-g) can reduced-sodium white beans, drained and rinsed
• ½ cup unsweetened raisins
• ¼ cup grated carrot
• ¼ cup water-packed roasted red pepper
• ¼ cup green olives with pimentos
• 3 tablespoon red-wine vinegar
• 2 tablespoons pine nuts, toasted
• 2 tablespoons capers, drained

Direction:
1. In a small bowl, cover the sun-dried tomatoes with water, and let sit for 5 to 7 minutes, or until soft. Drain, and chop the tomatoes.
2. In a medium bowl, combine the sun-dried tomatoes, beans, raisins, carrot, roasted red pepper, olives, vinegar, pine nuts, and capers. Using a wooden spoon or spatula, mix gently.
Nutrition: Calories: 182 | fat: 4g | protein: 8g | carbs: 32g | fiber: 7g

164.   Sesame-Tamari Portable Rice Balls

Preparation time: 20 minutes

Cooking time: 25 minutes
Serving: 18 rice balls
Ingredients:

- 3 cups water
- 3 cups white sushi rice, rinsed
- ½ cup toasted white or black sesame seeds
- 2 tablespoons raw sugar (optional)
- 2 tablespoons reduced-sodium gluten-free tamari, or to taste
- 1 teaspoon ume plum or rice vinegar
- 1 tablespoon toasted sesame oil (optional)

Direction:
1. Bring the water to a boil in a large saucepan, then lower the heat to medium-low and stir in the rice. Cook, stirring often, until soft, about 15 to 20 minutes. You want it to be moist (but not soggy) and very sticky and tender.
2. Transfer the cooked rice to a large bowl. Working quickly, add all but 2 tablespoons of the sesame seeds, the sugar, tamari, and vinegar. Stir thoroughly to combine and allow to cool slightly.
3. Wet your hands to prevent the rice from sticking. Scoop about ½ cup of the rice mixture into your hands. Form a ball, applying gentle but firm pressure. Repeat with the remaining rice; let sit for 5 minutes.
Nutrition: Calories: 341 | fat: 6g | protein: 9g | carbs: 67g | fiber: 3g

165.   Toast Points

Preparation time: 5 minutes
Cooking time: 20 minutes
Serving: 2 to 4
Ingredients:

- 8 whole-grain bread slices (thawed if frozen)
- Balsamic vinegar, for brushing (optional)
- Garlic powder, for seasoning

Direction:
1. Lay the bread flat on a parchment-lined baking sheet.
2. Brush the bread with a thin layer of vinegar (if using).
3. Sprinkle with garlic powder. 4. Transfer the baking sheet to a cold oven, and heat to 350ºF (180ºC).
5. When the oven reaches temperature, flip the bread over. Bake for another 5 to 15 minutes, or until crispy to your liking. Remove from the oven.
Nutrition: Calories: 165 | fat: 1g | protein: 8g | carbs: 31g | fiber: 6g

166.   Butter Carrots

Preparation time: 10 minutes
Cooking time: 10 minutes
Servings: 4
Ingredients:
- 2 cups baby carrots
- 1 tablespoon brown sugar
- ½ tablespoon vegan butter, melted
- A pinch each salt and black pepper
Directions:
1. Take a baking dish suitable to fit in your air fryer. Toss carrots with sugar, butter, salt and black pepper in the baking dish. Place the dish in the air fryer basket and seal the fryer.
2. Cook the carrots for 10 minutes at 350 degrees F on air fryer mode.
Nutrition: Calories: 270, Fat: 10 g, Carbs: 25 g, Protein: 5 g, Fiber:4 g

167.   Sweet Potato Nachos

Preparation Time: 10 minutes
Cooking Time: 20 minutes
Serving: 2
Ingredients:
For the Sweet Potato Rounds:
- 1 teaspoon of garlic powder
- 1 teaspoon of cumin
- 1 teaspoon of chili powder
- 1 large sweet potato
- 1–2 tablespoon of olive oil
- salt and pepper to taste
Toppings:
- 1/4 cup of sweet corn
- 1/4 cup of guacamole
- 1/4 cup of salsa
- 1/2 cup of cheddar jack cheese
- 1/4 cup of black beans
- 1/4 cup of plain Greek yogurt
- sprinkle of cilantro
Direction:
1. Preheat oven to 375 degrees F.
2. Slice 1 large sweet potato into thin rounds. Place on a baking sheet.
3. Drizzle with olive oil and season with cumin, garlic powder, salt, chili, and pepper.

4.   Bake for about 20 minutes, at 400 degrees f.
5.   Top with cheese once sweet potatoes are cooked.
6.   Then place back into the oven to melt the cheese for about 2 minutes.
7.   Top with black beans, corn, salsa, guacamole, yogurt, and cilantro.
8.   Serve and enjoy.

Nutrition: Calories: 381cal | Fat: 24g | Protein: 14g | Fiber: 6g | Sugar: 5g | Carbohydrate: 31g

168.   Roasted Bell Pepper and Goat Cheese Dip

Preparation Time: 5 minutes
Cooking Time: 0 minute
Serving: 8
Ingredients:
- 1 cup of nonfat Greek yogurt
- 1/2 cup of jarred roasted red-peppers, drained
- a squeeze of lemon juice (2 teaspoons)
- 1/2 teaspoon of garlic powder
- 1 tablespoon of fresh thyme
- 4 ounces of goat cheese
- 1/4 teaspoon of salt
- Optional toppings: chopped roasted red pepper, caramelized onion, and a sprinkle of thyme.

Direction:
1.   Place all of the ingredients into a high-speed food processor.
2.   Process until smooth.
3.   Serve and enjoy.

Nutrition: Calories: 140cal | Fat: 3g | Protein: 10g | Fiber: 3g | Sodium: 534.2mg | Sugar: 2g | Carbohydrate: 22g

169.   Strawberry Banana Fruit Leather

Preparation Time: 20 minutes
Cooking Time: 7 hours
Serving: 12
Ingredients:

- 1/4 cup of lemon juice
- 2 tablespoons of honey
- 1 pound of strawberries (4 cups, halved)
- 2 medium bananas (2 cups, sliced)
- pinch of salt

Direction:
1.   Preheat oven to 180 degrees F.
2.   Prep a rimmed baking sheet by covering it with parchment paper.
3.   In a food processor of a high-speed blender, place all ingredients. Process until everything is smooth and pureed together.
4.   Pour the strawberry banana mixture over the baking sheet.
5.   Spread into the corners using a spatula and lift the sheet up, then pound for some time to really make sure everything is even. This should be around 1/4 of an inch thick.
6.   Bake for about 6 to 8 hours at 180 degrees F.
7.   Fruit leather is done when it is not soft in any place and when it easily separates from the parchment paper. Do not overcook it!
8.   Use scissors to cut the fruit leather into 12-strips.
9.   Store in an airtight container, and place inside the refrigerator for about 2 to 4 weeks.
10.   Serve and enjoy.

Nutrition: Calories: 61cal | Fat: 0g | Protein: 1g | Fiber: 2g | Sodium: 1mg | Sugar: 10g | Carbohydrate: 16g

170.   Zucchini Fries

Preparation Time: 25 minutes
Cooking Time: 20 minutes
Serving: 1
Ingredients:
- 2 medium zucchinis
- 1 cup white whole-wheat flour
- 1 teaspoon salt
- ½ teaspoon seasoned salt
- 1 teaspoon paprika
- ¼ teaspoon ground black pepper
- 1 teaspoon red chili powder
- ½ cup almond milk, unsweetened
- 1 cup bread crumbs

Directions:
1.   Switch on the oven, then set it to 425 degrees F and let it preheat.

2. Cut the zucchini into fries, spread them on a baking tray, sprinkle with salt, and then let the fries sit for 20 minutes.

3. Meanwhile, take a shallow dish, place bread crumbs in it, add paprika, black pepper, and red chili powder and then stir until mixed.

4. Take a medium bowl and place flour in it.

5. Take a separate medium bowl and pour almond milk in it.

6. After 20 minutes, dredge each fry in flour, dip into the milk and then coat in bread crumbs.

7. Repeat with the fries, spread on the baking sheet, and then bake for 20 minutes until golden brown and crisp.

8. Serve straight away.

Nutrition: Calories: 70 Cal; Fat: 1.4 g; Protein: 3.8 g; Carbs: 11.6 g; Fiber: 3.4 g

171. Almond Energy Balls

Preparation Time: 20 minutes
Cooking Time: 0 minute
Serving: 25
Ingredients:
- 1/2 teaspoon of vanilla extract
- 1/8 teaspoon of sea salt
- 2 cups of almonds, raw and unsalted
- 1 cup of medjool dates, pitted (12)
- 1 cup of dried tart cherries
- 1 tablespoon of water

Direction:
1. In a food processor, place almonds and process until the almonds turn into a meal for about a minute.

2. Add in the tart cherries, pitted dates, sea salt vanilla, and water.

3. Process on high until you've created your dough for about 2 minutes.

4. Add 1/2 teaspoons of water until you have reached the preferred consistency if the mixture seems too dry.

5. Scoop out the heaping tablespoons of dough.

6. Roll in between your palms to make the balls.

7. Then store in an airtight container in the freezer or fridge.

8. Enjoy!

Nutrition: Calories: 122cal | Fat: 6g | Protein: 3g | Fiber: 2g | Sugar: 12g | Carbohydrate: 16g

172. Leeks with Butter

Preparation time: 10 minutes
Cooking time: 7 minutes
Servings: 4
Ingredients:
- 1 tablespoon vegan butter, melted
- 1 tablespoon lemon juice
- 4 leeks, washed and halved
- Salt and black pepper to taste

Directions:
1. Take a baking dish suitable to fit in your air fryer.

2. Toss the leeks with butter, salt, and black pepper in the dish. Place the dish in the air fryer basket.

3. Seal the fryer and cook the carrots for 7 minutes at 350 degrees F on air fryer mode.

4. Add a drizzle of lemon juice.

5. Mix well then serve.

Nutrition: Calories: 230, Fat: 9 g, Carbs: 20 g, Protein: 6 g, Fiber:8g

173. Juicy Brussel Sprouts

Preparation time: 10 minutes
Cooking time: 10 minutes
Servings: 4
Ingredients:
- 1-pound Brussels sprouts, trimmed
- ¼ cup green onions, chopped
- 6 cherry tomatoes, halved
- 1 tablespoon olive oil
- Salt and black pepper to taste

Directions:
1. Take a baking dish suitable to fit in your air fryer. Toss Brussels sprouts with salt and black pepper in the dish. Place this dish in the air fryer and seal the fryer.

2. Cook the sprouts for 10 minutes at 350 degrees F on air fryer mode.

3. Toss these sprouts with green onions, tomatoes, olive oil, salt, and pepper in a salad bowl.

Nutrition: Calories: 120, Fat: 3 g, Carbs: 23 g, Protein: 4 g, Fiber:9g

174.   Parsley Potatoes

Preparation time: 10 minutes
Cooking time: 10 minutes
Servings: 4
Ingredients
- 1-pound gold potatoes, sliced
- 2 tablespoons olive oil
- ¼ cup parsley leaves, chopped
- Juice from ½ lemon
- Salt and black pepper to taste

Directions
1. Take a baking dish suitable to fit in your air fryer.
2. Place the potatoes in it and season them liberally with salt, pepper, olive oil, and lemon juice.
3. Place the baking dish in the air fryer basket and seal it.
4. Cook the potatoes for 10 minutes at 350 degrees F on air fryer mode.
5. Serve warm with parsley garnishing.
6. Devour.

Nutrition: Calories: 280, Fat: 5 g, Carbs: 36 g, Protein: 4 g, Fiber3g

175.   Fried Asparagus

Preparation time: 10 minutes
Cooking time: 8 minutes
Servings: 4
Ingredients:
- 2 pounds' fresh asparagus, trimmed
- ½ teaspoon oregano, dried
- 4 ounces' vegan feta cheese, crumbled
- 4 garlic cloves, minced
- 2 tablespoons parsley, chopped
- ¼ teaspoon red pepper flakes
- ¼ cup olive oil
- Salt and black pepper to the taste
- 1 teaspoon lemon zest
- 1 lemon, juiced

Directions
1. Combine lemon zest with oregano, pepper flakes, garlic and oil in a large bowl.
2. Add asparagus, salt, pepper, and cheese to the bowl.
3. Toss well to coat then place the asparagus in the air fryer basket.

4. Seal the fryer and cook them for 8 minutes at 350 degrees F on Air fryer mode.
5. Garnish with parsley and lemon juice.
6. Enjoy warm.

Nutrition: Calories: 310, Fat: 10 g, Carbs: 32 g, Protein: 6 g, Fiber:9 g

176.   Balsamic Artichokes

Preparation time: 10 minutes
Cooking time: 7 minutes
Servings: 4
Ingredients:
- 4 big artichokes, trimmed
- ¼ cup olive oil
- 2 garlic cloves, minced
- 2 tablespoons lemon juice
- 2 teaspoons balsamic vinegar
- 1 teaspoon oregano, dried
- Salt and black pepper to the taste

Directions:
1. Season artichokes liberally with salt and pepper then rub them with half of the lemon juice and oil.
2. Add the artichokes to a baking dish suitable to fit in the air fryer.
3. Place the artichoke dish in the air fryer basket and seal it.
4. Cook them for 7 minutes at 360 degrees F on air fryer mode.
5. Whisk remaining lemon juice, and oil, vinegar, oregano, garlic, salt and pepper in a bowl.
6. Pour this mixture over the artichokes and mix them well. Enjoy.

Nutrition: Calories: 310, Fat: 10 g, Carbs: 25 g, Protein: 4 g, Fiber:9g

177.   Tomato Kebabs

Preparation time: 10 minutes
Cooking time: 6 minutes
Servings: 4
Ingredients:
- 3 tablespoons balsamic vinegar
- 24 cherry tomatoes
- 2 cups vegan feta cheese, sliced
- 2 tablespoons olive oil

- 3 garlic cloves, minced
- 1 tablespoon thyme, chopped
- Salt and black pepper to the taste

Ingredients for the Dressing
- 2 tablespoons balsamic vinegar
- 4 tablespoons olive oil
- Salt and black pepper to taste

Directions:
1. In a medium bowl combine oil, garlic cloves, thyme, salt, vinegar, and black pepper.
2. Mix well then add the tomatoes and coat them liberally.
3. Thread 6 tomatoes and cheese slices on each skewer alternatively.
4. Place these skewers in the air fryer basket and seal it.
5. Cook them for 6 minutes on air fryer mode at 360 degrees F.
6. Meanwhile, whisk together the dressing ingredients.
7. Place the cooked skewers on the serving plates.
8. Pour the vinegar dressing over them.
9. Enjoy.
Nutrition: Calories: 190, Fat: 6 g, Carbs: 18 g, Protein: 8 g, Fiber:6g

178.   Eggplant and Zucchini Snack

Preparation time: 10 minutes
Cooking time: 8 minutes
Servings: 4
Ingredients:
- 1 eggplant, cubed
- 3 zucchinis, cubed
- 2 tablespoons lemon juice
- 1 teaspoon oregano, dried
- 3 tablespoons olive oil
- 1 teaspoon thyme, dried
- Salt and black pepper to taste

Directions:
1. Take a baking dish suitable to fit in your air fryer.
2. Combine all ingredients in the baking dish.
3. Place the eggplant dish in the air fryer basket and seal it.
4. Cook them for 8 minutes at 360 degrees F on air fryer mode.

5. Enjoy warm.
Nutrition: Calories: 210, Fat: 4 g, Carbs: 16 g, Protein: 3 g, Fiber:9g

179.   Artichokes with Mayo Sauce

Preparation time: 10 minutes
Cooking time: 6 minutes
Servings: 4
Ingredients:
- 2 artichokes, trimmed
- 1 tablespoon lemon juice
- 2 garlic cloves, minced
- A drizzle olive oil

Ingredients for the Sauce
- 1 cup vegan mayonnaise
- ¼ cup olive oil
- ¼ cup coconut oil
- 3 garlic cloves

Directions:
1. Toss artichokes with lemon juice, oil and 2 garlic cloves in a large bowl.
2. Place the seasoned artichokes in the air fryer basket and seal it.
3. Cook the artichokes for 6 minutes at 350 degrees on air fryer mode.
4. Blend coconut oil with olive oil, mayonnaise and 3 garlic cloves in a food processor.
5. Place the artichokes on the serving plates.
6. Pour the mayonnaise mixture over the artichokes.
7. Enjoy fresh.
Nutrition: Calories: 230, Fat: 11 g, Carbs: 24 g, Protein: 6 g, Fiber:11 g

180.   Cranberry Vanilla Protein Bars

Preparation time: 15 minutes
Cooking time: 0 minutes
Serving: 4
Ingredients:
- 1 cup old-fashioned oats
- 2 cups vanilla flavor vegan protein powder
- ½ cup cashew butter

- ½ cup dried cranberries
- ¼ cup maple syrup (optional)
- ¼ cup chia seeds
- 1 tablespoon almond or soy milk
- 1 tablespoon pure vanilla extract

Direction:

1. Line a square 8x8" baking dish with parchment paper and set it aside.

2. Add the oats, protein powder, and shredded coconut to a food processor and blend until they resemble a fine powder. Transfer the blended ingredients to a large mixing bowl and add the remaining ingredients; mix with a spoon until everything is thoroughly combined. Move the dough to the baking dish and press it down evenly until flattened as much as possible. Place the dish into the freezer until set and firm, around 1½ hours.

3. To serve, slice the chunk into 8 even bars, and enjoy, share, or store!

Nutrition: Calories: 243 | fat: 10g | protein: 16g | carbs: 23g | fiber: 3g

181. Oatmeal Granola Bar Bites

Preparation time: 5 minutes
Cooking time: 25 minutes
Serving: 12
Ingredients:
- 1½ cups rolled oats
- ¼ cup unsweetened natural peanut butter
- 2 tablespoons ground flaxseed
- 1 tablespoon finely chopped pecans
- 1 tablespoon sliced almonds
- 1 tablespoon unsweetened raisins
- 1 tablespoon mini vegan chocolate chips

Direction:

1. Preheat the oven to 350ºF (180ºC). Line an 8-by-8-inch baking dish and a baking sheet with parchment paper.

2. In a large bowl, using a wooden spoon or rubber spatula, mix together the oats, applesauce, peanut butter, maple syrup, flaxseed, pecans, almonds, raisins, and chocolate chips.

3. Using the back of a measuring cup, firmly press the mixture into the prepared baking dish.

4. Lift the pressed mixture out, and cut into 12 equal pieces.

5. Place the cut pieces in single layer on the prepared baking sheet. 6. Transfer the baking sheet to the oven, and bake for 20 to 25 minutes, flipping halfway through, or until the bars are golden brown. Remove from the oven.

Nutrition: Calories: 98 | fat: 5g | protein: 3g | carbs: 12g | fiber: 2g

182. Grilled Watermelon

Preparation Time: 10 minutes
Cooking Time: 14 minutes
Servings: 4
Ingredients:
- 1 watermelon, peeled and cut into 1-inch-thick wedges
- 1 garlic clove, minced finely
- 2 tablespoons fresh lime juice
- Pinch of cayenne pepper
- Pinch of Salt

Direction:

1. Preheat the grill to high heat.

2. Grease the grill grate.

3. Arrange the watermelon pieces onto the grill and cook for about 2 minutes from both sides.

4. Meanwhile, in a small bowl mix together all ingredients.

5. Drizzle the watermelon slices with lemon mixture and serve.

Nutrition: Calories: 11 Fat: 0.1g Carbohydrates: 2.6g Dietary Fiber: 0.2g Sugar: 1.9g Protein: 0.2g

183. Kale Chips

Preparation Time: 10 minutes
Cooking Time: 15 minutes
Servings: 6
Ingredients:
- 1-pound fresh kale leaves, stemmed and torn
- ¼ teaspoon cayenne pepper
- Salt, as required
- 1 tablespoon olive oil

Direction:

1. Preheat your oven to 350 ºF.

2. Line a large baking sheet with parchment paper.

3.   Arrange the kale pieces onto the prepared baking sheet in a single layer.
4.   Sprinkle the kale with cayenne pepper and salt and drizzle with oil.
5.   Bake for approximately 10-15 minutes.
6.   Remove from the oven and let cool before serving.
Nutrition: Calories: 57 Fat: 2.3g Carbohydrates: 8g Dietary Fiber: 1.2g Sugar: 0g Protein: 26.3g

184.   Roasted Chickpeas

Preparation Time: 10 minutes
Cooking Time: 45 minutes
Servings: 8
Ingredients:
- 2 cups cooked chickpeas
- 1 garlic clove, minced
- ¼ teaspoon dried oregano, crushed
- ¼ teaspoon smoked paprika
- ¼ teaspoon ground cumin
- Salt, as required
- 1 tablespoon olive oil
Direction:
1.   Preheat your oven to 400 °F.
2.   Grease a large baking sheet.
3.   Place chickpeas onto the prepared baking sheet in a single layer.
4.   Roast for about 30 minutes, stirring the chickpeas after every 10 minutes.
5.   Meanwhile, in a small mixing bowl, mix together garlic, thyme and spices.
6.   Remove the baking sheet from oven.
7.   Place the garlic mixture and oil over the chickpeas and toss to coat well.
8.   Roast for approximately 10-15 minutes more.
9.   Now, turn the oven off but leave the baking sheet inside for about 10 minutes before serving.
Nutrition: Calories: 88 Fat: 2.5g Carbohydrates: 13.8g Dietary Fiber: 2.7g Sugar: 0g Protein: 3g

185.   Roasted Cashews

Preparation Time: 10 minutes
Cooking Time: 10 minutes
Servings: 8
Ingredients:
- 2 cups raw cashews

- ½ teaspoon ground cumin
- ¼ teaspoon cayenne pepper
- Pinch of salt
- 1 tablespoon fresh lemon juice
Direction:
1.   Preheat your oven to 400 °F.
2.   Line a large roasting pan with a piece of foil.
3.   In a large bowl, add the cashews and spices and toss to coat well.
4.   Transfer the cashews into prepared the roasting pan.
5.   Roast for approximately 8-10 minutes.
6.   Drizzle with lemon juice and serve.
Nutrition: Calories: 198 Fat: 15.9g Carbohydrates: 11.3g Dietary Fiber: 1.1g Sugar: 1.8g Protein: 5.3g

186.   Seed Crackers

Preparation Time: 15 minutes
Cooking Time: 20 minutes
Servings: 6
Ingredients:
- 3 tablespoons water
- 1 tablespoon chia seeds
- 3 tablespoons sunflower seeds
- 1 tablespoon quinoa flour
- 1 teaspoon ground turmeric
- Pinch of ground cinnamon
- Salt, as required
Direction:
1.   Preheat your oven to 345 °F.
2.   Line a baking sheet with parchment paper.
3.   In a bowl, add the water and chia seeds and soak for about 15 minutes.
4.   After 15 minutes, add the remaining ingredients and mix well.
5.   Spread the mixture onto prepared baking sheet.
6.   With a pizza slicer, slice into desired shapes.
7.   Bake for 20 minutes.
8.   Remove from the oven and place onto a wire rack to cool completely before serving.
Nutrition: Calories: 19 Fat: 1.3g Carbohydrates: 1.8g Dietary Fiber: 0.7g Sugar: 0.1g Protein: 0.8g

187.   Strawberry Gazpacho

Preparation Time: 15 minutes
Cooking time: 0 minutes
Servings: 4
Ingredients:
- 1½ pounds fresh strawberries, hulled and sliced, plus extra for garnishing
- ½ cup red bell pepper, seeded and chopped
- 1 small cucumber, peeled, seeded, and chopped
- ¼ cup onion, chopped
- ¼ cup fresh basil leaves
- 1 small garlic clove, chopped
- ¼ small jalapeño pepper, seeded and chopped
- 1 tablespoon olive oil
- 2 tablespoons apple cider vinegar

Direction:
1. In a high-powered blender, add 1½ pounds of the strawberries and remaining ingredients and pulse until well combined and smooth.
2. Transfer the gazpacho into a large serving bowl.
3. Cover the bowl and refrigerate for about 4 hours before serving.
4. Serve chilled with a garnish of strawberry slices.

Nutrition: Calories: 106 Fat: 4.2g Carbohydrates: 17.8g Dietary Fiber: 4.2g Sugar: 0.7g Protein: 1.9g

188. Avocado Guacamole

Preparation Time: 10 minutes
Cooking time: 0 minutes
Servings: 4
Ingredients:
- 12 medium ripe avocados, peeled, pitted, and chopped
- 1 small red onion, chopped
- 1 garlic clove, minced
- 1 Serrano pepper, seeded and chopped
- 1 tomato, seeded and chopped
- 2 tablespoons fresh cilantro leaves, chopped
- 1 tablespoon fresh lime juice
- Salt, as required

Direction:
1. In a large bowl, add avocado and mash it completely with a fork.

2. Add the remaining ingredients and gently stir to combine.
3. Serve immediately.

Nutrition: Calories: 217 Fat: 19.7g Carbohydrates: 11.3g Dietary Fiber: 7.4g Sugar: 1.7g Protein: 12.3g

189. Chickpeas Hummus

Nutrition: Calories: 129 Fat: 7.4g Carbohydrates: 12.2g Dietary Fiber: 3.3g Sugar: 1.2g Protein: 4.7g

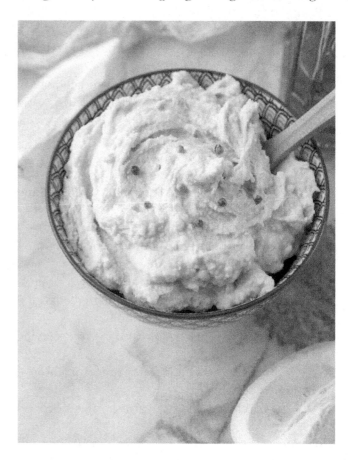

Preparation Time: 10 minutes
Cooking time: 0 minutes
Servings: 12
Ingredients:
• 2 (15-ounce) cans chickpeas, rinsed and drainer
• ½ cup tahini
• 1 garlic clove, chopped
• 2 tablespoons fresh lemon juice
• Salt, as required
• Filtered water, as needed
• 1 tablespoon olive oil
• Pinch of cayenne pepper
Direction:
1. In a high-powered blender, add all the ingredients and pulse until smooth.
2. Transfer the hummus into a large bowl and drizzle with oil.
3. Sprinkle with cayenne pepper and serve immediately.

Chapter 9. Smoothies and Drinks

190. Cucumber Watermelon Lemonade

Preparation time: 10 minutes
Cooking time: 0 minutes
Servings: 8
Ingredients:
- 5 large lemons, halved
- ¼ small watermelon, sliced
- ½ cucumber, peeled
- ¾ cup sugar
- 8 cups water

Direction:
1. Add all ingredients to a blender and blend until it is lump-free.
2. Strain and chill well to serve.
3. Enjoy.

Nutrition: Calories 148 Total Fat 13 g Saturated Fat 5 g Cholesterol 132 mg Sodium 297 mg Total Carbs 16 g Fiber 2 g Sugar 1.5 g Protein 2 g

191. Rice Horchata

Preparation time: 10 minutes
Cooking time: 0 minutes
Servings: 7
Ingredients:
- 7 cups rice milk
- 2 cups almond milk
- ½ cup sugar
- 3 cinnamon sticks
- 1 teaspoon vanilla extract

Direction:
1. Add all ingredients to a blender and blend until it is lump-free.
2. Chill well to serve.
3. Enjoy.

Nutrition: Calories 125 Total Fat 22 g Saturated Fat 11 g Cholesterol 122 mg Sodium 317 mg Carbs 15 g Fiber 2 g Sugar 2.1 g Protein 0.6 g

192. Winter Orange Tonic

Preparation time: 10 minutes
Cooking time: 10 minutes
Servings: 6:
Ingredients:
- 1 lemon, sliced
- 1 orange, sliced
- 1 tablespoon fresh ginger
- 4 cardamom pods
- ¼ teaspoon peppercorn
- 1 cinnamon stick
- 6 cups water

Direction:
1. Add all ingredients to a saucepan.
2. Steep the tea at a simmer for 10 minutes.
3. Strain and chill well.
4. Serve.

Nutrition: Calories 131 Total Fat 13 g Saturated Fat 8 g Cholesterol 212 mg Sodium 321 mg Total Carbs 9.7 g Fiber 3.1 g Sugar 1.8 g Protein 2 g

193. Cinnamon Hemp Seed Coffee

Preparation time: 10 minutes
Cooking time: 0 minutes
Servings: 2
Ingredients:
- 1 cup cold coffee
- ¼ cup almond milk
- A few pinches of cinnamon
- 2 tablespoons hemp seeds
- 1 splash of vanilla extract
- 1½ frozen bananas, sliced
- Handful of ice

Direction:
1. Add all of the ingredients to a blender and blend until it is lump-free.
2. Chill well to serve.
3. Enjoy.

Nutrition: Calories 141 Total Fat 9 g Saturated Fat 2.1 g Cholesterol 6 mg Sodium 23 mg Total Carbs 16 g Fiber 4 g Sugar 3 g Protein 3.1 g

194. Strawberry Smoothie

Preparation Time: 10 minutes
Cooking time: 0 minutes
Servings: 2
Ingredients:
- 1 cup frozen strawberries
- 1 banana, peeled and sliced
- ¼ teaspoon organic vanilla extract
- 2 cups chilled unsweetened almond milk
Direction:
1. Place all the ingredients in a high-powered blender and pulse until creamy.
2. Pour the smoothie into two glasses and serve immediately.
Nutrition: Calories: 131 Fat: 3.7g Carbohydrates: 25.3g Dietary Fiber: 4.8g Sugar: 14g Protein: 1.6g

195. Blackberry & Spinach Smoothie

Preparation Time: 10 minutes
Cooking time: 0 minutes
Servings: 2
Ingredients:
- ¾ cup fresh blackberries
- 2 cups fresh spinach leaves
- ¼ cup fresh mint leaves
- 1 tablespoon sunflower seeds
- 1 tablespoon pumpkin seeds
- 1½ cups unsweetened almond milk
- ¼ cup ice cubes
Direction:
1. Place all the ingredients in a high-powered blender and pulse until creamy.
2. Pour the smoothie into two glasses and serve immediately.
Nutrition: Calories: 97 Fat: 5.8g Carbohydrates: 9.8g Dietary Fiber: 5.3g Sugar: 2.9g Protein: 4.1g

196. Peach & Mango Smoothie

Preparation Time: 10 minutes
Cooking time: 0 minutes
Servings: 2
Ingredients:
- 1 cup fresh peach, pitted and chopped
- 1 cup frozen mango, peeled, pitted and cubed
- 1 teaspoon maple syrup
- 1½ cups unsweetened almond milk
Direction:
1. Place all the ingredients in a high-powered blender and pulse until creamy.
2. Pour the smoothie into two glasses and serve immediately.
Nutrition: Calories: 118 Fat: 3.2 Carbohydrates: 23.1g Dietary Fiber: 3.2g Sugar: 20.3g Protein: 2.1g

197. Carrot, Tomato & Celery Smoothie

Preparation Time: 10 minutes
Cooking time: 0 minutes
Servings: 2
Ingredients:
- 2 medium tomatoes
- 1 large carrot, peeled and chopped
- 1 celery stalk, chopped
- Pinch of salt
- ¼ teaspoon ground black pepper
- 2 teaspoons freshly squeezed lemon juice
- 1 cup ice cubes
Direction:
1. Place all the ingredients in a high-powered blender and pulse until creamy.
2. Pour the smoothie into two glasses and serve immediately.
Nutrition: Calories: 62 Fat: 0.6g Carbohydrates: 13.6g Dietary Fiber: 4.1g Sugar: 8.5g Protein: 2.6g

198. Kale & Avocado Smoothie

Preparation Time: 10 minutes
Cooking time: 0 minutes
Servings: 2
Ingredients:
- 3 stalks fresh kale, trimmed and chopped
- 1-2 celery stalks, chopped
- ½ of avocado, peeled, pitted, and chopped
- 1 (½-inch) piece ginger root, chopped
- 1 (½-inch) piece turmeric root, chopped
- 1½ cups unsweetened coconut milk
- ½ cup ice cubes

Direction:
1. Place all the ingredients in a high-speed blender and pulse until creamy.
2. Pour the smoothie into two glasses and serve immediately.
Nutrition: Calories: 248 Fat: 21.8g Carbohydrates: 11.3g Dietary Fiber: 4.2g Sugar: 0.5g Protein: 3.5g

199. Green Colada

Preparation time: 5 minutes
Cooking time: 0 minutes
Servings: 1
Ingredients:
- 1/2 cup frozen pineapple chunks
- 1/2 banana
- 1/2 teaspoon spirulina powder
- 1/4 teaspoon vanilla extract, unsweetened
- 1 cup of coconut milk

Directions:
1. Place all the ingredients in the order in a food processor or blender and then pulse for 2 to 3 minutes at high speed until smooth.
2. Pour the smoothie into a glass and then serve.
Nutrition: Calories: 127; Fat: 3g; Carbs: 25g; Fiber: 4g; Protein: 3g

200. Peach Crumble Shake

Preparation time: 5 minutes
Cooking time: 0 minutes

Servings: 1
Ingredients:
- 1 tablespoon chia seeds
- ¼ cup rolled oats
- 2 peaches, pitted, sliced
- ¾ teaspoon ground cinnamon
- 1 Medjool date, pitted
- ½ teaspoon vanilla extract, unsweetened
- 2 tablespoons lemon juice
- ½ cup of water
- 1 tablespoon coconut butter
- 1 cup coconut milk, unsweetened

Directions:
1. Place all the ingredients in the order in a food processor or blender and then pulse for 2 to 3 minutes at high speed until smooth.
2. Pour the smoothie into a glass and then serve.
Nutrition: Calories: 270; Fat: 4g; Carbs: 28g; Fiber: 3g; Protein: 25g

201. Wild Ginger Green Smoothie

Preparation time: 5 minutes
Cooking time: 0 minutes
Servings: 1
Ingredients:
- 1/2 cup pineapple chunks, frozen
- 1/2 cup chopped kale
- 1/2 frozen banana
- 1 tablespoon lime juice
- 2 inches' ginger, peeled, chopped
- 1/2 cup coconut milk, unsweetened
- 1/2 cup coconut water

Directions:
1. Place all the ingredients in the order in a food processor or blender and then pulse for 2 to 3 minutes at high speed until smooth.
2. Pour the smoothie into a glass and then serve.
Nutrition: Calories: 331; Fat: 14g; Carbs: 40g; Fiber: 9g; Protein: 16g

202. Red Veggie & Fruit Smoothie

Preparation Time: 10 minutes
Cooking time: 0 minutes

Servings: 2

Ingredients:

- ½ cup fresh raspberries
- ½ cup fresh strawberries
- ½ of red bell pepper, seeded and chopped
- ½ cup red cabbage, chopped
- 1 small tomato
- 1 cup water
- ½ cup ice cubes

Direction:

1. Place all the ingredients in a high-speed blender and pulse until creamy.
2. Pour the smoothie into two glasses and serve immediately.

Nutrition: Calories: 39 Fat: 0.4g Carbohydrates: 8.9g Dietary Fiber: 3.5g Sugar: 4.8g Protein: 1.3g

203. Avocado & Green Veggies Smoothie

Preparation Time: 10 minutes
Cooking time: 0 minutes
Servings: 2

Ingredients:

- 1 small avocado, peeled, pitted and chopped
- 1 small cucumber, peeled and chopped
- 1 small green bell pepper, seeded and chopped
- 2 cups fresh spinach, torn
- 2 tablespoons freshly squeezed lime juice
- 1 cup water
- ½ cup ice cubes

Direction:

1. Place all the ingredients in a high-powered blender and pulse until creamy.
2. Pour the smoothie into two glasses and serve immediately.

Nutrition: Calories: 254 Fat: 20g Carbohydrates: 19.8g Dietary Fiber: 8.9g Sugar: 6.1g Protein: 4.4g

204. Orange & Oats Smoothie

Preparation Time: 10 minutes
Cooking time: 0 minutes
Servings: 2

Ingredients:

- 2/3 cup rolled oats
- 2 oranges, peeled, seeded, and sectioned
- 2 large bananas, peeled and sliced
- 2 cups unsweetened almond milk
- 1 cup ice cubes, crushed

Direction:

1. Place all the ingredients in a high-powered blender and pulse until creamy.
2. Pour the smoothie into four glasses and serve immediately.

Nutrition: Calories: 175 Fat: 3g Carbohydrates: 36.6g Dietary Fiber: 5.9g Sugar: 17.1g Protein: 3.9g

205. Blueberry Smoothie

Preparation Time: 10 minutes
Cooking time: 0 minutes
Servings: 2

Ingredients:

- 2 cups frozen blueberries
- 1 small banana
- 1½ cups unsweetened almond milk
- ¼ cup ice cubes

Direction:

1. Add all the ingredients in a high-powered blender and pulse until smooth.
2. Pour the smoothie into two glasses and serve immediately.

Nutrition: Calories: 158 Fat: 3.3g Carbohydrates: 34g Dietary Fiber: 5.6g Sugar: 20.6g Protein: 2.4g

206. Raspberry & Tofu Smoothie

Preparation Time: 10 minutes
Cooking time: 0 minutes
Servings: 2

Ingredients:

- 1½ cups fresh raspberries
- 6 ounces' firm silken tofu, drained
- 1/8 teaspoon coconut extract
- 1 teaspoon powdered stevia
- 1½ cups unsweetened almond milk
- ¼ cup ice cubes, crushed

Direction:

1. Add all the ingredients in a high-powered blender and pulse until smooth.
2. Pour the smoothie into two glasses and serve immediately.
Nutrition: Calories: 131 Fat: 5.5g Carbohydrates: 14.6g Dietary Fiber: 6.8g Sugar: 5.2g Protein: 7.7g

207.   Chard, Lettuce, and Ginger Smoothie

Preparation time: 5 minutes
Cooking time: 0 minutes
Servings: 2
Ingredients:
- 10 Chard leaves, chopped
- 1-inch piece of ginger, chopped
- 10 lettuce leaves, chopped
- ½ teaspoon black salt
- 2 pears, chopped
- 2 teaspoons coconut sugar
- ¼ teaspoon ground black pepper
- ¼ teaspoon salt
- 2 tablespoons lemon juice
- 2 cups of water

Directions:
1. Place all the ingredients in the order to a food processor or blender and then pulse for 2 to 3 minutes at high speed until smooth.
2. Pour the smoothie into two glasses and then serve.
Nutrition: Calories: 514 Fat: 0g Carbs: 15g Protein: 4g Fiber: 4g

208.   Red Beet, Pear, and Apple Smoothie

Preparation time: 5 minutes
Cooking time: 0 minutes
Servings: 2
Ingredients:
- 1/2 of medium beet, peeled, chopped
- 1 tablespoon chopped cilantro
- 1 orange, juiced
- 1 medium pear, chopped
- 1 medium apple, cored, chopped
- 1/4 teaspoon ground black pepper
- 1/8 teaspoon rock salt

- 1 teaspoon coconut sugar
- 1/4 teaspoons salt
- 1 cup of water

Directions:
1. Place all the ingredients in the order to a food processor or blender and then pulse for 2 to 3 minutes at high speed until smooth.
2. Pour the smoothie into two glasses and then serve.
Nutrition: Calories: 132 Fat: 0g Carbs: 34g Protein: 1g Fiber: 5g

209.   Berry and Yogurt Smoothie

Preparation time: 5 minutes
Cooking time: 0 minutes
Servings: 2
Ingredients:
- 2 small bananas
- 3 cups frozen mixed berries
- 1(½) cup cashew yogurt
- 1/2 teaspoon vanilla extract, unsweetened
- 1/2 cup almond milk, unsweetened

Directions:
1. Place all the ingredients in the order to a food processor or blender and then pulse for 2 to 3 minutes at high speed until smooth.
2. Pour the smoothie into two glasses and then serve.
Nutrition: Calories: 326 Fat: 6.5g Carbs: 65.6g Protein: 8g Fiber: 8.4g

210.   Chocolate and Cherry Smoothie

Preparation time: 5 minutes
Cooking time: 0 minutes
Servings: 2
Ingredients:
- 4 cups frozen cherries
- 2 tablespoons cocoa powder
- 1 scoop of protein powder
- 1 teaspoon maple syrup
- 2 cups almond milk, unsweetened

Directions:

1. Place all the ingredients in the order to a food processor or blender and then pulse for 2 to 3 minutes at high speed until smooth.
2. Pour the smoothie into two glasses and then serve.

Nutrition: Calories: 324 Fat: 5g Carbs: 75.1g Protein: 7.2g Fiber: 11.3g

211. Strawberry and Chocolate Milkshake

Preparation time: 5 minutes
Cooking time: 0 minutes
Servings: 2
Ingredients:
• 2 cups frozen strawberries
• 3 tablespoons cocoa powder
• 1 scoop protein powder
• 2 tablespoons maple syrup
• 1 teaspoon vanilla extract, unsweetened
• 2 cups almond milk, unsweetened
Directions:
1. Place all the ingredients in the order to a food processor or blender and then pulse for 2 to 3 minutes at high speed until smooth.
2. Pour the smoothie into two glasses and then serve.

Nutrition: Calories: 199 Fat: 4.1g Carbs: 40.5g Protein: 3.7g Fiber: 5.5g

212. Trope-Kale Breeze

Preparation time: 5 minutes
Cooking time: 0 minutes
Servings: 3 to 4 cups.
Ingredients:
• 1 cup chopped pineapple (frozen or fresh)
• 1 cup chopped mango (frozen or fresh)
• ½ to 1 cup chopped kale
• ½ avocado
• ½ cup coconut milk
• 1 cup water, or coconut water
• 1 teaspoon matcha green tea powder (optional)
Directions:
1. Purée everything to a blender until smooth, adding more water (or coconut milk) if needed.

Nutrition: Calories: 566 Total fats: 36g Carbs: 66g Fiber: 12g Protein: 8g

213. Zobo Drink

Preparation time: 5 minutes
Cooking time: 10 minutes
Servings: 8
Ingredients:
• 2 cups dried hibiscus petals (zobo leaves), rinsed
• Pineapple rind from 1 pineapple
• 1 cup of granulated sugar
• 1 teaspoon fresh ginger, grated
• 10 cups of water
Directions:
1. Add water, ginger, and sugar into the pot and mix well.
2. Then add zobo leaves and pineapple rind.
3. Cover and cook on High for 10 minutes. Open and discard solids. Chill and serve.

Nutrition: Calories: 65 Carbs: 7g Fat: 2.6g Protein: 1.14g

214. Basil Lime Green Tea

Preparation time: 5 minutes
Cooking time: 4 minutes
Servings: 8
Ingredients:
• 8 cups of filtered water
• 10 bags of green tea
• ¼ cup of honey
• A pinch of baking soda
• Lime slices to taste
• Lemon slices to taste
• Basil leaves to taste
Directions:
1. Add water, honey, and baking soda to the pot and mix. Add the tea bags and cover. Cook on High for 4 minutes. Open and serve with lime slices, lemon slices, and basil leaves.

Nutrition: Calories: 32 Carbs: 8g Fat: 0g Protein: 0g

215. Berry Lemonade Tea

Preparation time: 5 minutes
Cooking time: 12 minutes
Servings: 4
Ingredients:
- 3 tea bags
- 2 cups of natural lemonade
- 1 cup of frozen mixed berries
- 2 cups of water
- 1 lemon, sliced

Directions:
1. Put everything in the Instant Pot and cover. Cook on High for 12 minutes. Open, strain, and serve.

Nutrition: Calories: 21 Carbs: 8g Fat: 0.2g Protein: 0.4g

216. Swedish Glögg

Preparation time: 5 minutes
Cooking time: 15 minutes
Servings: 1
Ingredients:
- ½ cup of orange juice
- ½ cup of water
- 1 piece of ginger cut into ½ pieces
- 1 whole clove
- 1 opened cardamom pods
- 2 tablespoons orange zest
- 1 cinnamon stick
- 1 whole allspice
- 1 vanilla bean

Directions:
1. Add everything in the pot. Cover and cook on High for 15 minutes. Open and serve.

Nutrition: Calories: 194 Carbs: 41g Fat: 3g Protein: 1.7g

217. Peach Smoothie

Preparation Time: 5 minutes
Cooking Time: 0 minute
Serving: 16 ounces of smoothie
Ingredients:
- 1 1/2 cups of frozen peaches

- 1 tablespoon of coconut sugar
- 1 cup of fresh spinach
- 8 ounces of kombucha
- 1/2 lime, juiced

Direction:
1. Blend kombucha and spinach together until no leafier chunks.
2. Add in the frozen peaches. Blend again until creamy.
3. Squeeze coconut sugar and lime juice onto a small shallow bowl/tray.
4. Dip rim of cup into lime juice. Then the sugar to coat the edges of the glass.
5. Use peach smoothie to fill the glass and enjoy it!

Nutrition: Calories: 219cal | Fat: 0.8g | Protein: 4g | Fiber: 4.6g | Sodium: 89.7mg | Sugar: 43.1g | Carbohydrate: 55.6g

218. Frozen Mojito

Preparation Time: 10 minutes
Cooking Time: 0 minute
Serving: 2
Ingredients:
- 2 tablespoons of freshly squeezed lime juice
- 1/2 cup 1/2 packed cup of fresh mint leaves plus sprigs for garnish
- 2-1/2 cups of ice cubes
- 3 ounces of white rum
- 3 tablespoons of simple syrup
- 1/4 cup of seltzer or club soda

Direction:
1. Add rum, lime juice, simple syrup, seltzer or club soda, and mint to a blender.
2. Blend until the mixture is slushy and ice is crushed.
3. Divide between 2 cocktail glasses.
4. Garnish with mint sprigs if you want.
5. Serve immediately.
6. Enjoy.

Nutrition: Calories: 153cal | Fat: 0.1g | Protein: 0.3g | Fiber: 0.6g | Sodium: 15.9mg | Sugar: 13g | Carbohydrate: 14.8g

219. Cassis Spritz

Preparation Time: 5 minutes
Cooking Time: 0 minute

Serving: 1
Ingredients:
- 2 ounces of dry white vermouth or dry white wine
- 1 cup of Sparkling water, chilled
- 1 cup of Ice
- 1-ounce of crème de cassis or black currant syrup
- 1 strip of orange zest for garnish

Direction:
1. Fill a tall glass with ice.
2. Add syrup or creme de cassis and wine or vermouth.
3. Top with sparkling water.
4. Garnish with orange zest.
5. Serve and enjoy.

Nutrition: Calories: 129cal | Fat: 0g | Protein: 0g | Fiber: 0g | Sodium: 9.6mg | Sugar: 16g | Carbohydrate: 17.4g

220. Strawberry Lime Margaritas

Preparation Time: 5 minutes
Cooking Time: 0 minute
Serving: 2
Ingredients:
- 2 cups of crushed ice, divided
- 2 tablespoons of fresh lemon juice
- 1/2 cup of frozen strawberries
- 3 ounces of tequila, divided
- 2 tablespoons of agave syrup, divided
- 2 tablespoons of fresh lime juice
- 1/4 cup of blueberries

Direction:
1. Add 1 tablespoon of agave, 1 1/2 ounces of tequila, 1 cup of crushed ice, and lime juice into a blender.
2. Blend until smooth—divide between 2 mason jars.
3. Rinse the blender, then add the rest of the tequila, lemon juice, 1 tablespoon of agave, lemon juice, 1 cup of crushed ice and strawberries.
4. Blend until smooth and divide between the two glasses, pouring slowly to create a layered effect.
5. Thread blueberries onto 2 skewers.
6. Garnish each cocktail with blueberries.
7. Serve and enjoy!

Nutrition: Calories: 191cal | Fat: 0.2g | Protein: 0.4g | Fiber: 1.4g | Sodium: 2.6mg | Sugar: 18.3g | Carbohydrate: 24.2g

221. Pina Colada in A Pineapple

Preparation Time: 10 minutes
Cooking Time: 0 minute
Serving: 2
Ingredients:
- 3 ounces of coconut cream, such as Coco Lopez
- 4 ounces of pineapple juice
- 1 pineapple
- 2 cups of ice cubes
- 3 ounces of white rum
- 2 cherries maraschino cherries for garnish

Direction:
1. Cut the top of the pineapple and discard; then reserve leaves for garnish if you want.
2. Run a knife just around the inside of the pineapple and scoop out the insides of the pineapple using a large spoon.
3. Reserve the flesh to thicken the drink if you want.
4. If desired, in a colander, place the pineapple flesh and mash it to extract as much juice as possible.
5. Place ice, coconut cream, rum, pineapple juice, and 1 cup of the reserved pineapple flesh into a blender.
6. Puree until smooth. Pour the mixture into the pineapple bowl.
7. Garnish with maraschino cherries and the reserved leaves.
8. Serve and enjoy.

Nutrition: Calories: 213cal | Fat: 9.1g | Protein: 1.1g | Fiber: 0.6g | Sodium: 7.2mg | Sugar: 6.2g | Carbohydrate: 9.2g

222. Kale Smoothie

Preparation time: 5 minutes
Cooking time: 0 minutes
Servings: 2
Ingredients:
- 2 cups chopped kale leaves
- 1 banana, peeled

- 1 cup frozen strawberries
- 1 cup unsweetened almond milk
- 4 Medjool dates, pitted and chopped

Directions:

1. Put all the ingredients to a food processor, then blitz until glossy and smooth.
2. Serve immediately or chill in the refrigerator for an hour before serving.

Nutrition: Calories: 663 Fat: 10.0g Carbs: 142.5g Fiber: 19.0g Protein: 17.4g

223. Hot Tropical Smoothie

Preparation time: 5 minutes
Cooking time: 0 minutes
Servings: 4
Ingredients:
- 1 cup frozen mango chunks
- 1 cup frozen pineapple chunks
- 1 small tangerine, peeled and pitted
- 2 cups spinach leaves
- 1 cup coconut water
- ¼ teaspoon cayenne pepper, optional

Directions:

1. Add all the ingredients to a food processor, then blitz until the mixture is smooth and combine well.
2. Serve immediately or chill in the refrigerator for an hour before serving.

Nutrition: Calories: 283 Fat: 1.9g Carbs: 67.9g Fiber: 10.4g Protein: 6.4g

224. Cranberry and Banana Smoothie

Preparation time: 5 minutes
Cooking time: 0 minutes
Servings: 4
- 1 cup frozen cranberries
- 1 large banana, peeled
- 4 Medjool dates, pitted and chopped
- 1(½) cup unsweetened almond milk

Directions:

1. Add all the ingredients to a food processor, then process until the mixture is glossy and well mixed.

2. Serve immediately or chill in the refrigerator for an hour before serving.

Nutrition: Calories: 616 Fat: 8.0g Carbs: 132.8g Fiber: 14.6g Protein: 15.7g

225. Cranberry and Protein Shake

Preparation time: 5 minutes
Cooking time: 0 minutes
Serving: 3
Ingredients:
- ¼ cup cranberries
- ¼ cup chia seeds, soaked in water for 20 minutes
- ¼ cup hemp seeds
- 2 cups unsweetened coconut milk
- 1 fresh banana
- 2 tablespoons vegan protein powder (chocolate or vanilla flavor)
- 4 ice cubes

Direction:

1. Put all the ingredients into a blender, and blend for 2 minutes until smooth and creamy.
2. Pour into three glasses and enjoy.

Nutrition: calories: 326 | fat: 16.7g | carbs: 19.8g | protein: 23.5g | fiber: 6.7g

226. Vegan Green Avocado Smoothie

Preparation time: 5 minutes
Cooking time: 10 minutes
Servings: 2
Ingredients
- 1 banana
- 1 c. water
- ½ avocado
- ½ lemon juice
- ½ c. coconut yogurt

Directions

1. Blend all ingredients until smooth.

Nutrition: Calories: 299. Fat: 1.1 g. Carbohydrates: 1.5 g. Protein: 7.9 g.

227. Super Smoothie

Preparation time: 5 minutes
Cooking time: 0 minutes
Servings: 4
Ingredients:
- 1 banana, peeled
- 1 cup chopped mango
- 1 cup raspberries
- ¼ cup rolled oats
- 1 carrot, peeled
- 1 cup chopped fresh kale
- 2 tablespoons chopped fresh parsley
- 1 tablespoon flaxseeds
- 1 tablespoon grated fresh ginger
- ½ cup unsweetened soy milk
- 1 cup water

Directions:
1. Put all the ingredients to a food processor, then blitz until glossy and smooth.
2. Serve immediately or chill in the refrigerator for an hour before serving.
Nutrition: Calories: 550 Fat: 39.0g Carbs: 31.0g Fiber: 15.0g Protein: 13.0g

228. Kiwi and Strawberry Smoothie

Preparation time: 5 minutes
Cooking time: 0 minutes
Servings: 3
Ingredients:
- 1 kiwi, peeled
- 5 medium strawberries
- ½ frozen banana
- 1 cup unsweetened almond milk
- 2 tablespoons hemp seeds
- 2 tablespoons peanut butter
- 1 to 2 teaspoons maple syrup
- ½ cup spinach leaves
- Handful broccoli sprouts

Directions:
1. Put all the ingredients to a food processor, then blitz until creamy and smooth.
2. Serve immediately or chill in the refrigerator for an hour before serving.
Nutrition: Calories: 562 Fat: 28.6g Carbs: 63.6g Fiber: 15.1g Protein: 23.3g

229. Banana and Chai Chia Smoothie

Preparation time: 5 minutes
Cooking time: 0 minutes
Servings: 3
Ingredients:
- 1 banana
- 1 cup alfalfa sprouts
- 1 tablespoon chia seeds
- ½ cup unsweetened coconut milk
- 1 to 2 soft Medjool dates, pitted
- ¼ teaspoon ground cinnamon
- 1 tablespoon grated fresh ginger
- 1 cup water
- Pinch ground cardamom

Directions:
1. Add all the ingredients to a blender, then process until the mixture is smooth and creamy. Add water or coconut milk if necessary. Serve immediately.
Nutrition: Calories:477 Fat: 41.0g Carbs: 31.0g Fiber: 14.0g Protein: 8.0g

230. Great Green Smoothie

Preparation: 5 minutes
Cooking time: 0 minutes
Servings: 4
Ingredients:
- 4 bananas, peeled
- 4 cups hulled strawberries
- 4 cups spinach
- 4 cups plant-based milk

Directions:
1. Preparing the Ingredients
Open 4 quart-size, freezer-safe bags. In each, layer in the following order: 1 banana (halved or sliced), 1 cup of strawberries, and 1 cup of spinach. Seal and place in the freezer.
2. Finish and Serve
To serve, take a frozen bag of Great Green Smoothie ingredients and transfer to a blender. Add 1 cup of plant-based milk, and blend until smooth. Place freezer bags in the freezer for up to 2 months.

Nutrition: Calories: 173; Protein: 4g; Total fat: 2g; Carbohydrates: 40g; Fiber: 7g

231. Smoothie Breakfast Bowl

Preparation: 10 minutes
Cooking time: 0 minutes
Servings: 4
Ingredients:
- 4 bananas, peeled
- 1 cup dragon fruit or fruit of choice
- 1 cup baked granola
- 2 cups fresh berries
- ½ cup slivered almonds
- 4 cups plant-based milk

Directions:
1. Preparing the Ingredients.
Open 4 quart-size, freezer-safe bags, and layer in the following order: 1 banana (halved or sliced) and ¼ cup dragon fruit. Into 4 small jelly jars, layer in the following order: ¼ cup granola, ½ cup berries, and 2 tablespoons slivered almonds.
2. Finish and Serve
To serve, take a frozen bag of bananas and dragon fruit and transfer to a blender. Add 1 cup of plant-based milk, and blend until smooth. Pour into a bowl. Add the contents of 1 jar of granola, berries, and almonds over the top of the smoothie and serve with a spoon. Place the freezer bags in the freezer for up to 2 months. Store the jars of berries, granola, and nuts in the refrigerator for up to 1 week.
Nutrition: Calories: 384; Protein: 6g; Total fat: 5g; Carbohydrates: 57g; Fiber: 8g

232. Max Power Smoothie

Preparation time: 5 minutes
Cooking time: 0 minutes
Servings: 4
Ingredients:
- 1 banana
- ¼ cup rolled oats, or 1 scoop plant protein powder
- 1 tablespoon flaxseed, or chia seeds
- 1 cup raspberries, or other berries

- 1 cup chopped mango (frozen or fresh)
- ½ cup non-dairy milk (optional)
- 1 cup water

Directions:
1. Purée everything in a blender until smooth, adding more water (or non-dairy milk) if needed.
2. Add none, some, or all the bonus boosters, as desired. Purée until blended.
Nutrition: Calories: 550 Fat: 9g Carbs: 116g Fiber: 29g Protein: 13g

233. Chai Chia Smoothie

Preparation time: 5 minutes
Cooking time: 0 minutes
Servings: 3
Ingredients:
- 1 banana
- ½ cup coconut milk
- 1 cup water
- 1 cup alfalfa sprouts (optional)
- 1 to 2 soft Medjool dates, pitted
- 1 tablespoon chia seeds, or ground flax or hemp hearts
- ¼ teaspoon ground cinnamon
- A pinch of ground cardamom
- 1 tablespoon grated fresh ginger, or ¼ teaspoon ground ginger

Directions:
1. Purée everything in a blender until smooth, adding more water (or coconut milk) if needed.
Nutrition: Calories: 477 Fat: 29g Carbs: 57g Fiber: 14g Protein: 8g

234. Cinnamon and Hemp Seed Coffee Shake

Preparation Time: 5 minutes
Cooking Time: 0 minutes
Serving: 1 glass
Ingredients:
- 1 ½ frozen bananas, sliced into coins
- 1/8 teaspoon ground cinnamon
- 2 tablespoons hemp seeds
- 1 tablespoon maple syrup
- ¼ teaspoon vanilla extract, unsweetened

- 1 cup regular coffee, cooled
- ¼ cup almond milk, unsweetened
- ½ cup of ice cubes

Directions:

1. Pour milk into a blender, add vanilla, cinnamon, and hemp seeds and then pulse until smooth.
2. Add banana, pour in the coffee, and then pulse until smooth.
3. Add ice, blend until well combined, blend in maple syrup and then serve.

Nutrition: Calories: 410 Cal; Fat: 19.5 g; Protein: 4.9 g; Carbs: 60.8 g; Fiber: 6.8 g;

235. Beet & Strawberry Smoothie

Preparation Time: 10 minutes
Cooking time: 0 minutes
Servings: 2
Ingredients:

- 2 cups frozen strawberries, pitted and chopped
- 2/3 cup roasted and frozen beet, chopped
- 1 teaspoon fresh ginger, peeled and grated
- 1 teaspoon fresh turmeric, peeled and grated
- ½ cup fresh orange juice
- 1 cup unsweetened almond milk

Direction:

1. Place all the ingredients in a high-powered blender and pulse until creamy.
2. Pour the smoothie into two glasses and serve immediately.

Nutrition: Calories: 258 Fat: 1.5g Carbohydrates: 26.7g Dietary Fiber: 4.9g Sugar: 18.7g Protein: 2.9g

236. Avocado & Spinach Smoothie

Preparation Time: 10 minutes
Cooking time: 0 minutes
Servings: 2
Ingredients:

- 2 cups fresh baby spinach
- ½ avocado, peeled, pitted and chopped
- 4-6 drops liquid stevia

- ½ teaspoon ground cinnamon
- 1 tablespoon hemp seeds
- 2 cups chilled water

Direction:

1. Add all the ingredients in a high-powered blender and pulse until smooth.
2. Pour the smoothie into two glasses and serve immediately.

Nutrition: Calories: 12 Fat: 11.7g Carbohydrates: 6.1g Dietary Fiber: 4.5g Sugar: 0.4g Protein: 3.1g

237. Cucumber & Greens Smoothie

Preparation Time: 10 minutes
Cooking time: 0 minutes
Servings: 2
Ingredients:

- 1 small cucumber, peeled and chopped
- 2 cups mixed fresh greens (spinach, kale, beet greens), trimmed and chopped
- ½ cup lettuce, torn
- ¼ cup fresh parsley leaves
- ¼ cup fresh mint leaves
- 2-3 drops liquid stevia
- 1 teaspoon fresh lemon juice
- 1½ cups filtered water
- ¼ cup ice cubes

Direction:

1. Add all the ingredients in a high-powered blender and pulse until smooth.
2. Pour the smoothie into two glasses and serve immediately.

Nutrition: Calories: 50 Fat: 0.5g Carbohydrates: 11.3g Dietary Fiber: 3.6g Sugar: 3.2g Protein: 2.5g

238. Maca Smoothie

Preparation time: 10 minutes
Cooking time: 0 minute
Servings: 2
Ingredients:

- 2 frozen bananas, peeled and sliced
- 2 tablespoons sunflower seeds
- 2 tablespoons sunflower butter
- 1 tablespoon maca powder
- 1 teaspoon ground cinnamon
- ½ teaspoon pure vanilla extract

- 1½ cups unsweetened almond milk

Direction:

1.   In a high-speed blender, place all ingredients and pulse until creamy.

2.   Pour into two glasses and serve immediately.

Nutrition: Calories 260 Total Fat 12.2 g Saturated Fat 1.3 g Cholesterol 0 mg Sodium 220 mg Total Carbs 36 g Fiber 5.2 g Sugar 15.2 g Protein 6.3 g

239.   Fruity Green Smoothie

Preparation time: 10 minutes

Cooking time: 0 minute

Servings: 2

Ingredients:

- 1 large sweet apple peeled, cored, and chopped roughly
- ½ cup frozen mango chunks
- 1 cup fresh baby spinach
- 1 cup cucumber, chopped
- ¾ cup celery stalk, chopped
- 2 tablespoons fresh mint leaves
- 3 tablespoons hemp hearts
- 1½ teaspoons virgin coconut oil
- ½ cup fresh red grapefruit juice
- ½ cup ice cubes

Direction:

1.   In a high-speed blender, place all ingredients and pulse until creamy.

2.   Pour into two glasses and serve immediately.

Nutrition: Calories 237 Total Fat 10.6 g Saturated Fat 4.2 g Cholesterol 0 mg Sodium 46 mg Total Carbs 31.8 g Fiber 7.1 g Sugar 22.7 g Protein 7.2 g

Green Smoothie

Preparation Time: 5 minutes

Cooking Time: 0 minutes

Serving: 1

Ingredients:

- ½ cup strawberries, frozen
- 4 leaves of kale
- ¼ of a medium banana
- 2 Medjool dates, pitted
- 1 tablespoon flax seed
- ¼ cup pumpkin seeds, hulled
- 1 cup of water

Directions:

1.   Place all the ingredients in the jar of a food processor or blender and then cover it with the lid.

2.   Pulse until smooth and then serve.

Nutrition: Calories: 204 Cal; Fat: 1.1 g; Protein: 6.5 g; Carbs: 48 g; Fiber: 8.3 g;

240.   Green Tofu Smoothie

Preparation time: 10 minutes

Cooking time: 0 minute

Servings: 2

Ingredients:

- 2 cups fresh spinach
- 1 banana, peeled and sliced
- 1 cup frozen mango chunks
- 1 kiwi, peeled and chopped roughly
- 6 ounces' silken tofu
- ½ teaspoon ground turmeric
- 1½ cups unsweetened almond milk
- ¼ cup ice cubes

Direction:

1.   In a high-speed blender, place all ingredients and pulse until creamy.

2.   Pour into two glasses and serve immediately.

Nutrition: Calories 224 Total Fat 7.1 g Saturated Fat 1.2 g Cholesterol 0 mg Sodium 172 mg Total Carbs 35.8 g Fiber 6.3 g Sugar 22.6 g Protein 10.4 g

241.   Pineapple Smoothie

Preparation time: 5 minutes

Cooking time: 0 minutes

Serving: 1 to 2

Ingredients:

- ¾ cup pineapple chunks
- ½ cup frozen strawberries
- ½ cup unsweetened apple juice

Direction:

1.   Put all the ingredients in a blender and pulse until smooth.

2.   Serve immediately.

Nutrition: Calories: 134 | fat: 0.2g | carbs: 32.4g | protein: 0.6g | fiber: 2.3g

242. Tropical Fruit Smoothie Bowl

Preparation time: 5 minutes
Cooking time: 0 minutes
Serving: 1 to 2
Ingredients:
- 2 cups frozen mango chunks
- 1 frozen banana
- ½ cup frozen pineapple chunks
- ½ to 1 cup plant-based milk
- ¼ cup chopped fruit of your choice
- 2 tablespoons chopped nuts of your choice

Toppings:
- 1½ tablespoons coconut shreds
- 1 tablespoon flaxseed meal

Direction:
1. Place all the ingredients except the toppings into a blender and process until smoothly blended.
2. Serve topped with the coconut shreds and flaxseed meal.

Nutrition: Calories: 343 | fat: 8.7g | carbs: 66.4g | protein: 6.8g | fiber: 7.0g

243. Berry Smoothie

Preparation time: 5 minutes
Cooking time: 0 minutes
Serving: 3
Ingredients:
- 1 cup strawberries
- 1 cup cranberries or raspberries
- 1 cup chopped melon (any kind)
- 1 cup water
- ½ cup unsweetened coconut milk
- 1 tablespoon chia seeds

Direction:
1. Blend all the ingredients in a blender until smoothly puréed. If you prefer a thinner smoothie, you can add more water or coconut milk if needed.
2. Serve immediately.

Nutrition: Calories: 175 | fat: 13.0g | carbs: 16.8g | protein: 3.1g | fiber: 5.3g

244. Golden Milk

Preparation time: 5 minutes
Cooking time: 5 minutes
Serving: 1
Ingredients:
- ½ teaspoon ground turmeric
- ½ teaspoon grated fresh ginger
- ¼ teaspoon ground cinnamon
- Pinch ground black pepper
- 1 cup canned full-fat coconut milk
- 1 tablespoon extra-virgin coconut oil (optional)
- 1 teaspoon maple syrup (optional)

Direction:
1. Combine the turmeric, ginger, cinnamon, and black pepper in a small saucepan over medium heat.
2. Add the milk, oil, and maple syrup (if desired) and whisk well.
3. Let the mixture heat for 5 minutes until very hot but not boiling.
4. Carefully pour hot milk into a blender and blend on low speed until it becomes frothy. Serve immediately.

Nutrition: Calories: 641 | fat: 61.9g | carbs: 16.7g | protein: 5.6g | fiber: 1.4g

245. Chia Fresca

Preparation time: 5 minutes
Cooking time: 0 minutes
Serving: 1
Ingredients:
- 1 cup unsweetened coconut water
- 1 tablespoon chia seeds
- 1 tablespoon fresh lime juice
- ½ teaspoon pure maple syrup (optional)
- ¼ cup strawberries
- ¼ cup diced peaches

Direction:
1. Stir together all the ingredients in a glass and allow to sit for 5 to 10 minutes, or until some liquid is absorbed, and the chia seeds become gelatinous.
2. Serve chilled.

Nutrition: Calories: 105 | fat: 3.1g | carbs: 22.2g | protein: 3.7g | fiber: 6.7g

246. Vanilla Milk Steamer

Preparation time: 5 minutes
Cooking time: 5 minutes
Serving: 1
Ingredients:
- 1 cup unsweetened almond milk
- 2 teaspoons pure maple syrup (optional)
- ½ teaspoon pure vanilla extract
- Pinch ground cinnamon

Direction:
1. Warm the almond milk in a small saucepan over medium heat for 5 minutes until steaming, stirring constantly (don't allow it to boil).
2. Carefully pour the hot milk into your blender and mix in the maple syrup (if desired) and vanilla. Blend on low speed for 10 seconds, then increase the speed to high and blend until well combined and frothy.
3. Serve sprinkled with the cinnamon.

Nutrition: Calories: 184 | fat: 7.9g | carbs: 20.7g | protein: 7.6g | fiber: 0g

247. Light Ginger Tea

Preparation time: 5 minutes
Cooking time: 10 to 15 minutes
Servings: 2
Ingredients:
- 1 small ginger knob, sliced into four 1-inch chunks
- 4 cups water
- Juice of 1 large lemon
- Maple syrup to taste

Directions:
1. Add the ginger knob and water in a saucepan, then simmer over medium heat for 10 to 15 minutes.
2. Turn off the heat, then mix in the lemon juice. Strain the liquid to remove the ginger, then fold in the maple syrup and serve.

Nutrition: Calories: 32 Fat: 0.1g Carbs: 8.6g Fiber: 0.1g Protein: 0.1g

248. Classic Switchel

Preparation time: 5 minutes
Cooking time: 0 minutes
Servings: 4
Ingredients:
- 1-inch piece ginger, minced
- 2 tablespoons apple cider vinegar
- 2 tablespoons maple syrup
- 4 cups water
- ¼ teaspoon sea salt, optional

Directions:
1. Combine all the ingredients in a glass. Stir to mix well.
2. Serve immediately or chill in the refrigerator for an hour before serving.

Nutrition: Calories: 110 Fat: 0g Carbs: 28.0g Fiber: 0g Protein: 0g

249. Lime and Cucumber Electrolyte Drink

Preparation time: 5 minutes
Cooking time: 0 minutes
Servings: 4
Ingredients:
- ¼ cup chopped cucumber
- 1 tablespoon fresh lime juice
- 1 tablespoon apple cider vinegar
- 2 tablespoons maple syrup
- ¼ teaspoon sea salt, optional
- 4 cups water

Directions:
1. Combine all the ingredients in a glass. Stir to mix well. Refrigerate overnight before serving.

Nutrition: Calories: 114 Fat: 0.1g Carbs: 28.9g Fiber: 0.3g Protein: 0.3g

250. Easy and Fresh

Preparation time: 5 minutes
Cooking time: 0 minutes
Servings: 4
Ingredients:
- 1 cup chopped mango

- 1 cup chopped peach
- 1 banana
- 1 cup strawberries
- 1 carrot, peeled and chopped
- 1 cup water

Directions:

1.   Put all the ingredients to a food processor, then blitz until glossy and smooth.

2.   Serve immediately or chill in the refrigerator for an hour before serving.

Nutrition: Calories: 376 Fat: 22.0g Carbs: 19.0g Fiber: 14.0g Protein: 5.0g

251.   Simple Date Shake

Preparation time: 10 minutes
Cooking time: 0 minutes
Servings: 2
Ingredients:
- 5 Medjool dates, pitted, soaked in boiling water for 5 minutes
- ¾ cup unsweetened coconut milk
- 1 teaspoon vanilla extract
- ½ teaspoon fresh lemon juice
- ¼ teaspoon sea salt, optional
- 1(½) cup ice

Directions:

1.   Put all the ingredients to a food processor, then blitz until it has a milkshake and smooth texture. Serve immediately.

Nutrition: Calories: 380 Fat: 21.6g Carbs: 50.3g Fiber: 6.0gProtein: 3.2g

252.   Beet and Clementine Protein Smoothie

Preparation time: 10 minutes
Cooking time: 0 minutes
Servings: 3
Ingredients:
- 1 small beet, peeled and chopped
- 1 clementine, peeled and broken into segments
- ½ ripe banana
- ½ cup raspberries
- 1 tablespoon chia seeds

- 2 tablespoons almond butter
- ¼ teaspoon vanilla extract
- 1 cup unsweetened almond milk
- 1/8 teaspoon fine sea salt, optional

Directions:

1.   Combine all the ingredients to a food processor, then pulse on high for 2 minutes or until glossy and creamy. Refrigerate for an hour and serve chilled.

Nutrition: Calories: 526 Fat: 25.4g Carbs: 61.9g Fiber: 17.3g Protein: 20.6g

253.   Matcha Limeade

Preparation time: 10 minutes
Cooking time: 0 minutes
Servings: 4
Ingredients:
- 2 tablespoons matcha powder
- ¼ cup raw agave syrup
- 3 cups water, divided
- 1 cup fresh lime juice
- 3 tablespoons chia seeds

Directions:

1.   Lightly simmer the matcha, agave syrup, and 1 cup of water in a saucepan over medium heat. Keep stirring until no matcha lumps.

2.   Pour the matcha mixture into a large glass, add the remaining ingredients, and mix well.

3.   Refrigerate for at least an hour before serving.

Nutrition: Calories: 152 Fat: 4.5g Carbs: 26.8g Fiber: 5.3g Protein: 3.7g

254.   Fruit Infused Water

Preparation time: 5 minutes
Cooking time: 0 minutes
Servings: 2
Ingredients:
- 3 strawberries, sliced
- 5 mint leaves
- ½ of orange, sliced
- 2 cups of water

Directions:

1.   Divide fruits and mint between two glasses, pour in water, stir until just mixed, and refrigerate for 2 hours.

2.   Serve straight away.
Nutrition: Calories: 5.4 Fat: 0.1g Carbs: 1.3g Protein: 0.1g Fiber: 0.4g

255.   Hazelnut and Chocolate Milk

Preparation time: 5 minutes
Cooking time: 0 minutes
Servings: 2
Ingredients:
*   2 tablespoons cocoa powder
*   4 dates, pitted
*   1 cup hazelnuts
*   3 cups of water
Directions:
1.   Place all the ingredients in the order to a food processor or blender and then pulse for 2 to 3 minutes at high speed until smooth.
2.   Pour the smoothie into two glasses and then serve.
Nutrition: Calories: 120 Fat: 5g Carbs: 19g Protein: 2g Fiber: 1g

256.   Banana Milk

Preparation time: 5 minutes
Cooking time: 0 minutes
Servings: 2
Ingredients:
*   2 dates
*   2 medium bananas, peeled
*   1 teaspoon vanilla extract, unsweetened
*   1/2 cup ice
*   2 cups of water
Directions:
1.   Place all the ingredients in the order to a food processor or blender and then pulse for 2 to 3 minutes at high speed until smooth.
2.   Pour the smoothie into two glasses and then serve.
Nutrition: Calories: 79 Fat: 0g Carbs: 19.8g Protein: 0.8g Fiber: 6g

257.   Apple, Carrot, Celery, and Kale Juice

Preparation time: 5 minutes
Cooking time: 0 minutes
Servings: 2
Ingredients:
*   5 curly kales
*   2 green apples, cored, peeled, chopped
*   2 large stalks celery
*   4 large carrots, cored, peeled, chopped
Directions:
1.   Process all the ingredients in the order in a juicer or blender and then strain it into two glasses.
2.   Serve straight away.
Nutrition: Calories: 183 Fat: 2.5g Carbs: 46g Protein: 13g Fiber: 3g

258.   Sweet and Sour Juice

Preparation time: 5 minutes
Cooking time: 0 minutes
Servings: 2
Ingredients:
*   2 medium apples, cored, peeled, chopped
*   2 large cucumbers, peeled
*   4 cups chopped grapefruit
*   1 cup mint
Directions:
1.   Process all the ingredients in the order in a juicer or blender and then strain it into two glasses.
2.   Serve straight away.
Nutrition: Calories: 90 Fat: 0g Carbs: 23g Protein: 0g Fiber: 9g

259.   Green Lemonade

Preparation time: 5 minutes
Cooking time: 0 minutes
Servings: 2
Ingredients:
*   10 large stalks of celery, chopped
*   2 medium green apples, cored, peeled, chopped
*   2 medium cucumbers, peeled, chopped
*   2 inches' piece of ginger
*   10 stalks of kale, chopped
*   2 cups parsley
Directions:

1.   Process all the ingredients in the order in a juicer or blender and then strain it into two glasses. Serve straight away.
Nutrition: Calories: 102.3 Fat: 1.1g Carbs: 26.2g Protein: 4.7g Fiber: 8.5g

260.   Pineapple and Spinach Juice

Preparation time: 5 minutes
Cooking time: 0 minutes
Servings: 2
Ingredients:
- 2 medium red apples, cored, peeled, chopped
- 3 cups spinach
- ½ of a medium pineapple, peeled
- 2 lemons, peeled

Directions:
1.   Process all the ingredients in the order in a juicer or blender and then strain it into two glasses.
2.   Serve straight away.
Nutrition: Calories: 131 Fat: 0.5g Carbs: 34.5g Protein: 1.7g Fiber: 5g

261.   Green Berry Drink

Preparation Time: 10 minutes
Cooking Time: 0 minutes
Serving: 2
Ingredients:
- 1 cup almond milk
- 1 pack natural sweetener
- ¼ cup raspberries
- 1 cup of water
- 1 tablespoon macadamia oil
- 1 cup spinach

Direction:
1.   Add listed ingredients to a blender
2.   Blend until you have a smooth and creamy texture
3.   Serve chilled and enjoy!
Nutrition: Calories: 292 Fat: 21g Carbohydrates: 17g Protein: 9g

262.   The Alkaline Strawberry Smoothie

Preparation Time: 5 minutes
Cooking Time:0 minute
Serving: 2
Ingredients
- ½ cup of organic strawberries/blueberries
- Half a banana
- 2 cups of coconut water
- ½ inch ginger
- Juice of 2 grapefruits

Direction:
1.   Add all the listed ingredients to a blender
2.   Blend on high until smooth and creamy
3.   Enjoy your smoothie
Nutrition: Calories: 200 Fat: 10g Carbohydrates: 14g Protein 2g

263.   Avocado and Blueberry Glass

Preparation Time: 10 minutes
Cooking Time: 0 minute
Serving: 2
Ingredients:
- 1 cup unsweetened milk, vanilla
- 1 tablespoon cashew cream
- ½ avocado, peeled, pitted and sliced
- 1 scoop coconut zero carb protein powder
- 14 cups frozen blueberries, unsweetened
- Liquid Stevia

Direction:
1.   Add listed ingredients to a blender
2.   Blend until you have a smooth and creamy texture
3.   Serve chilled and enjoy!
Nutrition: Calories: 385 Calories: 372 Fat: 22g Carbohydrates: 4g Protein: 32g

264. Coconut and Hazelnut Chilled Glass

Preparation Time: 10 minutes
Cooking time: 0 minute
Serving: 1
Ingredients:
- ½ cup of coconut milk
- ¼ cup hazelnuts, chopped
- 1 ½ cups of water
- 1 pack Stevia

Directions:
1. Add listed ingredients to a blender
2. Blend until you have a smooth and creamy texture
3. Serve chilled and enjoy!

Nutrition: Calories: 457 Fat: 46g Carbohydrates: 12g Protein: 7g

265. Strawberry Lover's Drink

Preparation Time: 10 minutes
Cooking Time: 0 minute
Serving: 2
Ingredients:
- 16 ounces unsweetened almond milk, vanilla
- 1 teaspoon natural sweetener, such as maple syrup
- 4 ounces' almond cream
- 1 scoop vanilla whey protein
- ¼ cup frozen strawberries, unsweetened

Direction:
1. Add listed ingredients to a blender
2. Blend until you have a smooth and creamy texture
3. Serve chilled and enjoy!

Nutrition: Calories: 304 Fat: 25g Carbohydrates: 7g Protein: 15g

266. The Unique Smoothie Bowl

Preparation Time: 10 minutes
Cooking Time: 0 minute
Serving: 2
Ingredients:
- 2 cups baby spinach leaves
- 1 cup of coconut milk
- ¼ cup cashew cream
- 2 tablespoons flaxseed oil
- 2 tablespoons chia seeds
- 2 tablespoons walnuts, roughly chopped
- A handful of fresh berries

Directions:
1. Add spinach leaves, coconut milk, cream and flaxseed oil to a blender
2. Blitz until smooth
3. Pour smoothie into serving bowls
4. Sprinkle chia seeds, berries, walnuts on top
5. Serve and enjoy!

Nutrition: Calories: 380 Fat: 36g Carbohydrates: 12g Protein: 5g

267. Minty Smoothie

Preparation Time: 10 minutes
Cooking time: 0 minute
Serving: 1
Ingredients:
- 1 stalk celery
- 2 cups of water
- 2 ounces' almonds
- 1 packet Stevia
- 1 cup of spinach
- 2 mint leaves

Directions:
1. Add listed ingredients to a blender
2. Blend until you have a smooth and creamy texture
3. Serve chilled and enjoy!

Nutrition: Calories: 417 Fat: 43g Carbohydrates: 10g Protein: 5.5g

268.   Pineapple Kefir Smoothie

Preparation time: 4 minutes
Cooking time: 0 minutes
Servings: 2
Ingredients:
- 1 cup kefir
- 1 slice pineapple
- Ice to taste

Direction:
1. Cut the pineapple slice into small pieces, removing the heart.
2. Put the small glass of the blender, add the kefir and blend.
3. Serve with ice to taste.

Nutrition: Calorie: 111 Protein: 3.7g Fat: 2.7g Carbohydrates: 17.9g

269.   Green Smoothie with Fruits and Vitamins

Preparation time: 4 minutes
Cooking time: 0 minutes
Servings: 2
Ingredients:
- ½ cucumber
- 3 tsp of maca powder
- Celery
- 1 cup of water
- 1 green apple
- 3 tsp of chia seeds

Direction:
1. Pour all the ingredients in the blender and process them until you get a homogeneous drink.
2. Consume it as part of breakfast, or 30 minutes before breakfast.

Nutrition: Calorie: 184.2 Protein: 4.3g Fat: 1.3g Carbohydrates: 44.6g

270.   Banana-Raspberry Smoothie Bowl

Preparation time: 10 minutes
Cooking time: 0 minute
Serving: 4
Ingredients:
- 6 cups frozen banana chunks
- 1 cup frozen raspberries
- 2 tablespoons nut butter of choice
- 1 heaping tablespoon ground flaxseed
- ½ teaspoon almond extract
- ½ cup unsweetened plant-based milk

Direction:
1. In a food processor, pulse the banana chunks until they have a crumbly texture.
2. Add the raspberries, nut butter, flaxseed, and almond extract and process to combine.
3. While the food processor is running, slowly add the milk. As the liquid mixes in, the frozen mixture should begin to form a ball. Scrape the sides of the food processor and continue to blend until no chunks remain and the mixture has a thick smoothie or soft-serve ice cream texture. Serve.

Nutrition: Calories: 297.5; Total fat: 7g; Total carbs: 60g; Fiber: 10g; Sugar: 30g; Protein: 6g; Sodium: 19mg

271.   Pumpkin Chai Smoothie

Preparation Time: 5 minutes
Cooking Time: 0 minutes
Serving: 1 glass
Ingredients:
- 1 cup cooked pumpkin
- ¼ cup pecans
- 1 frozen banana
- ¼ teaspoon ground cinnamon
- ¼ teaspoon cardamom
- ¼ teaspoon ground nutmeg
- 2 teaspoons maple syrup
- 1 cup of water, cold
- ½ cup of ice cubes

Directions:
1. Place pecans in a small bowl, cover with water, and then let them soak for 10 minutes.

2. Drain the pecans, add them into a blender, and then add the remaining ingredients.

3. Pulse for 1 minute until smooth, and then serve.

Nutrition: Calories: 157.5 Cal; Fat: 3.8 g; Protein: 3 g; Carbs: 32.3 g; Fiber: 4.5 g;

272. Orange Smoothie

Preparation Time: 5 minutes
Cooking time: 0 minute
Servings: 1
Ingredients:
- 1 cup chopped zucchini rounds, frozen
- 1 cup spinach
- 1 small peeled navel orange, frozen
- 1 small chopped beet
- 1 scoop of vanilla protein powder
- 1 cup almond milk, unsweetened

Direction:
1. Put the whole shopping list: in the order in a food processor or a blender and then blend for 2 or 3 minutes on high speed until smooth.
2. Pour the smoothie into a glass and serve.

Nutrition: Calories: 253 Cal Fat: 5 g Carbs: 44.6 g Protein: 3 g Fiber: 8 g

273. Green Honeydew Smoothie

Preparation Time: 5 minutes
Cooking Time: 15 minutes
Serving: 4
Ingredients:
- 1 large banana
- 6 large leaves of basil
- ½ cup frozen pineapple
- 1 teaspoon lime juice
- 1 cup pieces of honeydew melon
- 1 teaspoon green tea matcha powder
- ¼ cup almond milk, unsweetened

Directions:
1. Place all the ingredients in the jar of a food processor or blender and then cover it with the lid.
2. Pulse until smooth and then serve.

Nutrition: Calories: 223.5 Cal; Fat: 2.7 g; Protein: 20.1 g; Carbs: 32.7 g; Fiber: 5.2 g;

274. Veggie Smoothie

Preparation time: 5 minutes
Cooking time: 0 minutes
Servings: 2
Ingredients:
- 2 cups coconut water, unsweetened
- 2/3 cup broccoli florets
- 2 cups honeydew melon pieces
- One lime, peeled, deseeded, halved
- ½ cup kale, destemmed, rinsed
- 2 Medjool dates pitted
- ½ cup mint leaves
- 1 cup of ice cubes

Direction:
1. Collect the whole shopping list:
2. Connect a high-powder blender, then add the whole Shopping List: in the order shown in the Shopping List: List.
3. Blend for 45-60 seconds or longer depending on the blender, until well blended and smooth, then distribute the smoothie between two glasses.
4. Serve immediately.

Nutrition: Calories: 220 Cal Total Fat: 1 g Saturated Fat: 0.6 g Carbohydrates: 46 g Fiber: 8.6 g Sugars: 39 g Protein: 5.4 g

275. Peanut Butter & Pumpkin Shake

Preparation time: 5 minutes
Cooking time: 0 minute
Servings: 1
Ingredients:
- 1/2 cup peach slices, frozen
- 2 teaspoon ground ginger
- 1/2 frozen banana
- 1 teaspoon cinnamon
- 1 scoop of vanilla protein powder
- 4 tablespoon powdered peanut butter
- 5 drops liquid stevia
- 1 cup almond milk, unsweetened
- 1/2 cup pumpkin puree

Direction:
1. Put the whole shopping list: in the order in a food processor or a blender and then blend for 2 or 3 minutes on high speed until smooth.
2. Pour the smoothie into a glass and serve.

Nutrition: Calories: 366 Cal Fat: 7.8 g Carbs: 47 g Protein: 33 g Fiber: 13 g

276. Avocado Smoothie

Preparation time: 5 minutes
Cooking time: 0 minutes
Servings: 3
Ingredients:
- 1 Avocado
- 1 cup Coconut Milk
- 2 cups Ice Cubes
- 2 tbsp Erythritol
- ½ tsp Powdered Cardamom
- 1 tbsp Vanilla Extract

Direction:
1. Combine the whole shopping list: in one bowl. Mix until well combined.
2. Press the mixture into a rectangular silicone mold and freeze for one hour to set.
3. Slice to serve.
Nutrition: Calories 305 Carbohydrates 9 g Fats 29 g Protein 3 g

277. Butternut Smoothie

Preparation time: 5 minutes
Cooking time: 0 minutes
Servings: 2
Ingredients:
- 2 cups almond milk, unsweetened
- ½ cup of water
- 1 cup butternut squash pieces, frozen
- Two bananas, peeled, frozen
- 1 cup raspberries, frozen
- Two tablespoons hemp seeds
- Two tablespoons chia seeds
- One teaspoon ground cinnamon
- 1/4 cup peanut butter

Direction:
1. Collect the whole shopping list.
2. Connect a high-powder blender, then add the whole Shopping List: in the order shown in the Shopping List: List.
3. Blend for 45-60 seconds or longer depending on the blender, until well blended and smooth, then distribute the smoothie between two glasses.
4. Serve immediately.
Nutrition: Calories: 520 Cal Total Fat: 26.1 g Saturated Fat: 4.4 g Carbohydrates: 56.2 g Fiber: 15.8 g Sugars: 22.8 g Protein: 14.1 g

278. Tropical Fruit Smoothie

Preparation time: 10 minutes
Cooking time 0 minute
Serving: 2
Ingredients:
- ½ cup pineapple chunks
- ½ cup mango chunks
- 1 banana, peeled and sliced
- 1 tablespoon fresh lemon juice
- 1½ cups unsweetened coconut milk

Direction:
1.   In a blender, place all the ingredients and pulse until smooth.
2.   Place the smoothie into glasses and serve immediately.
Meal Prep Tip:
1.   In 2 zip lock bags, divide the banana, pineapple and mango chunks. Seal the bags and store in the freezer for about 2-3 days.
2.   Just before serving, remove from the freezer and transfer into a blender with coconut milk and lemon juice and pulse until smooth.
Nutrition: Calories: 370, Fats: 25.2g, Carbs: 29.7g, Fiber: 2.8g, Sugar: 21.6g, Proteins: 3.5g, Sodium: 59mg

Chapter 10. Sides, Salads and Sauces

279.   Parsley Arugula Pesto

Preparation time: 5 minutes
Cooking time: 0 minutes
Servings: 12
Ingredients:

* 1 clove garlic
* 1 cup parsley
* 1 cup arugula
* ¼ cup walnuts
* ¼ teaspoon salt
* 1 tablespoon olive oil
* 1 tablespoon lemon juice

Direction:
1.   Add all the ingredients to a blender.
2.   Press the pulse button and blend until it is lump-free.
3.   Serve.

Nutrition: Calories 22 Total Fat 1.5 g Saturated Fat 0.6 g Cholesterol 3 mg Sodium 126 mg Total Carbs 6.3 g Sugar 5.1 g Fiber 0.7 g Protein 0.6 g

280.   Basil Peanut Salad Dressing

Preparation time: 10 minutes
Cooking time: 0 minutes
Servings: 6
Ingredients:

* 3 cups basil leaves
* 1 cup peanuts
* ½ cup olive oil
* ¾ cup water
* Juice from ½ of a lemon
* 1 pinch each of salt, pepper, red chili flakes, to taste

Direction:
1.   Add all the ingredients to a blender.
2.   Press the pulse button and blend until it is lump-free.
3.   Serve.

Nutrition: Calories 86 Total Fat 1.8 g Saturated Fat 0.8 g Cholesterol 3 mg Sodium 537 mg Total Carbs 7 g Sugar 1.7 g Fiber 0.5 g Protein 4.6 g

281.   Roasted Red Salsa

Preparation time: 10 minutes
Cooking time: 0 minutes
Servings: 4
Ingredients:

* ½ yellow onion, quartered
* 4 ripe roma tomatoes, halved
* 1 jalapeno pepper, halved
* 3 cloves of garlic, peeled
* 1 tablespoon brown sugar
* ½ teaspoon salt
* 1 teaspoon apple cider vinegar
* ¼ cup fresh cilantro, chopped

Direction:
1.   Add all the ingredients to a blender.
2.   Press the pulse button and chop the ingredients into a chunky salsa.
3.   Serve.

Nutrition: Calories 93 Total Fat 0.2 g Saturated Fat 0 g Cholesterol 0 mg Sodium 738 mg Total Carbs 11.3 g Sugar 0.2 g Fiber 0.5 g Protein 0.3 g

282.   Black Bean Lime Dip

Preparation Time: 5 minutes
Cooking Time: 6 minutes
Servings: 4
Ingredients:

* 15.5 ounces cooked black beans
* 1 teaspoon minced garlic
* 1/2 of a lime, juiced
* 1 inch of ginger, grated
* 1/3 teaspoon salt
* 1/3 teaspoon ground black pepper
* 1 tablespoon olive oil

Directions:
1.   Add oil to a frying pan. When hot, add garlic and ginger. Cook for 1 minute until fragrant.

2.   Then add beans, splash with some water and fry for 3 minutes until hot.

3.   Season beans with salt and black pepper, drizzle with lime juice, remove the pan from heat and mash the beans until smooth pasta comes together.

4.   Serve the dip with whole-grain bread sticks or vegetables.

Nutrition: Calories: 100 Fat: 8g Carbohydrates: 5g Protein: 2g

283.   Beetroot Hummus

Preparation Time: 10 minutes
Cooking Time: 20 minutes
Servings: 4
Ingredients:
- 15 ounces cooked chickpeas
- 3 small beets
- 1 teaspoon minced garlic
- 1/2 teaspoon smoked paprika
- 1 teaspoon of sea salt
- 1/4 teaspoon red chili flakes
- 2 tablespoons olive oil
- 1 lemon, juiced
- 2 tablespoon tahini
- 1 tablespoon chopped almonds
- 1 tablespoon chopped cilantro

Directions:
1.   Drizzle oil over beets, season with salt, wrap beets in foil, and bake for 10 minutes at 425 degrees F until tender.

2.   When done, let beet cool for 10 minutes, peel and dice them and place them in a food processor.

3.   Add the last ingredients and process for 2 minutes until smooth, tip the hummus in a bowl, drizzle with some more oil, and then serve straight away.

Nutrition: Calories: 50.1 Fat: 2.5 g Carbohydrates: 5 g Protein: 2 g

284.   Buffalo Dip

Preparation time: 5 minutes
Cooking time: 25 minutes
Servings: 4
Ingredients:
- 2 cups cashews
- 2 teaspoons garlic powder
- 1 1/2 teaspoons salt

- 2 teaspoons onion powder
- 3 tablespoons lemon juice
- 1 cup buffalo sauce
- 1 cup of water
- 14-ounce artichoke hearts, packed in water, drained

Directions:
1.   Switch on the oven, then set it to 375 degrees F and let it preheat.

2.   Meanwhile, pour 3 cups of boiling water in a bowl, add cashews, and let soak for 5 minutes.

3.   Then drain the cashew, transfer them into the blender, pour in water, add lemon juice and all the seasoning and blend until smooth.

4.   Add artichokes and buffalo sauce, process until chunky mixture comes together, and transfer the dip to an ovenproof dish.

5.   Bake for 20 minutes and then serve.

Nutrition: Calories: 100 Fat: 3g Carbohydrates: 3g Protein: 1g

285.   Cashew Yogurt

Preparation time: 5 minutes
Cooking time: 5 minutes
Servings: 8
Ingredients:
- 3 probiotic supplements
- 2 2/3 cups cashews, unsalted, soaked in warm water for 15 minutes
- 1/4 teaspoon sea salt
- 4 tablespoon lemon juice
- 1 1/2 cup water

Directions:
1.   Drain the cashews, add them into the food processor, then add remaining ingredients, except for probiotic supplements, and pulse for 2 minutes until smooth.

2.   Tip the mixture in a bowl, add probiotic supplements, stir until mixed, then cover the bowl with a cheesecloth and let it stand for 12 hours in a dark and cool room.

3.   Serve straight away.

Nutrition: Calories: 110 Fat: 7g Carbohydrates: 9g Protein: 3g

286. Nacho Cheese Sauce

Preparation time: 15 minutes
Cooking time: 5 minutes
Servings: 12
Ingredients:
- 2 cups cashews, unsalted
- 2 teaspoons salt
- 1/2 cup nutritional yeast
- 1 teaspoon garlic powder
- 1/2 teaspoon smoked paprika
- 1/2 teaspoon red chili powder
- 1 teaspoon onion powder
- 2 teaspoons Sriracha
- 3 tablespoons lemon juice
- 4 cups water, divided

Directions:
1. Leave the cashews in warm water for 15 minutes.
2. Drain the cashews, transfer them to a food processor, add remaining ingredients, reserve 3 cups water, and pulse for 3 minutes until smooth.
3. Tip the mixture in a saucepan, place it over medium heat, and cook until the sauce thickens and bubbles, whisking constantly.
4. When done, taste the sauce to adjust seasoning and then serve.
Nutrition: Calories: 110 Fat: 10g Carbohydrates: 8g Protein: 5g

287. Spicy Red Wine Tomato Sauce

Preparation time: 10 minutes
Cooking time: 1 hour
Servings: 4
Ingredients:
- 28 ounces' puree of whole tomatoes, peeled
- 4 cloves of garlic, peeled
- 1 tablespoon dried basil
- 1/4 teaspoon ground black pepper
- 1 tablespoon dried oregano
- 1/4 teaspoon red pepper flakes
- 1 tablespoon dried sage
- 1 tablespoon dried thyme
- 3 teaspoon coconut sugar
- 1/2 of lemon, juice
- 1/4 cup red wine

Directions:
1. Take a large saucepan, place it over medium heat, add tomatoes and remaining ingredients.
2. Stir and simmer for 1 hour or more until thickened and cooked.
3. Serve sauce over pasta.
Nutrition: Calories: 110 Fat: 2.5 g Carbohydrates: 9 g Protein: 2 g

288. Hot Sauce

Preparation time: 10 minutes
Cooking time: 20 minutes
Servings: 6
Ingredients:
- 4 Serrano peppers, destemmed
- 1/2 of medium white onion, chopped
- 1 medium carrot, chopped
- 10 habanero chilies, destemmed
- 6 cloves of garlic, unpeeled
- 2 teaspoons sea salt
- 1 cup apple cider vinegar
- 1/2 teaspoon brown rice syrup
- 1 cup of water

Directions:
1. Take a skillet pan, place it on medium heat, add garlic, and cook for 15 minutes until roasted, frequently turning garlic, set aside to cool.
2. Meanwhile, take a saucepan, place it over medium-low heat, add remaining ingredients in it, except for salt and syrup, stir, and cook for 12 minutes until vegetables are tender.
3. When the garlic has roasted and cooled, peel them, and add them to a food processor.
4. Then add cooked saucepan along with remaining ingredients, and pulse for 3 minutes until smooth.
5. Let sauce cool and then serve straight away
Nutrition: Calories: 137 Fat: 0 g Carbohydrates: 30 g Protein: 4 g

289. Bolognese Sauce

Preparation time: 15 minutes
Cooking time: 45 minutes
Servings: 8
Ingredients:

- 1/2 of small green bell pepper, sliced
- 1 stalk of celery, chopped
- 1 small carrot, chopped
- 1 medium white onion, peeled, chopped
- 2 teaspoons minced garlic
- 1/2 teaspoon crushed red pepper flakes
- 3 tablespoons olive oil
- 8-ounce tempeh, crumbled
- 8 ounces' white mushrooms, chopped
- 1/2 cup dried red lentils
- 28-ounce crushed tomatoes
- 28-ounce whole tomatoes, chopped
- 1 teaspoon dried oregano
- 1/2 teaspoon fennel seed
- 1/2 teaspoon ground black pepper
- 1/2 teaspoon salt
- 1 teaspoon dried basil
- 1/4 cup chopped parsley
- 1 bay leaf
- 6-ounce tomato paste
- 1 cup dry red wine

Directions:

1.   Take an oven, place it over medium heat, add oil, and when hot, add the first six ingredients, stir, and cook for 5 minutes until sauté.

2.   Then switch heat to medium-high level, add two ingredients after olive oil, stir, and Cooking Time: for 3 minutes.

3.   Switch heat to medium-low level, stir in tomato paste, and continue cooking for 2 minutes.

4.   Add remaining ingredients except for lentils, stir, and bring the mixture to boil.

5.   Switch heat to the low level, simmer sauce for 10 minutes, cover the pan partially, add lentils, and continue cooking for 20 minutes until tender.

6.   Serve sauce with cooked pasta.

Nutrition: Calories: 161 Fat: 8g Carbohydrates: 14g Protein: 7g

290.   Mushroom Gravy

Preparation time: 10 minutes
Cooking time: 15 minutes
Servings: 10
Ingredients:
- 2 cups sliced fresh mushrooms
- 1 1/2 cups mushroom broth (extra 2 tablespoons)
- 2 tablespoons dry red or white wine
- 1/4 cup minced yellow onion

- 1/2 teaspoon ground dried thyme
- 1/4 teaspoon ground sage
- Salt and freshly ground black pepper
- 1/2 to 1 teaspoon vegan gravy browner

Directions:

1.   Combine the onion and 2 tablespoons of broth in the open instant pot on low and simmer until the onion softens.

2.   Add the mushrooms and soften more before adding the sage, thyme, and wine.

3.   Add half the broth and boil.

4.   Reduce the heat and simmer 5 minutes.

5.   Add the remaining broth, then put it into a blender and make it smooth.

6.   Put back into the instant pot, salt, and pepper, then seal and cook for 10 minutes.

7.   Depressurize naturally and serve hot.

Nutrition: Calories: 30 Fat: 2g Carbohydrates: 3g Protein: 0g

291.   Pumpkin Butter

Preparation time: 10 minutes
Cooking time: 30 minutes
Servings: 2
Ingredients:
- 1 - 15 Ounce can Pure Pumpkin
- 1 Tablespoon Lemon Juice
- 1/4 Teaspoon Cinnamon
- 1/8 Teaspoon Ground Cloves
- 1/4 Cup Maple Syrup or Agave
- 2/3 Cup Coconut Sugar, muscovado sugar, or maple sugar
- 1 Cup Water- For the bottom of instant pot

Directions:

1.   Mix pumpkin, lemon juice, cinnamon, cloves, and syrup or agave in an oven-safe bowl.

2.   Add coconut sugar or other sugar and cover the bowl with foil.

3.   Place the steam rack into the instant pot and fill it with water.

4.   Place the oven-safe bowl on the steam rack - cook for 25 minutes on high pressure.

5.   Quick release or let pressure dissolve on its own.

6.   Remove foil and stir. Add more spices if needed.

7.   For thicker butter spread, remove the steam rack and in the empty instant pot, pour in contents

and sauté on low setting, stirring occasionally until it thickens.

8.   Use as a spread for bread, pancakes, or oatmeal topping. Enjoy!

Nutrition: Calories: 59 Fat: 0g Carbohydrates: 15g Protein: 1g

292.   Almond Sage Sauce

Preparation Time: 4 hours
Cooking Time: 5 minutes
Servings: 1
Ingredients:
- 1/2 cup raw, unsalted almonds
- 3/4 cup non-dairy milk
- 1 tsp. nutritional yeast flakes
- 3/4 tsp. ground culinary sage
- 1/4 tsp. salt
- 1/4 tsp. black pepper
- 1/8 tsp. garlic powder
- 1/8 tsp. onion powder

Directions:
1.   Soaked almonds for 4 hours, then drained and rinsed
2.   Set all ingredients in a food processor and process until smooth and creamy.
3.   Serve immediately.

Nutrition: Calories: 90 Fat: 9g Carbohydrates: 2g Protein: 2g

293.   Chipotle Sauce

Preparation Time: 5 minutes
Cooking Time: 5 minutes
Servings: 1
Ingredients:
- 1/2 cup raw cashews
- 1/2 cup non-dairy milk
- 1 tsp. chipotle powder
- 1 tsp. lemon juice
- 1/2 tsp. paprika
- 1/4 tsp. salt
- 1/8 tsp. garlic powder
- 1/8 tsp onion powder

Directions:
1.   Prepare and process all ingredients in a food processor until smooth and creamy.

2.   Serve immediately.

Nutrition: Calories: 100 Fat: 10g Carbohydrates: 1g Protein: 3g

294.   Cilantro Chili Cheese Sauce

Preparation Time: 10 minutes
Cooking Time: 5 minutes
Servings:
Ingredients:
- 1/2 cup raw cashews
- 1/2 cup non-dairy milk
- 1/4 cup fresh cilantro
- 3 tbsp. nutritional yeast flakes
- 1 tbsp. chili powder
- 1 tsp. lemon juice
- 1/4 tsp. salt
- 1/4 tsp. pepper
- 1/8 tsp. onion powder
- 1/8 tsp. garlic powder

Directions:
1.   Wash and chop the cilantro.
2.   Prepare and process all ingredients in a food processor until smooth and creamy.
3.   Serve and enjoy!

Nutrition: Calories: 90 Fat: 9g Carbohydrates: 2g Protein: 2g

295.   Sun-Dried Tomato Spread

Preparation Time: 5 minutes
Cooking Time: 5 minutes
Servings: 1
Ingredients:
- 1 cup canned white kidney beans
- 1/2 cup sun-dried tomatoes, still in the oil
- 1/4 cup fresh basil leaves, washed thoroughly
- 3 tbsp. raw almond butter
- 1 tbsp. nutritional yeast
- 2-3 garlic cloves
- Salt and pepper to taste

Directions:
1.   Set and process all ingredients in a food processor until blended to your preference.

2. Scrape spread out of the food processor and serve.

Nutrition: Calories: 79 Fat: 6g Carbohydrates: 5g Protein: 1g

296. Raw Salsa

Preparation Time: 5 minutes
Cooking Time: 5 minutes
Servings: 1
Ingredients:
- 2 ripe red tomatoes, roughly chopped
- 3/4 cup roughly torn fresh cilantro, thoroughly washed
- 1/2 cup onion, roughly chopped
- 1 clove fresh garlic, minced
- 1 tbsp. extra virgin olive oil
- 1 tsp. fresh lemon or lime juice
- 1/4 tsp. salt
- 1/4 tsp. cayenne pepper

Directions:
1. Prepare ingredients into a food processor and process until the tomatoes have been broken down and your salsa mixture is nice and thick.
2. Graze mixture into a serving bowl and serve.

Nutrition: Calories: 100 Fat: 0g Carbohydrates: 20g Protein: 4g

297. Raw Marinara

Preparation Time: 5 minutes
Cooking Time: 5 minutes
Servings: 1
Ingredients:
- 1/2 cup sun-dried tomatoes in oil
- 1/2 of raw red bell pepper, chopped
- 1 raw tomato, chopped
- 1/4 cup fresh basil, thoroughly washed
- 3 tbsp. hemp seeds
- 1 clove of garlic
- 1/4 tsp. pepper

Directions:
1. Set and process all ingredients in a food processor.
2. Blend until thoroughly mixed. The finished product will be chunky and thick.
3. Serve and enjoy.

Nutrition: Calories: 52 Fat: 1g Carbohydrates: 11g Protein: 2g

298. Roasted Red Pepper Dip

Preparation Time: 10 minutes
Cooking Time: 5 minutes
Servings: 1
Ingredients:
- 1 can (15-ounce) red kidney beans
- 1/2 cup roasted red bell pepper
- 1/4 cup fresh cilantro, washed thoroughly
- 1 tbsp. lemon juice
- 1 tbsp. extra virgin olive oil
- 1 small clove garlic
- 1 tsp. chili powder
- 1/2 tsp. cumin
- 1/2 tsp. coriander
- 1/4 tsp. cayenne pepper
- 1/8 tsp. salt

Directions:
1. Rinse and drain the red kidney beans.
2. Process all ingredients in a food processor.
3. Blend until thoroughly mix.
4. Scrape out of processor into a bowl and serve.

Nutrition: Calories: 80 Fat: 7g Carbohydrates: 3g Protein: 1g

299. Sunflower Seed Dip

Preparation Time: 5 minutes
Cooking Time: 5 minutes
Servings: 1
Ingredients:
- 1/2 cup sunflower seeds
- 1/4 cup walnuts
- 2 tbsp. maple syrup
- 2 tbsp. filtered water
- 1 tsp. lemon juice
- pinch of cinnamon to taste

Directions:
1. Set and process all ingredients into a food processor.
2. Blend until walnuts are thoroughly chopped.
3. You may need to use a cake spatula to scrape down the sides of the container before giving it another blend.
4. Prepare mixture into a bowl and serve.

Nutrition: Calories: 100 Fat: 10g Carbohydrates: 2g Protein: 2g

300. Red Pepper Hemp Dressing

Preparation Time: 10 minutes
Cooking Time: 5 minutes
Servings: 1
Ingredients:
- 5 tbsp. hemp seeds
- 1/4 cup roasted red peppers
- 1/4 cup filtered water
- 1 tbsp. lemon juice
- 1 tbsp. extra virgin olive oil
- 1/2 tsp. dried basil
- 1/4 tsp. salt
- 1/4 tsp. maple syrup
- 1/8 tsp. garlic powder
- 1/8 tsp onion powder

Directions:
1. Put and process all ingredients in a food processor.
2. Blend until completely smooth.
3. Serve immediately.
Nutrition: Calories: 60 Fat: 6g Carbohydrates: 3g Protein: 0g

301. Garlic Tahini Dressing

Preparation Time: 5 minutes
Cooking Time: 5 minutes
Servings: 1
Ingredients:
- 1/3 cup tahini
- 1/3 cup plus 2 tbsp. filtered water
- 2 tbsp. lemon juice
- 1 clove garlic
- 1/4 tsp. salt
- 1/4 tsp. pepper
- 1/8 tsp. paprika
- 1/8 tsp. cayenne

Directions:
1. Set and process all ingredients in a food processor and blend until smooth.
2. Serve and enjoy.

Nutrition: Calories: 45 Fat: 3g Carbohydrates: 4g Protein: 2g

302. Sweet Almond Sauce

Preparation Time: 4 hours
Cooking Time: 5 minutes
Servings: 1
Ingredients:
- 1/2 cup raw almonds
- 1/2 cup non-dairy milk
- 2 tbsp. maple syrup
- 1/2 tsp. vanilla extract
- 1/4 tsp. powdered cinnamon
- squeeze of lemon juice (to taste)

Directions:
1. Soak almonds for 4 hours, then rinse and drain.
2. Process to combine all ingredients in a food processor until smooth.
3. Serve and enjoy.
Nutrition: Calories: 150 Fat: 7g Carbohydrates: 19g Protein: 2g

303. Raspberry Sauce

Preparation Time: 5 minutes
Cooking Time: 5 minutes
Servings: 1
Ingredients:
- 1/2 cup raspberries (can use fresh or frozen. frozen raspberries do not need to be thawed beforehand.)
- 1/4 cup filtered water
- 3 tbsp. maple syrup
- 2 tbsp. non-dairy milk

Directions:
1. Prepare all ingredients in a food processor and blend until smooth.
2. Finished product will have a whipped-like consistency.
3. Serve immediately.
Nutrition: Calories: 46 Fat: 0g Carbohydrates: 11g Protein: 1g

304. Sweet Cashew Cream

Preparation Time: 5 minutes
Cooking Time: 5 minutes
Servings: 1
Ingredients:
- 1/2 cup raw cashews
- 1/2 cup non-dairy milk
- 1 tbsp. maple syrup
- 1/2 tsp. vanilla extract

Directions:
1. Prepare all ingredients in a food processor and blend until smooth.
2. Serve and enjoy.

Nutrition: Calories: 59 Fat: 5g Carbohydrates: 3g Protein: 2g

305. Pumpkin Pie Sauce

Preparation Time: 5 minutes
Cooking Time: 5 minutes
Servings: 1
Ingredients:
- 1 cup Full-Fat coconut milk (in a can)
- 1/2 cup pumpkin puree
- 3 tbsp. maple syrup
- 1 tsp. vanilla extract
- 1/2 tsp. cinnamon
- 1/8 tsp. nutmeg
- 1/8 tsp. ground cloves

Directions:
1. Prepare and process all ingredients in a food processor.
2. Blend until smooth.
3. Serve and enjoy.

Nutrition: Calories: 100 Fat: 0g Carbohydrates: 26g Protein: 1g

306. Tofu with Thai Slaw

Preparation Time: 15 minutes
Cooking Time: 10 minutes
Serving: 4
Ingredients:

- 1 (16-oz) block extra-firm tofu, cubed
- Salt, to taste
- 1 tablespoon olive oil
- Black pepper, to taste

Salad:
- ¼ cup cashew butter
- 2 tablespoons white miso paste
- 2 tablespoons lime juice
- 1 teaspoon sesame oil
- 1 teaspoon grated ginger
- 5 tablespoons water
- 7 cups red cabbage, shredded
- 2 scallions, chopped
- ½ cup cilantro, chopped
- ½ cup fresh basil
- 2 Thai chiles pepper, diced
- Salt, to taste
- ¼ cup toasted peanuts

Directions:
1. At 400 degrees F, preheat your Air Fryer.
2. Toss tofu with black pepper, salt and oil in a bowl.
3. Spread the tofu cubes in the Air Fryer basket.
4. Air fry them for 10 minutes and shake once cooked halfway through.
5. Meanwhile, toss all the salad ingredients in a suitable salad bowl.
6. Mix well and top the salad with tofu cubes.
7. Serve fresh.

Nutrition: Calories 195; Fat 13.8g; Cholesterol 0mg; Carbohydrate 14.8g; Sugars 4.5g; Protein 6.9g

307. Tofu Broccoli Salad

Preparation Time: 15 minutes
Cooking Time: 10 minutes
Serving: 4
Ingredients:
- 1-pound broccoli crowns
- 1 (16-oz) block extra-firm tofu, cubed
- Salt, to taste
- 1 tablespoon olive oil
- Black pepper, to taste

Salad:
- 3 tablespoons olive oil
- 3 tablespoons mayo
- 1½ tablespoons apple cider vinegar
- 2 teaspoon Dijon mustard
- 1 teaspoon choc zero maple syrup
- 1 garlic clove, minced

- 1/3 cup diced red onions
- 1/3 cup dried cranberries

Directions:

1. At 350 degrees F, preheat your Air Fryer.
2. Toss tofu with broccoli, black pepper, salt and oil in a bowl.
3. Spread the tofu cubes in the Air Fryer basket.
4. Air fry them for 10 minutes and shake once cooked halfway through.
5. Meanwhile, toss all the salad ingredients in a suitable salad bowl.
6. Mix well and toss in tofu and broccoli.
7. Serve fresh.

Nutrition: Calories 157; Fat 9g; Cholesterol 3mg; Carbohydrate 13.6g; Sugars 1.8g; Protein 6.7g

308. Brussels Sprout Salad

Preparation Time: 15 minutes
Cooking Time: 7 minutes
Serving: 4
Ingredients:

- 4 cups Brussels sprouts
- 1 onion, shredded
- ¼ cup olive oil
- ¼ cup fresh lemon juice
- ½ cup pine nuts, toasted
- 1/3 cup dried cranberries
- 1/3 cup chopped chives
- Salt and black pepper, to taste

Directions:

1. At 400 degrees F, preheat your Air Fryer.
2. Toss Brussel sprouts with 2 tablespoons oil in a bowl.
3. Spread the Brussel sprouts in the Air Fryer basket.
4. Air fry them for 7 minutes and shake once cooked halfway through.
5. Meanwhile, toss all the salad ingredients in a suitable salad bowl.
6. Mix well and top the salad with tofu cubes.
7. Serve fresh.

Nutrition: Calories 281; Fat 24.7g; Cholesterol 0mg; Carbohydrate 14.1g; Sugars 4.4g; Protein 5.9g

309. Tofu Kale Salad

Preparation Time: 15 minutes
Cooking Time: 10 minutes
Serving: 4
Ingredients:

- 1 (16-oz) block extra-firm tofu, cubed
- Salt, to taste
- 1 tablespoon olive oil
- Black pepper, to taste

Salad:

- ¼ teaspoon salt
- 1 big bunch curly green kale, chopped
- ½ cup raw sliced almonds
- 1/3 cup dried cherries, chopped
- 4 oz. vegan feta cheese, crumbled

Vinaigrette:

- 1/3 cup olive oil
- 1 tablespoon sherry vinegar
- 1 tablespoon Dijon mustard
- 2 garlic cloves, minced
- ¼ teaspoon salt

Directions:

1. At 400 degrees F, preheat your Air Fryer.
2. Toss tofu with black pepper, salt and oil in a bowl.
3. Spread the tofu cubes in the Air Fryer basket.
4. Air fry them for 10 minutes and shake once cooked halfway through.
5. Meanwhile, toss all the salad ingredients in a suitable salad bowl.
6. Mix well and top the salad with tofu cubes.
7. Serve fresh.
8. Enjoy.

Nutrition: Calories 262; Fat 27.3g; Cholesterol 0mg; Carbohydrate 3.6g; Sugars 0.7g; Protein 4.4g

310. Tofu Greek Salad

Preparation Time: 15 minutes
Cooking Time: 10 minutes
Serving: 2
Ingredients:

- 4 medium zucchinis, peeled and sliced
- 2 tbsp. olive oil
- 2 tbsp. lemon juice
- 2 small garlic cloves, chopped
- 2 tbsp. parsley, chopped
- ¼ tsp. salt

Directions:

1. At 400 degrees F, preheat your Air Fryer.

2. Toss zucchini with lemon juice, garlic, salt and oil in a bowl.
3. Spread the zucchini in the Air Fryer basket.
4. Air fry them for 10 minutes and shake once cooked halfway through.
5. Add parsley on top and mix well.
6. Serve fresh.
Nutrition: Calories 192; Fat 14.9g; Cholesterol 0mg; Carbohydrate 14.7g; Sugars 7.2g; Protein 5.2g

311. Eggplant Arugula Salad

Preparation Time: 15 minutes
Cooking Time: 11 minutes
Serving: 4
Ingredients:
- 1½ cups cherry tomatoes, sliced in half
- 3-4 small eggplant, sliced
- Olive oil for drizzling
- 1 garlic clove, minced
- ½ cup pine nuts, toasted
- 1 handful of arugulas
- 1 handful of torn basil
- Generous splashes of sherry vinegar
- Salt and black pepper, to taste
Directions:
1. At 400 degrees F, preheat your Air Fryer.
2. Toss eggplant with oil in a bowl.
3. Spread the eggplant in the Air Fryer basket.
4. Air fry them for 11 minutes and shake once cooked halfway through.
5. Meanwhile, toss all the salad ingredients in a suitable salad bowl.
6. Mix well and top the salad with eggplant.
7. Serve fresh.
Nutrition: Calories 267; Fat 2.3g; Cholesterol 0mg; Carbohydrate 60.7g; Sugars 34g; Protein 11.6g

312. Cauliflower Salad

Preparation Time: 10 minutes
Cooking Time: 10 minutes
Serving: 4
Ingredients:
- 1 large cauliflower head, cut into florets
- 2 tbsp olive oil
- 1/2 tsp salt
- 1/2 tsp black pepper
Salad:
- 1 celery stalk, sliced
- 1/3 cup hazelnuts, raw, skin on
- 1/2 pomegranate, seeds only
- 1 cup parsley leaves, chopped
Dressing:
- 2 tbsp olive oil
- 1/3 tsp cinnamon powder
- 1/3 tsp allspice
- 1 tbsp sherry vinegar
- 1 1/2 tsp maple syrup
- 1/4 tsp salt
- 1/4 tsp black pepper
Directions:
1. At 400 degrees F, preheat your Air Fryer.
2. Toss cauliflower florets with black pepper, salt and oil in a bowl.
3. Spread cauliflower florets in the Air Fryer basket.
4. Air fry them for 10 minutes and shake once cooked halfway through.
5. Meanwhile, toss all the salad and dressing ingredients in a suitable salad bowl.
6. Mix well and toss in air fried cauliflower florets then mix well.
7. Serve fresh.
Nutrition: Calories 178; Fat 11.2g; Cholesterol 0mg; Carbohydrate 18.5g; Sugars 9.6g; Protein 5.7g

313. Kale Sprouts Salad

Preparation Time: 15 minutes
Cooking Time: 8 minutes
Serving: 4
Ingredients:
- 1 bunch of curly green kale
- 12 Brussels sprouts
- ¼ cup sliced almonds
- ¼ cup shaved vegan Parmesan
- Salt, to taste
Tahini-maple dressing:
- ¼ cup tahini
- 2 tablespoons white wine vinegar
- 2 teaspoons white miso
- 2 teaspoon choc zero maple syrup
- Pinch of red pepper flakes
- ¼ cup water
Directions:
1. At 400 degrees F, preheat your Air Fryer.

2. Toss brussels sprouts with salt in a bowl.
3. Spread the brussels sprouts in the Air Fryer basket.
4. Air fry them for 8 minutes and shake once cooked halfway through.
5. Meanwhile, toss all the salad ingredients in a suitable salad bowl.
6. Mix well and stir in brussels sprouts.
7. Serve fresh.
Nutrition: Calories 221; Fat 14.6g; Cholesterol 10mg; Carbohydrate 15g; Sugars 1.8g; Protein 12.1g

314. Broccoli Salad

Preparation Time: 5 minutes
Cooking Time: 6 minutes
Serving: 6
Ingredients:
• 2 heads of broccoli, cut into florets
• 2 teaspoons olive oil
• 1/2 teaspoon salt
• 1/2 cup almonds
• 1/4 cup dried cranberries
• 1 tablespoon fresh dill, chopped
• 4 very thin slices of lemon
Lemony Dressing:
• 1/4 cup lemon juice
• 1 tablespoon maple syrup
• 1 teaspoon Dijon mustard
• 1 teaspoon balsamic vinegar
• 1 garlic clove, grated
• 2 tablespoons olive oil
Directions:
1. At 350 degrees F, preheat your Air Fryer.
2. Toss broccoli florets with oil and salt in the Air Fryer basket.
3. Air fry them for 6 minutes in the air fryer basket.
4. Mix lemon juice, maple syrup, Dijon mustard, vinegar, garlic and olive oil in a salad bowl.
5. Toss in broccoli, almond, dill, cranberries and lemon slices.
6. Mix well and serve.
Nutrition: Calories 203; Fat 10.3g; Cholesterol 0mg; Carbohydrate 25.9g; Sugars 12.9g; Protein 7.6g

315. Tempeh Caprese Salad

Preparation Time: 5 minutes
Cooking Time: 10 minutes
Serving: 4
Ingredients:
• 1 (16-oz) block tempeh, diced
• Salt, to taste
• 1 tablespoon olive oil
• Black pepper, to taste
Salad:
• 4 ripe tomatoes, cubed
• 4 oz. vegan mozzarella cheese, cubed
• 2 avocados, peeled, pitted, and cubed
• 3 tablespoons balsamic vinegar
• 3 tablespoons red wine vinegar
• ½ teaspoon dried basil
• salt and ground black pepper to taste
Directions:
1. At 370 degrees F, preheat your Air Fryer.
2. Toss tempeh with black pepper, salt and oil in a bowl.
3. Spread the tempeh cubes in the Air Fryer basket.
4. Air fry them for 10 minutes and shake once cooked halfway through.
5. Meanwhile, toss all the salad ingredients in a suitable salad bowl.
6. Mix well and top the salad with tempeh cubes.
7. Serve fresh.
Nutrition: Calories 303; Fat 23.9g; Cholesterol 0mg; Carbohydrate 18.6g; Sugars 2.5g; Protein 12.6g

316. Mango & Avocado Salad

Preparation Time: 15 minutes
Cooking time: 0 minutes
Servings: 6
Ingredients:
• 2½ cups mango, peeled, pitted and cubed
• 2½ cups avocado, peeled, pitted and cubed
• 1 red onion, sliced
• 6 cups fresh lettuce, torn
• ¼ cup fresh mint leaves, chopped
• 2 tablespoons fresh orange juice
• Salt, as required
Direction:
1. Place all the ingredients in a salad bowl and gently, toss to combine.
2. Cover and refrigerate to chill before serving.

Nutrition: Calories: 182 Fat: 12.3g Carbohydrates: 18.8g Dietary Fiber: 6.2g Sugar: 11.3g Protein: 2.6g

317.   Apple & Spinach Salad

Preparation Time: 10 minutes
Cooking time: 0 minutes
Servings: 4
Ingredients:
• 4 large apples, cored and sliced
• 6 cups fresh baby spinach
• 3 tablespoons extra-virgin olive oil
• 2 tablespoons apple cider vinegar
Direction:
1. In a salad bowl, add all the ingredients and toss to coat well.
2. Serve immediately.
Nutrition: Calories: 218 Fat: 11.1g Carbohydrates: 32.5g Dietary Fiber: 6.4g Sugar: 23.4g Protein: 1.9g

318.   Mixed Berries Salad

Preparation Time: 15 minutes
Cooking time: 0 minutes
Servings: 4
Ingredients:
• 1 cup fresh strawberries, hulled and sliced
• ½ cup fresh blackberries
• ½ cup fresh blueberries
• ½ cup fresh raspberries
• 6 cups fresh arugula
• 2 tablespoons olive oil
• Salt, as required
Direction:
1. In a salad bowl, place all ingredients and toss to coat well.
2. Serve immediately.
Nutrition: Calories: 105 Fat: 7.6g Carbohydrates: 10.1g Dietary Fiber: 3.6g Sugar: 5.7g Protein: 1.6g

319.   Beet & Spinach Salad

Preparation Time: 15 minutes
Cooking Time: 1 hour
Servings: 2
Ingredients:
• 3 medium beets, trimmed
• 1 tablespoon extra-virgin olive oil
• 1 tablespoon balsamic vinegar
• 1 teaspoon maple syrup
• Salt and ground black pepper, as required
• 4 cups fresh spinach, torn
• ¼ cup walnuts, chopped
Direction:
1. Preheat your oven to 400 °F.
2. With a piece foil, wrap each beet completely.
3. Arrange the foil packets onto a baking sheet and roast for about 1 hour.
4. Remove from the oven and carefully, open the foil packets.
5. Set aside to cool slightly.
6. With a paper towel, remove the peel of beets and then cut into chunks.
7. In a serving bowl, add the oil, vinegar, maple syrup, salt and black pepper and beat well.
8. Add beet chunks, spinach and walnuts and toss to coat well.
9. Serve immediately.
Nutrition: Calories: 247 Fat: 16.7g Carbohydrates: 21g Dietary Fiber: 5.4g Sugar: 14.4g Protein: 8g

320.   Cucumber & Tomato Salad

Preparation Time: 15 minutes
Cooking time: 0 minutes
Servings: 4
Ingredients:
• 2 cups plum tomatoes, chopped
• 2 cups cucumbers, chopped
• 2 cups mixed fresh lettuce, torn
• 2 cups fresh baby spinach
• 2 tablespoons extra virgin olive oil
• 2 tablespoons fresh lime juice
• Salt, as required
Direction:

1. Place all the ingredients in a salad bowl and gently, toss to combine.
2. Serve immediately.
Nutrition: Calories: 96 Fat: 7.4g Carbohydrates: 7.9g Dietary Fiber: 1.8g Sugar: 4.8g Protein: 2g

321. Zucchini & Tomato Salad

Preparation Time: 15 minutes
Cooking time: 0 minutes
Servings: 4
Ingredients:
- 2 medium zucchinis, sliced thinly
- 2 cups plum tomatoes, sliced
- 2 tablespoons olive oil
- 2 tablespoons fresh key lime juice
- Pinch of Salt

Direction:
1. In a salad bowl, place all ingredients and gently toss to combine.
2. Serve immediately.
Nutrition: Calories: 93 Fat: 7.4g Carbohydrates: 6.9g Dietary Fiber: 2.2g Sugar: 4.1g Protein: 2g

322. Quinoa, Bean, & Mango Salad

Preparation Time: 20 minutes
Cooking Time: 20 minutes
Servings: 6
Ingredients:
- 1¾ cups vegetable broth
- 1 cup quinoa, rinsed
- Salt, as required
- 1½ cups canned black beans, rinsed and drained
- 2 medium bell peppers, seeded and chopped
- 2 cucumbers, chopped
- ½ cup scallion (green part), chopped
- 1 tablespoon olive oil
- 2 tablespoons fresh cilantro leaves, chopped

Direction:
1. In a saucepan, add the broth over high heat and bring to a boil.
2. Add the quinoa and salt and cook until boiling.

3. Now, lower the heat to low and simmer, covered for about 15-20 minutes or until all the liquid is absorbed.
4. Remove from the heat and set aside, covered for about 5-10 minutes.
5. Uncover and with a fork, fluff the quinoa.
6. In a large serving bowl, place the quinoa with the remaining ingredients and gently, toss to coat.
7. Serve immediately.
Nutrition: Calories: 218 Fat: 4.9g Carbohydrates: 34.8g Dietary Fiber: 7.1g Sugar: 3g Protein: 10.4g

323. Quinoa & Veggie Salad

Preparation Time: 15 minutes
Cooking Time: 20 minutes
Servings: 6
Ingredients:
For Quinoa:
- 1 cup quinoa, rinsed
- 1 (15-ounce) can unsweetened coconut milk
- ½ cup water
For Dressing:
- 2 tablespoons balsamic vinegar
- 2 tablespoons extra-virgin olive oil
- 2 tablespoons fresh lime juice
- 1 tablespoon maple syrup
- ½ teaspoon Dijon mustard
- Salt and ground black pepper, as required
For Salad:
- 1½ cups frozen shelled edamame, thawed
- 1½ cups tomato, chopped
- 1½ cups cucumber, chopped
- 1 cup fresh baby spinach leaves, chopped
- 2 tablespoons fresh mint leaves, chopped
- 2 tablespoons fresh cilantro, chopped

Direction:
1. For quinoa: in a medium saucepan, add all ingredients over medium-high heat and bring to a boil.
2. Now, lower the heat to low and simmer, covered for about 20 minutes or until all the liquid is absorbed.
3. Remove the saucepan of quinoa from heat and set aside, covered for about 5 minutes.
4. With a fork, fluff the quinoa and let it cool completely.

5. For dressing: in a bowl, add all ingredients and beat until well combined.

6. In a large salad bowl, add the quinoa, salad ingredients and dressing and toss to coat well.

Nutrition: Calories: 276 Fat: 15.1g Carbohydrates: 32.2g Dietary Fiber: 6g Sugar: 3.6g Protein: 14.1g

324. Red Beans & Corn Salad

Preparation Time: 15 minutes
Cooking time: 0 minutes
Servings: 6
Ingredients:
For Dressing:
- 5 tablespoons olive oil
- 4 tablespoons fresh lime juice
- 1 tablespoon apple cider vinegar
- 3 tablespoons agave nectar
- Salt and ground black pepper, as required

For Salad:
- 3 (15-ounce) cans red kidney beans, drained and rinsed
- 1 (15¼-ounce) can corn, drained and rinsed
- 2 cups cherry tomatoes, halved
- 1¼ cups onion, sliced
- 1/3 cup fresh cilantro, minced
- 8 cups lettuce, torn

Direction:
1. For dressing: add all ingredients in a small bowl and beat until well combined.
2. In a large serving bowl, add beans, corn, cilantro and lettuce and mix.
3. Add dressing and toss to coat well.
4. Serve immediately.

Nutrition: Calories: 396 Fat: 12.6g Carbohydrates: 59.9g Dietary Fiber: 21g Sugar: 13g Protein: 17.1g

325. Chickpeas & Veggie Salad

Preparation Time: 15 minutes
Cooking time: 0 minutes
Servings: 4
Ingredients:
For Salad:
- 3 cups cooked chickpeas

- 2 cups, cucumber, chopped
- 1 cup cherry tomatoes, halved
- 1 cup radishes, trimmed and sliced
- 6 cups fresh baby arugula
- 4 tablespoons scallion greens, chopped
- 4 tablespoons fresh parsley leaves, chopped

For Dressing:
- 1 garlic clove, minced
- 3 tablespoons extra-virgin olive oil
- 1 tablespoon balsamic vinegar
- 1 tablespoon fresh lemon juice
- Salt and ground black pepper, as required

Instructions:
1. For salad: in a large serving bowl, add all the ingredients and mix.
2. For dressing: in another bowl, add all the ingredients and beat until well combined.
3. Pour dressing over salad and gently toss to coat well.
4. Serve immediately.

Nutrition: Calories: 338 Fat: 13g Carbohydrates: 46.7g Dietary Fiber: 10.1g Sugar: 3.2g Protein: 11.7g

326. Peaches, Peas, and Beans Summer Salad

Preparation time: 15 minutes
Cooking time: 5 minutes
Serving: 6
Ingredients:
Dressing:
- 1 tablespoon balsamic vinegar
- 1 teaspoon Dijon mustard
- 1 teaspoon gluten-free tamari soy sauce
- 2 tablespoons coconut oil (optional)
- Salt and pepper, to taste (optional)

Salad:
- ¾ pound (340 g) young green, yellow or burgundy string beans, trimmed
- 2 ripe and firm peaches
- 1 small shallot, peeled and sliced paper thin
- Large handful of snap peas, trimmed and sliced down the middle
- Salt and pepper, to taste (optional)
- ¼ cup chopped fresh basil leaves
- ¼ cup whole toasted almonds, coarsely chopped

Direction:

1. Make the Dressing: In a small jar with a tight-fitting lid, combine the balsamic vinegar, Dijon mustard, tamari, oil, salt, and pepper, if using. Tightly secure the lid, and shake the jar vigorously until the dressing has a smooth consistency. Set aside.

2. Make the Salad: Bring a medium saucepan of water to a boil. Salt the water and then throw in the trimmed green beans. Blanch the beans for 3 minutes or until tender and crisp. Drain the beans and place them in a bowl of ice water to cool immediately.

3. Remove the pits from the peaches and cut the fruit into thin slices. In a large bowl, combine the sliced peaches, shallots, and snap peas. Drain the green beans and lightly dry them. Add the beans to the large bowl. Season the salad with salt and pepper, if using.

4. Pour the dressing over the vegetables and peaches, and toss lightly to combine. Scatter the chopped basil and almonds over the top, and serve.

Nutrition: Calories: 132 | fat: 8g | protein: 4g | carbs: 13g | fiber: 4g

327. Shaved Root Salad with Crispy Lentils

Preparation time: 20 minutes
Cooking time: 30 minutes
Serving: 6
Ingredients:
Dressing:
- 2 tablespoons virgin olive oil (optional)
- 1 tablespoon pure maple syrup (optional)
- 1 tablespoon grainy mustard
- 1 tablespoon filtered water
- 1 tablespoon sherry vinegar or apple cider vinegar
- 1 teaspoon prepared horseradish
- 1 clove garlic, grated
- Salt and pepper, to taste (optional)
Salad:
- 1/3 cup French or black beluga lentils, rinsed
- ½ teaspoon virgin olive oil (optional)
- Salt and pepper, to taste (optional)
- 2 small beets, peeled
- 2 medium carrots, peeled
- 1 small celery root, peeled
- 2 tablespoons chopped fresh dill, for garnish
Direction:

1. Preheat the oven to 400°F (205°C).

2. Make the Dressing: In a jar with a tight-fitting lid, combine the olive oil, maple syrup, mustard, water, sherry vinegar, horseradish, garlic, salt, and pepper, if using. Tightly secure the lid, and shake the jar vigorously until the dressing has a creamy and smooth consistency. Set aside.

3. Make the Salad: Bring a medium saucepan of water to a boil. Drop in the lentils and a big pinch of salt, if using. Bring to a boil again, and then reduce heat to a simmer until lentils are just tender, about 20 minutes. Drain the lentils and spread them out on a kitchen towel to dry.

4. Transfer the dried lentils to a baking sheet. Toss the lentils with the olive oil, salt, and pepper, if using. Slide the baking sheet into the oven, and roast the lentils until they have dried and browned slightly, about 8 minutes. Remove from the oven and set aside.

5. Using a mandoline, slice the beets paper thin and place them in a large bowl. Slice the carrots with the mandoline, and add them to the bowl. Cut the celery root down the middle lengthwise. Slice each half of the celery root with the mandoline, and add the slices to the bowl.

6. Season all the sliced vegetables with salt and pepper, if using, and toss.

7. Toss the sliced vegetables with 2/3 of the dressing. Transfer the dressed vegetables to a serving platter. Scatter the crispy lentils over the vegetables. Pour the remaining dressing over the lentils. Garnish the salad with the fresh dill, and serve immediately.

Nutrition: Calories: 80 | fat: 5g | protein: 1g | carbs: 8g | fiber: 2g

328. Lentil, Lemon and Mushroom Salad

Preparation time: 10 minutes
Cooking time: 25 minutes
Serving: 2
Ingredients:
- ½ cup dry lentils of choice
- 2 cups vegetable broth
- 3 cups mushrooms, thickly sliced
- 1 cup sweet or purple onion, chopped
- 4 teaspoons extra virgin olive oil (optional)

- 2 tablespoons garlic powder or 3 garlic cloves, minced
- ¼ teaspoon chili flakes
- 1 tablespoon lemon juice
- 2 tablespoons cilantro, chopped
- ½ cup arugula
- Salt and pepper to taste (optional)

Direction:

1. Sprout the lentils for 2 to 3 days.

2. Place the vegetable stock in a deep saucepan and bring it to a boil. Add the lentils to the boiling broth, cover the pan, and cook for about 5 minutes over low heat until the lentils are a bit tender. Remove the pan from heat and drain the excess water. Add the mushrooms to the frying pan and mix in thoroughly. Continue cooking until the onions are completely translucent and the mushrooms have softened; remove the pan from the heat. Mix the lentils, onions, mushrooms, and garlic in a large bowl. Add the lemon juice and the remaining olive oil. Toss or stir to combine everything thoroughly.

4. Serve the mushroom and onion mixture over some arugula in bowl, adding salt and pepper to taste, if desired, or, store and enjoy later!

Nutrition: Calories: 262 | fat: 10g | protein: 16g | carbs: 28g | fiber: 15g

329. Bulgur Lettuce Cups

Preparation time: 10 minutes
Cooking time: 20 minutes
Serving: 2 to 4
Ingredients:
Sauce:
- 1/2 cup unsweetened natural peanut butter
- 1/4 cup soy sauce
- 3 tablespoons seasoned rice vinegar
- 2 tablespoons lime juice
- 1 teaspoon liquid aminos
- 1 teaspoon sriracha
Cups:
- 1 cup bulgur
- 1/4 cup seasoned rice vinegar
- 1/2 teaspoon garlic powder
- 1/2 teaspoon ground ginger
- 1 cup shredded carrots

- 1 cup shredded cabbage
- 1/2 cup sliced scallions, green and white parts
- 1 head red leaf lettuce or Bibb lettuce

Direction:

Make the Sauce: 1. In a small bowl, combine the peanut butter, soy sauce, vinegar, lime juice, liquid aminos, and sriracha. Whisk until well combined.

Make the Cups:

2. In a medium saucepan, cook the bulgur for about 12 minutes. Remove from the heat. Drain any excess water after cooking.

3. In a small bowl, combine the soy sauce, vinegar, garlic powder, ginger, and red pepper flakes. Mix well.

4. Add the carrots, cabbage, scallions, and soy sauce mixture to the cooked bulgur. Mix thoroughly.

5. Serve the filling scooped into individual lettuce leaves, topped with a drizzle of peanut sauce.

Nutrition: Calories: 532 | fat: 17g | protein: 25g | carbs: 79g | fiber: 18g

330. Quinoa, Corn and Black Bean Salad

Preparation time: 25 minutes
Cooking time: 0 minutes
Serving: 4
Ingredients:
- 2½ cups cooked quinoa
- 3 ears corn, kernels removed (about 2 cups)
- 1 red bell pepper, roasted, seeded, and diced
- 1/2 small red onion, peeled and diced
- 2 cups cooked black beans, or 1 (15-ounce / 425-g) can, drained and rinsed
- 1 cup finely chopped cilantro
- 6 green onions (white and green parts), thinly sliced
- 1 jalapeño pepper, minced (for less heat, remove the seeds)
- Zest of 1 lime and juice of 2 limes
- 1 tablespoon cumin seeds, toasted and ground
- Salt, to taste (optional)

Direction:

1. Combine all ingredients in a large bowl and mix well. Chill for 1 hour before serving

Nutrition: Calories: 366 | fat: 3g | protein: 16g | carbs: 70g | fiber: 14g

331. Mango Black Bean Salad

Preparation time: 25 minutes
Cooking time: 0 minutes
Serving: 4
Ingredients:
- 4 cups cooked black beans, or 2 (15-ounce / 425-g) cans, drained and rinsed
- 2 mangoes, peeled, halved, pitted, and diced
- 1 medium red bell pepper, seeded and diced small
- 1 bunch green onions (green and white parts), thinly sliced
- 1/2 cup finely chopped cilantro
- 1 jalapeño pepper, minced (for less heat, remove the seeds)
- 1/2 cup red wine vinegar
- Zest and juice of 1 orange
- Zest and juice of 1 lime

Direction:
1. Combine all ingredients in a large bowl and mix well. Chill for 1 hour before serving.

Nutrition: Calories: 299 | fat: 1g | protein: 16g | carbs: 56g | fiber: 17g

332. Thanksgiving Panzanella Salad with Delicata Squash

Preparation time: 25 minutes
Cooking time: 50 minutes
Serving: 6
Ingredients:
Dressing:
- 2 tablespoons balsamic vinegar
- Salt and pepper, to taste
- 1 small clove garlic, finely minced or grated
- 1 teaspoon Dijon mustard
- 2 teaspoons pure maple syrup (optional)
- 1/4 cup plus 1 tablespoon virgin olive oil (optional)
Salad:
- 1 standard delicata squash
- 2 to 3 shallots, peeled
- 1 tablespoon plus 2 teaspoons virgin olive oil, divided (optional)
- 1 tablespoon minced fresh rosemary
- 2 teaspoons minced fresh thyme leaves
- Salt and pepper, to taste (optional)
- 4 cups cubed whole-grain sourdough bread
- 2 cups sliced Lacinato kale
- 1/3 cup pomegranate seeds
- 2 stalks celery, thinly sliced
- 1/4 cup leaves from the heart of a celery bunch or flat-leaf parsley, for garnish

Direction:
1. Line two baking sheets with parchment paper and set aside.
2. Make the Dressing: In a medium bowl, whisk together the balsamic vinegar, salt, pepper, if using, minced garlic, Dijon mustard, maple syrup, and olive oil, if using. Set aside.
3. Make the Salad: Cut the delicata squash down the middle lengthwise. Scoop out the seeds and discard them. Cut the squash halves into ¼-inch slices, and then transfer those slices to one of the parchment-lined baking sheets.
4. trying to preserve the root end for intact pieces. Place them on the baking sheet with the delicata squash.
5. Right on the baking sheet, toss the squash and shallots with the 1 tablespoon of olive oil and the minced rosemary, thyme, salt, and pepper, if using. Once the vegetables are evenly coated, slide the baking sheet into the oven. Roast the squash and shallots for approximately 45 minutes, stirring and flipping the vegetables a couple of times, or until all pieces are golden brown and soft. Let the vegetables cool completely.
6. While the vegetables are roasting, transfer the bread cubes to the other parchment-lined baking sheet. Toss the bread cubes with the remaining 2 teaspoons of olive oil and the salt and pepper, if using. Once the bread is evenly coated, slide the baking sheet into the oven. Bake the bread pieces, stirring and flipping a couple of times, until evenly golden brown on all sides, about 12 to 14 minutes.
7. In a large serving bowl, combine the cooled roasted squash and shallots, the toasted bread pieces, and the sliced kale, pomegranate seeds, and chopped celery. Drizzle the dressing over top and toss evenly to combine. Let the salad sit for 5 to 10 minutes before serving, so that some of the dressing can permeate

the crisp pieces of bread. Roughly chop the celery leaves to garnish the top of the salad. Serve immediately.

Nutrition: Calories: 333 | fat: 13g | protein: 12g | carbs: 43g | fiber: 8g

333. Rice Salad with Fennel, Orange and Chickpeas

Preparation time: 15 minutes
Cooking time: 50 minutes
Serving: 4
Ingredients:
- 1½ cups brown basmati rice
- 2 cups cooked chickpeas, or 1 (15-ounce / 425-g) can, drained and rinsed
- 1 fennel bulb, trimmed and diced
- 1 orange, zested, peeled, and segmented (zest and segments reserved)
- 1/4 cup plus 2 tablespoons white wine vinegar
- 1/2 teaspoon crushed red pepper flakes
- 1/4 cup finely chopped parsley

Direction:
1. Rinse the rice under cold water and drain. Add it to a pot with 3 cups of cold water. Bring it to a boil over high heat, reduce the heat to medium, and cook, covered, for 45 to 50 minutes, or until the rice is tender.
2. While the rice cooks, combine the chickpeas, fennel, orange zest and segments, white wine vinegar, crushed red pepper flakes, and parsley in a large bowl and mix well. When the rice is finished, add the rice to the bowl and mix well.

Nutrition: Calories: 317 | fat: 11g | protein: 14g | carbs: 54g | fiber: 18g

334. Warm Sweet Potato and Brussels Sprout Salad

Preparation time: 20 minutes
Cooking time: 30 minutes
Serving: 4
- 3 sweet potatoes, peeled and cut into ¼-inch dice
- 1 teaspoon dried thyme
- 1 teaspoon garlic powder
- 1/2 teaspoon onion powder
- 1 pound (454 g) Brussels sprouts
- 1 cup walnuts, chopped
- 1/4 cup reduced-sugar dried cranberries
- 2 tablespoons balsamic vinegar
- Freshly ground black pepper, to taste

Direction:
1. Preheat the oven to 450ºF (235ºC). Line a baking sheet with parchment paper.
2. Place the sweet potatoes in a colander and rinse. Shake the colander to remove excess water. Sprinkle the damp sweet potatoes with the thyme, garlic powder, and onion powder. Toss to coat evenly with the spices. Transfer to the prepared baking sheet and spread the sweet potatoes in a single layer.
3. Bake for 20 minutes. Flip the sweet potatoes and bake for 10 minutes more, until fork-tender.
4. In a large bowl, toss together the Brussels sprouts, sweet potatoes, walnuts, and cranberries. Drizzle with the vinegar and season with pepper.

Nutrition: Calories: 360 | fat: 20g | protein: 10g | carbs: 44g | fiber: 12g

335. Bean and Corn Salad

Preparation time: 15 minutes
Cooking time: 0 minutes
Serving: 6
- 1 (15-ounce / 425-g) can pinto beans, drained and rinsed
- 1 (15-ounce / 425-g) can chickpeas, drained and rinsed

- 3/4 cup diced tomato
- 1/4 cup chopped cilantro
- 3 to 4 tablespoons lemon or lime juice
- Salt, to taste (optional)

Direction:

1. In a large bowl, mix together all the ingredients. The salad can be served chilled or at room temperature.

Nutrition: Calories: 200 | fat: 30g | protein: 10g | carbs: 38g | fiber: 9g

336. Mexican-Inspired Salad and Sweet Vinaigrette

Preparation time: 10 minutes
Cooking time: 0 minutes
Serving: 4
Ingredients:
Salad:

- 3 cups chopped spinach
- 1/2 cup cilantro leaves
- 1/3 cup chopped raw pecans or walnuts
- 1/3 cup dried cranberries or raisins

Dressing:

- 2 tablespoons balsamic vinegar
- 1 tablespoon olive oil (optional)

Direction:

1. In a large bowl, combine the spinach, cilantro, onion, pecans (or walnuts), and dried cranberries (or raisins).

2. In a separate small bowl, whisk together the balsamic vinegar, maple syrup, and olive oil, if desired.

3. Pour the dressing over the salad and toss together to coat thoroughly.

Nutrition: Calories: 126 | fat: 8g | protein: 2g | carbs: 11g | fiber: 2g

337. Zingy Melon and Mango Salad

Preparation time: 5 minutes
Cooking time: 0 minutes
Serving: 2
Ingredients:

- 1 large mango, peeled, pitted, and cut into 1-inch pieces (about 1 cup)
- 1/2 small cantaloupe or watermelon, peeled and cut into 1-inch pieces (about 2 cups)
- Juice of 1 lime
- 1/4 cup chopped fresh cilantro
- 1 teaspoon chili powder

Direction:

1. In a large bowl, combine the mango and cantaloupe. Add the lime juice and cilantro and gently toss until combined. To serve, spoon into bowls and sprinkle with chili powder.

Nutrition: Calories: 171 | fat: 1g | protein: 3g | carbs: 42g | fiber: 5g

338. White Beans Summer Salad

Preparation time: 10 minutes
Cooking time: 0 minutes
Serving: 2
Ingredients:

- 2 cups cooked or canned white beans
- 1/2 cubed cucumber
- 8 sun-dried tomatoes, minced
- 4 tangerines
- 1 tablespoon fresh or dried thyme

Optional Toppings:

- Black pepper
- Tahini

Direction:

1. When using dry white beans, soak and cook 2/3 cup of dry white beans if necessary.

2. Transfer the white beans to a large bowl, and add the minced sun-dried tomatoes, cucumber cubes and thyme. If using fresh thyme, chop it finely before adding it to the bowl.

3. Stir thoroughly using a spatula and make sure everything is mixed evenly.

4. Peel and section the tangerines and set them aside to garnish the salad.

5. Divide the white beans salad between two bowls, garnish with the tangerine and the optional toppings, serve and enjoy!

6. Store the salad in an airtight container in the fridge, and consume within 2 days. Alternatively, store in the

freezer for a maximum of 30 days and thaw at room temperature. The salad can be served cold.
Nutrition: Calories: 376 | fat: 2g | protein: 22g | carbs: 68g | fiber: 17g

339.   Larb Salad

Preparation time: 15 minutes
Cooking time: 5 minutes
Serving: 4
Ingredients:
- 1 teaspoon canola oil (optional)
- 3 tablespoons lime juice, divided
- 2½ tablespoons minced cilantro
- 2 tablespoons soy sauce
- 1 green onion, sliced
- 1/4 cup thinly sliced red, white, or yellow onion
- 2 tablespoons minced mint
- 8 iceberg or romaine lettuce leaves

Direction:
1. Heat the oil (if desired) in a saucepan over medium heat. Add the tofu and 1 tablespoon of the lime juice, and sauté for 4 to 5 minutes or until the tofu is light brown. 2. Place the tofu in a medium bowl and combine with the remaining 2 tablespoons lime juice, cilantro, soy sauce, green onion, jalapeño, onion, and mint. Mix well. 3. Serve in the lettuce leaves.
Nutrition: Calories: 245 | fat: 10g | protein: 18g | carbs: 26g | fiber: 9g

340.   Southwestern Black Bean Pasta Salad

Preparation time: 15 minutes
Cooking time: 15 minutes
Serving: 4
Ingredients:
- 8 ounces (227 g) whole wheat rotini pasta
- 1 large avocado, halved and pitted
- 2 tablespoons freshly squeezed lime juice
- 1½ teaspoons chili powder
- 1 teaspoon smoked paprika
- 1 garlic clove, chopped
- 1 small red bell pepper, diced
- 1-pint cherry tomatoes, halved
- 1/4 cup chopped red onion
- 1/2 cup chopped fresh cilantro

Direction:
1. Cook the pasta according to package instructions. Drain, rinse lightly, and let cool.
2. Scoop the avocado flesh into a blender and add the lime juice, chili powder, paprika, cumin, and garlic. Blend until smooth.
3. In a large bowl, toss together the pasta, corn, black beans, bell pepper, tomatoes, red onion, cilantro, and dressing until well mixed. Refrigerate for at least 1 hour before serving or, for best results, up to 1 day.
Nutrition: Calories: 478 | fat: 10g | protein: 18g | carbs: 84g | fiber: 17g

341.   Sweet Potato Bisque

Preparation time: 15 minutes
Cooking time: 45 minutes
Servings: 4
Ingredients:
- 2 sweet potatoes, peeled and sliced
- 2 cups frozen butternut squash
- 2(14.5-ounce) cans full-fat coconut milk
- 1 medium yellow onion, sliced
- 1 teaspoon minced garlic (2 cloves)
- 1 tablespoon dried basil
- 1 tablespoon chili powder
- 1 tablespoon ground cumin
- 1/2 cup water
- Pinch salt
- Freshly ground black pepper to taste

Directions:
1.   Combine the sweet potatoes, butternut squash, coconut milk, onion, garlic, dried basil, chili powder, cumin, and water in a slow cooker; mix well.
2.   Cook on low heat.
3.   Blend the soup until it's nice and creamy.
4.   Season with salt and pepper.
Nutrition: Calories: 447 Total fats: 8g Protein: 72g Sodium: 346g Fat: 19g

342. Chickpea Medley

Preparation time: 5 minutes
Cooking time: 15 minutes
Servings: 4
Ingredients:
- 2 tablespoons tahini
- 2 tablespoons coconut amines
- 1(15-ounce) can chickpeas or 1(1/2) cup cooked chickpeas, rinsed and drained
- 1 cup finely chopped lightly packed spinach
- 3 big Carrot, peeled and grated

Directions:
1. Merge together the tahini and coconut amines in a bowl.
2. Add the chickpeas, spinach, and carrot to the bowl. Stir well and serve at room temperature.
3. Simple swap: Coconut amines are almost like a sweeter, mellower version of soy sauce. However, if you want to use regular soy sauce or tamari, just use 1(1/2) tablespoon and add a dash of maple syrup or agave nectar to balance out the saltiness.

Nutrition: Calories: 437 Total fats: 8g Protein: 92g Sodium: 246 Fat: 19g

343. Pasta with Lemon and Artichokes

Preparation time: 10 minutes
Cooking time: 20 minutes
Servings: 4
Ingredients:
- 16 ounces' linguine or angel hair pasta
- 1/4 cup extra-virgin olive oil
- 8 garlic cloves, finely minced or pressed
- 2(15-ounce) jars water-packed artichoke hearts, drained and quartered
- 2 tablespoons freshly squeezed lemon juice
- 1/4 cup thinly sliced fresh basil
- 1 teaspoon sea salt
- Freshly ground black pepper to taste

Directions:
1. Use a large pot of water to a boil over high heat and cook the pasta until al dente according to the directions on the package.
2. While the pasta is cooking, heat the oil in a skillet over medium heat and cook the garlic, stirring often for 1 to 2 minutes until it just begins to brown. Toss the garlic with the artichokes in a large bowl.
3. When the pasta is done, drain it and add it to the artichoke mixture, then add the lemon juice, basil, salt, and pepper. Gently stir and serve.

Nutrition: Calories: 237 Total fats: 7g Protein: 52g Sodium: 346 Fat: 19g

344. Roasted Pine Nut Orzo

Preparation time: 10 minutes
Cooking time: 15 minutes
Servings: 3
Ingredients:
- 16 ounces' orzo
- 1 cup diced roasted red peppers
- 1/4 cup pitted, chopped Klamath olives
- 4 garlic cloves, minced or pressed
- 3 tablespoons olive oil
- 1(1/2) tablespoon squeezed lemon juice
- 2 teaspoons balsamic vinegar
- 1 teaspoon sea salt
- 1/4 cup pine nuts
- 1/4 cup packed thinly sliced or torn fresh basil

Directions:
1. Use a large pot of water to a boil over medium-high heat and add the orzo. Cook, stirring often for 10 minutes, or until the orzo has a chewy and firm texture. Drain well.
2. While the orzo is cooking, in a large bowl, combine the peppers, olives, garlic, olive oil, lemon juice, vinegar, and salt. Stir well.
3. In a dry skillet toasts the pine nuts over medium-low heat until aromatic and lightly browned, shaking the pan often so that they cook evenly
4. Upon reaching the desired texture and add it to the sauce mixture within a minute or so, to avoid clumping.

Nutrition: Calories: 537 Total fats: 7g Protein: 72g Sodium: 246g Fat: 19g

345. Banana and Almond Butter Oats

Preparation time: 10 minutes

Cooking time: 5 minutes
Servings: 2
Ingredients:
- 1 cup gluten-free moved oats
- 1 cup almond milk
- 1 cup of water
- 1 teaspoon cinnamon
- 2 tablespoons almond spread
- 1 banana, cut

Directions:
1.   Mix the water and almond milk in a bubble in a little pot. Add the oats and diminish to a stew.
2.   Cook until oats have consumed all fluid. Blend in cinnamon. Top with almond spread and banana and serve.

Nutrition: Calories: 112 Fat: 10g Protein: 9g Carbohydrates: 54g Fiber: 15g Sugar: 5g Sodium: 180mg

346.   Red Tofu Curry

Preparation time: 15 minutes
Cooking time: 65 minutes
Servings: 4
Ingredients:
- 1(½) tablespoon canola oil
- 1 package extra-firm tofu
- 3 cups baby carrots
- 2 cups peeled red
- 2 onions,
- 3 teaspoons garlic
- 1-piece ginger
- 1(1/2) cup water
- 1 cup canned unsweetened coconut milk
- 1(1/2) tablespoon red curry paste
- 1 vegetable bouillon cube
- 1/2 teaspoon salt
- Cooked rice for serving
- Fresh cilantro for garnish

Directions:
1.   Heat the oil in a skillet. Place the tofu and brown.
2.   Merge all the ingredients and mix well.
3.   Cook on low heat
4.   Present over rice and garnished with cilantro.

Nutrition: Calories: 617 Total fats: 2g Protein: 32g Sodium: 563mg Fiber: 10g

347.   Spicy Tomato-Lentil Stew

Preparation time: 15 minutes
Cooking time: 60 minutes
Servings: 5
Ingredients:
- 2 cups dry brown
- 1 can crushed tomatoes
- 1 can diced tomatoes
- 2 cups peeled potatoes
- 1 yellow onion
- 1/2 cup carrot
- 1/2 cup celery
- 2 tablespoons hot sauce
- 2 teaspoons garlic
- 2 teaspoons cumin
- 1 teaspoon chili
- 1/2 teaspoon coriander
- 1/4 teaspoon paprika
- 1(1/4) bay leaf
- Pepper to taste
- 4 bouillon cubes

Directions:
1.   Merge all the ingredients and mix well.
2.   Cook on low heat
3.   Ready to serve.

Nutrition: Calories: 517 Total fats: 2g Protein: 32g Sodium: 1,063mg Fiber: 38g

348.   Mixed-Bean Chili

Preparation time: 10 minutes
Cooking time: 60 minutes
Servings: 4
Ingredients:
- 5(15-ounce) cans of your choice beans, drained and rinsed
- 1(15-ounce) can diced tomatoes with juice
- 1 (6-ounce) can tomato paste
- 1 cup water
- 1 green bell pepper, diced
- 2 cups stemmed and chopped kale
- 1/2 medium yellow onion, diced
- 2 tablespoons ground cumin
- 1 tablespoon chili powder
- 1 teaspoon minced garlic (2 cloves)
- 1 teaspoon cayenne pepper

- Pinch salt

Directions:

1. Place the beans, diced tomatoes, tomato paste, water, bell pepper, kale, onion, cumin, chili powder, garlic, and cayenne pepper in a slow cooker.

2. Season with salt and serve.

Nutrition: Calories: 417 Total fats: 2g Protein: 72g Sodium: 463mg Fiber: 10g

349.   Split-Pea Soup

Preparation time: 10 minutes
Cooking time: 65 minutes
Servings: 5
Ingredients:

- 1-pound dried green split peas, rinsed
- 6 cups water
- 3 carrots, diced
- 3 celery stalks, diced
- 1 medium russet potato, peeled and diced
- 1 small yellow onion, diced
- 1(1/2) teaspoon minced garlic (3 cloves)
- 5 vegetable bouillon cubes
- 1 bay leaf
- Freshly ground black pepper to taste

Directions:

1. Combine the split peas, water, carrots, celery, potato, onion, garlic, bouillon cubes, and bay leaf in a slow cooker; mix well.

2. Cook on low heat and season with pepper.

Nutrition: Calories: 817 Total fats: 2g Protein: 82g Sodium: 363mg Fiber: 10g

350.   Tomato Bisque

Preparation time: 10 minutes
Cooking time: 65 minutes
Servings: 4
Ingredients:

- 2 (28-ounce) cans crushed tomatoes
- 1 (28-ounce) can whole peeled tomatoes with juice
- 1 (15-ounce) can white beans, drained and rinsed
- 1/2 cup cashew pieces
- 2 vegetable bouillon cubes
- 1 tablespoon dried basil
- 2 teaspoons minced garlic (4 cloves)
- 3 cups water

- Pinch salt
- Freshly ground black pepper to taste

Directions:

1. Combine the crushed tomatoes, whole peeled tomatoes, white beans, cashew pieces, bouillon cubes, dried basil, garlic, and water in a slow cooker.

2. Cook on low heat.

3. Blend the soup until smooth. Season with salt and pepper.

Nutrition: Calories: 817 Total fats: 2g Protein: 82g

351.   Cheesy Potato-Broccoli Soup

Preparation time: 15 minutes
Cooking time: 70 minutes
Servings: 4
Ingredients:

- 2 pounds red or Yukon potatoes, chopped
- 1(10-ounce) bag frozen broccoli
- 2 cups unsweetened nondairy milk
- 1 small yellow onion, chopped
- 1(1/2) teaspoon minced garlic (3 cloves)
- 3 vegetable bouillon cubes
- 4 cups water
- 1 cup melts able vegan Cheddar-cheese shreds (such as Diana or Follow Your Heart)
- Pinch salt
- Freshly ground black pepper to taste

Directions:

1. Combine the potatoes, broccoli, nondairy milk, onion, garlic, bouillon cubes, and water in a slow cooker; mix well.

2. Cook on low heat.

3. Forty-five minutes before serving, use an immersion blender (or a regular blender, working in batches) to blend the soup until it's nice and creamy.

4. Stir in the vegan cheese, cover, and cook for another 45 minutes.

5. Season with salt and pepper.

Nutrition: Calories: 517 Total fats: 2g Protein: 92g

352.   Vegetable Stew

Preparation time: 15 minutes
Cooking time: 65 minutes
Servings: 4
Ingredients:

- 1(28-ounce) can diced tomatoes with juice
- 1 can white beans
- 1 cup diced green beans
- 2 medium potatoes, diced
- 1 cup frozen carrots and peas mix
- 1 small yellow onion, diced
- 1(1-inch) piece ginger, peeled and minced
- 1 teaspoon minced garlic (2 cloves)
- 3 cups vegetable broth
- 2 teaspoons ground cumin
- 1/2 teaspoon red pepper flakes
- Juice of 1/2 lemon
- Pinch salt
- Freshly ground black pepper to taste
- Pesto for serving

Directions:
1. Combine the diced tomatoes, white beans, green beans, potatoes, carrots, and peas mix, onion, ginger, garlic, vegetable broth, cumin, red pepper flakes, and lemon juice in a slow cooker.
2. Cook on low heat.
3. Pour with salt and pepper and serve with a dollop of pesto.

Nutrition: Calories: 617 Total fats: 2g Protein: 92g Sodium: 356 Fat: 16g

353. Frijoles De La Olla

Preparation time: 15 minutes
Cooking time: 65 minutes
Servings: 4
Ingredients:
- 1-pound dry pinto beans, rinsed
- 1 small yellow onion, diced
- 1 jalapeno pepper, seeded and finely chopped
- 1(1/2) teaspoon minced garlic (3 cloves)
- 1 tablespoon ground cumin
- 1/2 teaspoon Mexican oregano (optional)
- 1 teaspoon red pepper flakes (optional)
- 4 cups water
- 2 tablespoons salt

Directions:
1. Place the beans, onion, jalapeno, garlic, cumin, oregano (if using), red pepper flakes (if using), water, and salt in a slow cooker. Cook on low heat.

Nutrition: Total fat: 2g Protein: 82g Sodium: 346 Fat: 16g

354. Vegetable Hominy Soup

Preparation time: 15 minutes
Cooking time: 30 minutes
Servings: 4
Ingredients:
- 1(28-ounce) can hominy, drained
- 1(28-ounce) can diced tomatoes with green chills
- 5 medium red or Yukon potatoes, diced
- 1 large yellow onion, diced
- 2 cups chopped carrots
- 2 celery stalks, chopped
- 2 teaspoons minced garlic (4 cloves)
- 2 tablespoons chopped cilantro
- 1(1/2) tablespoon ground cumin
- 1(1/2) tablespoon seasoned salt
- 1 tablespoon chili powder
- 1 bay leaf
- 4 vegetable bouillon cubes
- 5 cups water
- Pinch salt
- Freshly ground black pepper to taste

Directions:
1. Combine the hominy, diced tomatoes, potatoes, onion, carrots, celery, garlic, cilantro, cumin, seasoned salt, chili powder, bay leaf, vegetable bouillon, and water in a slow cooker; mix well. Cook on low heat.
2. . Remove the bay leaf. Season with salt and pepper.

Nutrition: Calories: 417 Total fats: 2g Protein: 72g Sodium: 346 Fat: 16g

355. Lentil-Quinoa Chili

Preparation time: 15 minutes
Cooking time: 30 minutes
Servings: 4
Ingredients:
- 1/2 cup dry green lentils
- 1 can black beans
- 1/3 cup uncooked quinoa, rinsed
- 1 small yellow onion, diced
- 2 medium carrots, diced
- 2 teaspoons ground cumin
- 2 teaspoons chili powder

- 1(1/2) teaspoon minced garlic (3 cloves)
- 1 teaspoon dried oregano
- 3 vegetable bouillon cubes
- 1 bay leaf
- 4 cups water
- Pinch salt

Directions:

1. Place the lentils, black beans, quinoa, onion, carrots, cumin, chili powder, garlic, oregano, bouillon cubes, bay leaf, and water in a slow cooker; mix well.
2. Cook on low heat.
3. Remove the bay leaf, season with salt, and serve.

Nutrition: Calories: 617 Total fats: 2g Protein: 72g Sodium: 346 Fat: 16g

356.   Eggplant Curry

Preparation time: 15 minutes
Cooking time: 35 minutes
Servings: 5
Ingredients:
- 5 cups chopped eggplant
- 4 cups chopped zucchini
- 2 cups stemmed and chopped kale
- 1(15-ounce) can full-fat coconut milk
- 1(14.5-ounce) can diced tomatoes, drained
- 1(6-ounce) can tomato paste
- 1 medium yellow onion, chopped
- 2 teaspoons minced garlic (4 cloves)
- 1 tablespoon curry powder
- 1 tablespoon gram masala
- 1/4 teaspoon cayenne pepper
- 1/4 teaspoon ground cumin
- 1 teaspoon salt
- Cooked rice for serving

Directions:

1. Combine the eggplant, zucchini, kale, coconut milk, diced tomatoes, tomato paste, onion, garlic, curry powder, gram masala, cayenne pepper, cumin, and salt in a slow cooker; mix well.
2. Cook on low heat.

Nutrition: Calories: 417 Total fats: 2g Protein: 72g Sodium: 346 Fat: 19g

357.   Creamy Artichoke Soup

Preparation time: 5 minutes
Cooking time: 40 minutes
Servings: 4
Ingredients:
- 1 can artichoke hearts, drained
- 3 cups vegetable broth
- 2 tablespoons lemon juice
- 1 small onion, finely cut
- 2 cloves garlic, crushed
- 3 tablespoons olive oil
- 2 tablespoons flour
- 1/2 cup vegan cream

Directions:

1. Gently sauté the onion and garlic in some olive oil.
2. Add the flour, whisking constantly, and then add the hot vegetable broth slowly, while still whisking. Cook for about 5 minutes.
3. Blend the artichoke, lemon juice, salt, and pepper until smooth. Add the puree to the broth mix, stir well, and then stir in the cream.
4. Cook until heated through. Garnish with a swirl of vegan cream or a sliver of artichoke.

Nutrition: Calories: 211 Carbs: 12g Fat: 7g Protein: 11g

358.   Super Radish Avocado Salad

Preparation time: 10 minutes
Cooking time: 25 minutes
Servings: 2
Ingredients:
- 6 shredded carrots
- 6 ounces diced radishes
- 1 diced avocado
- 1/3 cup ponzu

Directions:

1. Bring all the above ingredients together in a serving bowl and toss.
2. Enjoy!

Nutrition: Calories: 211 Carbs: 9g Fat: 7g Protein: 12g

359. Beauty School Ginger Cucumbers

Preparation time: 10 minutes
Cooking time: 5 minutes
Servings: 2
Ingredients:
- 1 sliced cucumber
- 3 teaspoons rice wine vinegar
- 1(1/2) tablespoon sugar
- 1 teaspoon minced ginger

Directions:
1. Bring all the above ingredients together in a mixing bowl and toss the ingredients well.
2. Enjoy!

Nutrition: Calories: 210 Carbs: 14g Fat: 7g Protein: 19g

360. Mushroom Salad

Preparation time: 10 minutes
Cooking time: 20 minutes
Servings: 2
Ingredients:
- 1 tablespoon butter
- 1/2-pound cremini mushrooms, chopped
- 2 tablespoons extra-virgin olive oil
- Salt and black pepper to taste
- 2 bunches arugula
- 4 slices prosciutto
- 1 tablespoon apple cider vinegar
- 4 sundried tomatoes in oil, drained and chopped
- Fresh parsley leaves, chopped

Directions:
1. Heat a pan with butter and half of the oil.
2. Add the mushrooms, salt, and pepper. Stir-fry for 3 minutes. Reduce heat. Stir again, and cook for 3 minutes more.
3. Add the rest of the oil and vinegar. Stir and cook for 1 minute.
4. Place arugula on a platter, add prosciutto on top, add the mushroom mixture, sundried tomatoes, more salt and pepper, parsley, and serve.

Nutrition: Calories: 191 Carbs: 6g Fat: 7g Protein: 17g

361. October Potato Soup

Preparation time: 5 minutes
Cooking time: 20 minutes
Servings: 3
Ingredients:
- 4 minced garlic cloves
- 2 teaspoons coconut oil
- 3 diced celery stalks
- 1 diced onion
- 2 teaspoons yellow mustard seeds
- 5 diced Yukon potatoes
- 6 cups vegetable broth
- 1 teaspoon oregano
- 1 teaspoon paprika
- 1/2 teaspoon cayenne pepper
- 1 teaspoon chili powder
- Salt and pepper to taste

Directions:
1. Begin by sautéing the garlic and the mustard seeds together in the oil in a large soup pot.
2. Next, add the onion and sauté the mixture for another five minutes.
3. Add the celery, the broth, the potatoes, and all the spices, and continue to stir.
4. Allow the soup to simmer for thirty minutes without a cover.
5. Next, Position about three cups of the soup in a blender, and puree the soup until you've reached a smooth consistency. Pour this back into the big soup pot, stir, and serve warm. Enjoy.

Nutrition: Calories: 203 Carbs: 12g Fat: 7g Protein: 9g

362. Rice with Asparagus and Cauliflower

Preparation time: 5 minutes
Cooking time: 20 minutes
Servings: 2
Ingredients:
- 3 ounces' asparagus
- 3 ounces' cauliflower, chopped
- 2 ounces' tomato sauce
- 1/2 cup of brown rice
- 3/4 cup of water

- 1/3 teaspoon salt
- 1/4 teaspoon ground black pepper
- 1/4 teaspoon garlic powder
- 1 tablespoon olive oil

Directions:

1. Take a medium saucepan, place it over medium heat, add oil, and add asparagus and cauliflower and then sauté for 5 to 7 minutes until golden-brown.

2. Season with garlic powder, salt, and black pepper, stir in tomato sauce and then cook for 1 minute.

3. Add rice, pour in water, stir until mixed, cover with a lid and cook for 10 to 12 minutes until rice has absorbed all the liquid and become tender.

4. When done, remove the pan from heat, fluff rice with a fork, and then serve.

Nutrition: Calories: 257 Carbs: 4g Fat: 4g Protein: 40g

363. Spaghetti with Tomato Sauce

Preparation time: 5 minutes
Cooking time: 15 minutes
Servings: 2
Ingredients:

- 4 ounces' spaghetti
- 2 green onions, greens, and whites separated
- 1/8 teaspoon coconut sugar
- 3 ounces' tomato sauce
- 1 tablespoon olive oil
- 1/3 teaspoon salt
- 1/4 teaspoon ground black pepper

Directions:

1. Prepare the spaghetti, and for this, cook it according to the directions on the packet and then set aside.

2. Then take a skillet pan, place it over medium heat, add oil and when hot, add white parts of green onions and cook for 2 minutes until tender.

3. Add tomato sauce, season with salt, and black pepper and bring it to a boil.

4. Switch heat to medium-low level, simmer sauce for 1 minute, then add the cooked spaghetti and toss until mixed.

5. Divide the spaghetti between two plates and then serve.

Nutrition: Calories: 265 Carbs: 8g Fat: 2g Protein: 7g

364. Crispy Cauliflower

Preparation time: 5 minutes
Cooking time: 15 minutes
Servings: 2
Ingredients:

- 6 ounces of cauliflower florets
- 1/2 of zucchini, sliced
- 1/2 teaspoon of sea salt
- 1/2 tablespoon curry powder
- 1/4 teaspoon maple syrup
- 2 tablespoons olive oil

Directions:

1. Switch on the oven, then set it to 450°F and let it preheat.

2. Meanwhile, take a medium bowl, add cauliflower florets and zucchini slices, add the remaining ingredients reserving 1 tablespoon oil, and toss until well coated.

3. Take a medium skillet pan, place it over medium-high heat, add the remaining oil and wait until it gets hot.

4. Spread cauliflower and zucchini in a single layer and sauté for 5 minutes, tossing frequently.

5. Then transfer the pan into the oven and then bake for 8 to 10 minutes until vegetables have turned golden-brown and thoroughly cooked, stirring halfway.

Nutrition: Calories: 161 Carbs: 2g Fat: 2g Protein: 7g

365.   Green Onion Soup

Preparation time: 5 minutes
Cooking time: 12 minutes
Servings: 2
Ingredients:
- 6 green onions, chopped
- 7 ounces diced potatoes
- 1/3 teaspoon salt
- 2 tablespoons olive oil
- 1/4 cup vegetable broth
- 1/4 teaspoon ground white pepper
- 1/4 teaspoon ground coriander

Directions:
1.   Take a small pan, place potato in it, cover with water, and then place the pan over medium heat.
2.   Boil the potato until cooked and tender, and when done, drain the potatoes and set aside until required.
3.   Return saucepan over low heat, add oil and add green onions and cook for 5 minutes until cooked.
4.   Season with salt, pepper, and coriander, add potatoes, pour in vegetable broth, stir until mixed and bring it to simmer.
5.   Then remove the pan from heat and blend the mixture by using an immersion blender until creamy.
6.   Taste to adjust seasoning, then ladle soup into bowls and then serve.

Nutrition: Calories: 191 Carbs: 1g Fat: 1g Protein: 15g

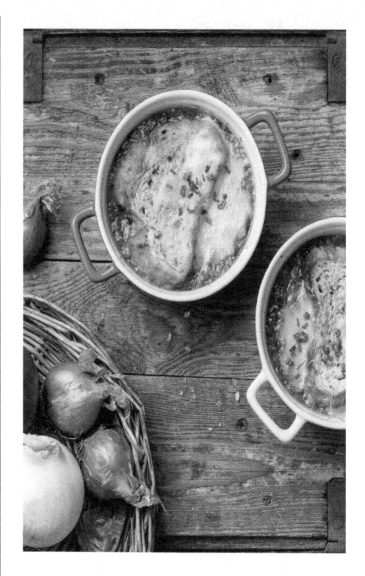

Chapter 11. Main Dishes

366. Asparagus Soup

Preparation Time: 15 minutes
Cooking Time: 40 minutes
Servings: 4
Ingredients:
- 1 tablespoon olive oil
- 3 scallions, chopped
- 1½ pounds fresh asparagus, trimmed and chopped
- 4 cups vegetable broth
- 2 tablespoons freshly squeezed lemon juice
- Salt and ground black pepper, as required
- 2 tablespoons coconut cream

Direction:
1. In a large saucepan, heat the oil over medium heat and sauté the scallion for 4-5 minutes.
2. Stir in the asparagus and broth and bring to a boil.
3. Now adjust the heat to low and simmer, covered for 25-30 minutes.
4. Remove from the heat and set aside to cool slightly.
5. Now, transfer the soup into a high-speed blender in 2 batches and pulse until smooth.
6. Return the soup into the same pan over medium heat and simmer for 4-5 minutes.
7. Stir in the lemon juice, salt, and black pepper and remove from the heat.
8. Serve hot with a topping of coconut cream.
Nutrition: Calories: 125 Fat: 6.9g Carbohydrates: 8.9g Dietary Fiber: 4.1g Sugar: 4.6g Protein: 9g

367. Mushroom Soup

Preparation Time: 15 minutes
Cooking Time: 25 minutes
Servings: 4
Ingredients:
- 2 teaspoons avocado oil
- 1¼ cups fresh Portobello mushrooms, sliced
- 1¼ cups fresh button mushrooms, sliced
- ½ cup white onion, chopped
- 1 garlic clove, crushed
- ½ teaspoon dried thyme
- Salt and cayenne powder, as required
- 1¾ cups unsweetened coconut milk
- 1½ cups water

Direction:
1. In a soup pan, heat the avocado oil over medium-high heat and cook the mushrooms, onions, garlic, thyme, salt and black pepper for about 5-6 minutes.
2. Add in the coconut milk and water and bring to a boil.
3. Now, adjust the heat to medium-low and simmer for about 10-15 minutes, stirring occasionally.
4. Serve hot.
Nutrition: Calories: 177 Fat: 14.9g Carbohydrates: 5.9g Dietary Fiber: 0.9g Sugar: 4g Protein: 2.9g

368. Beans & Veggie Burgers

Preparation Time: 20 minutes
Cooking Time: 25 minutes
Servings: 8
Ingredients:
- ½ cup walnuts
- 1 carrot, peeled and chopped
- 1 celery stalk, chopped
- 4 scallions, chopped
- 5 garlic cloves, chopped
- 2¼ cups canned black beans, rinsed and drained
- 2½ cups sweet potato, peeled and grated
- ½ teaspoon red pepper flakes, crushed
- ¼ teaspoon cayenne pepper
- Salt and ground black pepper, as required

Direction:
1. Preheat your oven to 400 °F.
2. Line a baking sheet with parchment paper.
3. In a food processor, add the walnuts and pulse until finely ground.
4. Add the carrot, celery, scallion and garlic and pulse until chopped finely.
5. Transfer the vegetable mixture into a large bowl.
6. In the same food processor, add the beans and pulse until chopped.
7. Add 1½ cups of the sweet potato and pulse until a chunky mixture forms.
8. Transfer the bean mixture into the bowl with vegetable mixture.
9. Stir in remaining sweet potato and spices and mix until well combined.
10. Make 8 equal-sized patties from the mixture.

11.   Arrange the patties onto the prepared baking sheet in a single layer.
12.   Bake for approximately 25 minutes.
13.   Serve hot.

Nutrition: Calories: 300 Fat: 5.5g Carbohydrates: 49.8g Dietary Fiber: 11.4g Sugar: 5.9g Protein: 15.3g

369.   Mixed Veggies Burgers

Preparation Time: 15 minutes
Cooking Time: 6 minutes
Servings: 4
Ingredients:
• ½ cup fresh kale, tough ribs removed and chopped
• ½ cup green bell peppers, seeded and chopped
• ½ cup onions, chopped
• 1 plum tomato, chopped
• 2 teaspoons fresh oregano, chopped
• 2 teaspoons fresh basil, chopped
• 1 teaspoon dried dill
• 1 teaspoon onion powder
• ½ teaspoon ginger powder
• ½ teaspoon cayenne powder
• Salt, as required
• 1 cup chickpeas flour
• ¼-½ cup water
• 2 tablespoons olive oil
• 4 cups fresh arugula
Direction:
1.   In a bowl, add all vegetables, herbs, spices and salt and mix well.
2.   Add the flour and mix well.
3.   Slowly, add the water and mix until a thick mixture is formed.
4.   Make desired-sized patties from the mixture.
5.   In a skillet, heat the oil over medium-high heat and cook the patties for about 2-3 minutes per side.
6.   Divide the arugula onto serving plates and top each with 2 burgers.
7.   Serve immediately.

Nutrition: Calories: 177 Fat: 8.7g Carbohydrates: 19.2g Dietary Fiber: 4.1g Protein: 6.6g

370.   Burgers with Mushroom Sauce

Preparation Time: 25 minutes
Cooking Time: 30 minutes
Servings: 4
Ingredients:
For Patties:
• ½ cup millet, rinsed
• 1 cup hot water
• 1 (14-ounce) can chickpeas, rinsed, drained and mashed roughly
• 1 carrot, peeled and grated finely
• ½ of red bell pepper, seeded and chopped
• ½ of yellow onion, chopped
• 1 garlic clove, minced
• ½ tablespoon fresh cilantro, chopped
• ½ teaspoon curry powder
• Salt and ground black pepper, as required
• 4 tablespoons chickpea flour
• 2 tablespoons canola oil
For Mushroom Sauce:
• 2¼ cups unsweetened soy milk
• 2 tablespoons arrowroot flour
• 1 tablespoon low-sodium soy sauce
• Pinch of ground black pepper
• 1 teaspoon olive oil
• 1 cup fresh button mushrooms, chopped
• 1 garlic clove, minced
Direction:
1.   For patties: heat a small non-stick pan over medium heat and toast the millet for about 5 minutes, stirring continuously.
2.   Add the hot water and bring to a rolling boil.
3.   Now adjust the heat to low and simmer, covered for about 15 minutes.
4.   Remove from the heat and set aside, covered for about 10 minutes.
5.   Uncover the pan and let the millet cool completely.
6.   After cooling, fluff the millet with a fork.
7.   In a large bowl, add the millet and remaining ingredients except for chickpea flour and oil and mix until well combined.
8.   Slowly, add the chickpea flour, 1 tablespoon at a time and mix well.
9.   Make 4 equal-sized patties from the mixture.
10.   In a non-stick frying pan, heat the oil over medium heat and cook the patties for about 3-4 minutes per side or until golden brown.

11.   Meanwhile, for mushroom sauce: in a bowl, add the soy milk, flour, soy sauce and black pepper and beat until smooth. Set aside.

12.   Heat the oil in a skillet over medium heat and sauté the mushrooms and garlic for about 3 minutes.

13.   Stir in the soy milk mixture and cook for about 8 minutes, stirring frequently.

14.   Place 1 patty onto each serving plate and serve with the topping of mushroom sauce.

Nutrition: Calories: 497 Fat: 15.4g Carbohydrates: 69.9g Dietary Fiber: 10.3g Sugar: 16.1g Protein: 21g

371.   Beans Balls with Salad

Preparation Time: 20 minutes
Cooking Time: 20 minutes
 Servings: 2
Ingredients:
For Beans Balls:
•   1 (15-ounce) can pinto beans, drained and rinsed
•   ½ of carrot, peeled and minced
•   2 tablespoons fresh cilantro, minced
•   ½ of garlic clove, minced
•   ¼ cup whole-wheat breadcrumbs
•   1 tablespoon Italian seasoning
•   Salt and ground black pepper, as required
•   ½ tablespoon vegetable oil
For Salad:
•   3 cups fresh mixed salad greens
•   1 tomato, chopped
Direction:
1.   Preheat your oven to 375 °F.
2.   Line a baking sheet with parchment paper.
3.   For patties: in a large bowl, place all ingredients and mix well.
4.   Now, with a potato masher, mash until a sticky mixture is formed.
5.   With your hands, make 1-inch balls from the mixture.
6.   Arrange the balls onto the prepared baking sheet in a single layer.
7.   Bake for approximately 20 minutes or until desired doneness of balls, flipping once halfway through.
8.   Meanwhile, for salad: in a bowl, add all ingredients and toss to coat well.

9.   Divide the salad onto serving plates and top with balls evenly.
10.   Serve immediately.
Nutrition: Calories: 455 Fat: 7.8g Carbohydrates: 75.9g Dietary Fiber: 20.5g Sugar: 3.8g Protein: 24.1g

372.   Veggie Balls in Tomato Sauce

Preparation Time: 20 minutes
Cooking Time: 15 minutes
Servings: 8
Ingredients:
•   1½ cups cooked chickpeas
•   2 cups fresh button mushrooms
•   ½ cup onions, chopped
•   ¼ cup green bell peppers, seeded and chopped
•   2 teaspoons oregano
•   2 teaspoons fresh basil
•   1 teaspoon savory
•   1 teaspoon dried sage
•   1 teaspoon dried dill
•   1 tablespoon onion powder
•   ½ teaspoon cayenne powder
•   ½ teaspoon ginger powder
•   Salt, as required
•   ½-1 cup chickpea flour
•   6 cups homemade tomato sauce
•   2 tablespoons olive oil
Direction:
1.   In a food processor, add the chickpeas, veggies, herbs and spices and pulse until well combined.
2.   Transfer the mixture into a large bowl with flour and mix until well combined.
3.   Make desired-sized balls from the mixture.
4.   In a skillet, heat the grapeseed oil over medium-high heat and cook the balls in 2 batches for about 4-5 minutes or until golden brown from all sides.
5.   In a large pan, add the tomato sauce and veggie balls over medium heat and simmer for about 5 minutes.
6.   Serve hot.
Nutrition: Calories: 247 Fat: 6.6g Carbohydrates: 38.8g Dietary Fiber: 10.7g Sugar: 13.6g Protein: 11.8g

373. Veggie Kabobs

Preparation Time: 20 minutes
Cooking Time: 10 minutes
Servings: 4
Ingredients:
For Marinade:
- 2 garlic cloves, minced
- 2 teaspoons fresh basil, minced
- 2 teaspoons fresh oregano, minced
- ½ teaspoon cayenne pepper
- Salt and ground black pepper, as required
- 2 tablespoons freshly squeezed lemon juice
- 2 tablespoons olive oil

For Veggies:
- 2 large zucchinis, cut into thick slices
- 8 large button mushrooms, quartered
- 1 yellow bell pepper, seeded and cubed
- 1 red bell pepper, seeded and cubed

Direction:
1. For marinade: in a large bowl, add all the ingredients and mix until well combined.
2. Add the vegetables and toss to coat well.
3. Cover and refrigerate to marinate for at least 6-8 hours.
4. Preheat the grill to medium-high heat. Generously, grease the grill grate.
5. Remove the vegetables from the bowl and thread onto pre-soaked wooden skewers.
6. Grill for about 8-10 minutes or until done completely, flipping occasionally.
Nutrition: Calories: 122 Fat: 7.8g Carbohydrates: 12.7g Dietary Fiber: 3.5g Sugar: 6.8g Protein: 4.3g

374. Nutty Brussels Sprout

Preparation Time: 10 minutes
Cooking Time: 15 minutes
Servings: 2
Ingredients:
- ½ pound Brussels sprouts, halved
- 1 tablespoon olive oil
- 2 garlic cloves, minced
- ½ teaspoon red pepper flakes, crushed
- Salt and ground black pepper, as required
- 1 tablespoon freshly squeezed lemon juice
- 2 tablespoons pine nuts

Direction:
1. In a large saucepan of the boiling water, arrange a steamer basket.
2. Place the asparagus in steamer basket and steam, covered for about 6-8 minutes.
3. Drain the asparagus well.
4. In a large skillet, heat the oil over medium heat and sauté the garlic and red pepper flakes for about 40 seconds.
5. Stir in the Brussels sprouts, salt and black pepper and sauté for about 4-5 minutes.
6. Stir in lemon juice and sauté for about 1 minute more.
7. Stir in the pine nuts and remove from the heat.
8. Serve hot.
Nutrition: Calories: 146 Fat: 10.5g Carbohydrates: 12.3g Dietary Fiber: 4.6g Sugar: 2.8g Protein: 4.8g

375. Kale with Cranberries & Pine Nuts

Preparation Time: 10 minutes
Cooking Time: 14 minutes
Servings: 6
Ingredients:
- 2 pounds' fresh kale, tough ribs removed and chopped
- 3 tablespoons extra-virgin olive oil
- 1 tablespoon garlic, minced
- ½ cup dried unsweetened cranberries
- Salt and ground black pepper, as required
- 1/3 cup pine nuts

Direction:
1. In a large saucepan of boiling salted water, cook the kale for about 5-7 minutes.
2. In a colander, drain the kale and immediately transfer into an ice bath.
3. Drain the kale and set aside.
4. In a skillet, heat the oil over medium heat and sauté the garlic for about 1 minute.
5. Add kale, cranberries, salt and black pepper and cook for about 4-6 minutes, tossing frequently with tongs.
6. Stir in the pine nuts and serve hot.
Nutrition: Calories: 196 Fat: 12.2g Carbohydrates: 19.3g Dietary Fiber: 2.9g Sugar: 1.3g Protein: 5.6g

376. Squash with Fruit

Preparation Time: 15 minutes
Cooking Time: 40 minutes
Servings: 4
Ingredients:
- ¼ cup water
- 1 medium butternut squash, halved and seeded
- ½ tablespoon olive oil
- ½ tablespoon balsamic vinegar
- Salt and ground black pepper, as required
- 4 large dates, pitted and chopped
- 4 fresh figs, chopped
- 3 tablespoons pistachios, chopped
- 2 tablespoons pumpkin seeds

Direction:
1. Preheat your oven to 375 °F.
2. Place the water in the bottom of a baking dish.
3. Arrange the squash halves in in a large baking dish, hollow side up and drizzle with oil and vinegar.
4. Sprinkle with salt and black pepper.
5. Spread the dates, figs and pistachios on top.
6. Bake for approximately 40 minutes or until squash becomes tender.
7. Serve hot with the garnishing of pumpkin seeds.
Nutrition: Calories: 227 Fat: 5.5g Carbohydrates: 46.4g Dietary Fiber: 7.5g Sugar: 19.6g Protein: 5g

377. Curried Mushroom

Preparation Time: 15 minutes
Cooking Time: 15 minutes
Servings: 4
Ingredients:
- 2 tablespoons olive oil
- 2 onions, chopped
- 3 garlic cloves, minced
- ½ pound fresh button mushrooms, chopped
- ¼ pound fresh shiitake mushrooms, chopped
- ¼ pound fresh Portobello mushrooms, chopped
- Salt and ground black pepper, as required
- ¼ cup vegetable broth
- ½ cup unsweetened coconut milk
- 2 tablespoons fresh parsley, chopped

Direction:

1. In a large skillet, heat oil over medium heat and sauté the onion and garlic for 4-5 minutes.
2. Add the mushrooms, salt, and black pepper and cook for 4-5 minutes.
3. Add the broth and coconut milk and bring to a gentle boil.
4. Simmer for 4-5 minutes or until desired doneness.
5. Stir in the cilantro and remove from heat.
6. Serve hot.
Nutrition: Calories: 182 Fat: 14.7g Carbohydrates: 11.5g Dietary Fiber: 3.1g Sugar: 5g Protein: 5.4g

378. Curried Pumpkin

Preparation Time: 15 minutes
Cooking Time: 35 minutes
Servings: 4
Ingredients:
For Roasted Pumpkin:
- 1 medium sugar pumpkin, peeled and cubed
- Salt, as required
- 1 teaspoon olive oil
For Curry:
- 1 teaspoon olive oil
- 1 onion, chopped
- 1 tablespoon fresh ginger, minced
- 1 tablespoon garlic, minced
- 1 cup unsweetened coconut milk
- 2 cups vegetable broth
- 1 tablespoon curry powder
- 1 teaspoon ground cumin
- ½ teaspoon ground turmeric
- Salt and ground black pepper, as required
- 1 tablespoon freshly squeezed lime juice
- 2 tablespoons fresh parsley, chopped

Direction:
1. Preheat your oven to 400 °F.
2. Line a large baking sheet with parchment paper.
3. In a large bowl, add all ingredients for the roasted pumpkin and toss to coat well.
4. Place pumpkin onto prepared baking sheet in a single layer.
5. Roast for 20-25 minutes, flipping once halfway through.
6. Meanwhile, in a large pan, heat oil for the curry on medium-high heat.
7. Add onion and sauté for 4-5 minutes.

8. Add ginger and garlic and sauté for about 1 minute.

9. Add coconut milk, broth, spices, salt, and black pepper and bring to a boil.

10. Now adjust the heat to low and simmer for 10 minutes.

11. Stir in the roasted pumpkin and simmer for 10 more minutes.

12. Serve hot with a garnish of parsley.

Nutrition: Calories: 263 Fat: 18.3g Carbohydrates: 23.3g Dietary Fiber: 7.8g Sugar: 9.3g Protein: 6.6g

379. Braised Cauliflower & Broccoli

Preparation Time: 15 minutes
Cooking Time: 30 minutes
Servings: 3
Ingredients:
- 2 tablespoons olive oil
- 1 large onion, chopped
- 2 garlic cloves, minced
- ¼ teaspoon fresh ginger, grated finely
- 1 teaspoon ground cumin
- 1 teaspoon cayenne pepper
- Salt and ground black pepper, as required
- 2 cups vegetable broth
- 1½ cups small broccoli florets
- 1½ cups small cauliflower florets
- 1 tablespoon freshly squeezed lemon juice
- 1 cup cashews
- 1 teaspoon fresh lemon zest, grated finely

Direction:
1. In a large saucepan, heat oil over medium heat and sauté the onion for about 3-4 minutes.
2. Add the garlic, ginger and spices and sauté for about 1 minute.
3. Add 1 cup of the broth and bring to a boil.
4. Add the vegetables and again bring to a boil.
5. Cover the soup pan and cook for about 15-20 minutes, stirring occasionally.
6. Stir in the lemon juice and remove from the heat.
7. Serve hot with the topping of cashews and lemon zest.

Nutrition: Calories: 425 Fat: 32g Carbohydrates: 27.6g Dietary Fiber: 5.2g Sugar: 7.1g Protein: 13.4g

380. 3-Veggies Combo

Preparation Time: 15 minutes
Cooking Time: 25 minutes
Servings: 4
Ingredients:
- 1 tablespoon olive oil
- 1 small yellow onion, chopped
- 1 teaspoon fresh thyme, chopped
- 1 garlic clove, minced
- 8 ounces' fresh button mushroom, sliced
- 1 pound Brussels sprouts
- 3 cups fresh spinach
- 4 tablespoons walnuts
- Salt and ground black pepper, as required

Direction:
1. In a large skillet, heat the oil over medium heat and sauté the onion for about 3-4 minutes.
2. Add the thyme and garlic and sauté for about 1 minute.
3. Add the mushrooms and cook for about 15 minutes or until caramelized.
4. Add the Brussels sprouts and cook for about 2-3 minutes.
5. Stir in the spinach and cook for about 3-4 minutes.
6. Stir in the walnuts, salt and black pepper and remove from the heat.
7. Serve hot.

Nutrition: Calories: 153 Fat: 8.8g Carbohydrates: 15.8g Dietary Fiber: 6.3g Sugar: 8.3g Protein: 8.5g

381. Quinoa with Mushrooms

Preparation Time: 15 minutes
Cooking Time: 30 minutes
Servings: 4
Ingredients:
- ½ tablespoon avocado oil
- 1 cup uncooked quinoa, rinsed
- 12 ounces fresh white mushrooms, sliced
- 3 garlic cloves, minced
- 1¾ cup water
- ¼ teaspoon cayenne powder
- Salt, as required
- ¼ cup fresh cilantro, chopped

Direction:

1.   In a medium saucepan, heat avocado oil over medium-high heat and sauté the garlic for about 30-40 seconds.
2.   Add the mushrooms and cook on for about 5-6 minutes, stirring frequently.
3.   Stir in the quinoa and cook for about 2 minutes, stirring continuously.
4.   Add the water, cayenne and salt and bring to a boil.
5.   Now, adjust the heat to low and simmer, covered for about 15-18 minutes or until almost all the liquid is absorbed.
6.   Serve hot with the garnishing of cilantro.

Nutrition: Calories: 181 Fat: 3.1g Carbohydrates: 31g Dietary Fiber: 4g Sugar: 1.5g Protein: 8.9g

382.   Couscous Stuffed Bell Peppers

Preparation Time: 15 minutes
Cooking Time: 40 minutes
 Servings: 4
Ingredients:
• 1 cup water
• ½ cup uncooked couscous
• 4 bell peppers, tops removed and seeded
• 2 tablespoons fresh parsley, chopped
• 1 tablespoon olive oil
• 1 tablespoon freshly squeezed lemon juice
• Salt and ground black pepper, as required
Direction:
1.   In a saucepan, add the water over medium-high heat and bring to a rolling boil.
2.   Stir in the couscous and immediate, cover the pan.
3.   Remove from the heat and set the pan aside, covered for about 10 minutes.
4.   With a fork, fluff the couscous and let it cool completely.
5.   Preheat your oven to 350 °F.
6.   Light, grease a baking sheet.
7.   Arrange the bell peppers onto the prepared baking sheet.
8.   In a large bowl, add the cooled couscous and remaining ingredients and mix until well combined.
9.   Stuff each bell pepper with couscous mixture.
10.   Bake for approximately 35 minutes or until bell peppers are tender.

11.   Serve hot
Nutrition: Calories: 151 Fat: 4g Carbohydrates: 26g Dietary Fiber: 2.8g Sugar: 6.1g Protein: 4.1g

383.   Tofu with Spinach

Preparation Time: 15 minutes
Cooking Time: 10 minutes
Servings: 2
Ingredients:
• 1 tablespoon extra-virgin olive oil
• ½ pound tofu, pressed, drained and cubed
• 1 teaspoon fresh ginger, minced
• 1 garlic clove, minced
• ¼ teaspoon red pepper flakes, crushed
• 6 ounces' fresh spinach, chopped
• 1 tablespoon low-sodium soy sauce
Direction:
1.   Heat the olive oil in a large non-stick wok over medium-high heat and stir-fry the tofu for about 3-3 minutes.
2.   Add the ginger, garlic and red pepper flakes and cook for about 1 minute, stirring continuously.
3.   Stir in the spinach and soy sauce and stir-fry for about 4-5 minutes.
4.   Serve hot.
Nutrition: Calories: 190 Fat: 10.8g Carbohydrates: 12.6g Dietary Fiber: 2.5g Sugar: 1.3g Protein: 12.5g

384.   Tofu with Peas

Preparation Time: 15 minutes
Cooking Time: 20 minutes
Servings: 5
Ingredients:
• 3 tablespoons low-sodium soy sauce
• 2 tablespoons canola oil, divided
• 1 (16-ounce) package extra-firm tofu, drained, pressed and cubed
• 1 cup yellow onion, chopped
• 1 tablespoon fresh ginger, minced
• 2 garlic cloves, minced
• 2 large tomatoes, chopped finely
• 5 cups frozen peas, thawed
• 2 tablespoons fresh cilantro, chopped
Direction:
1.   In a large skillet, heat 1 tablespoon of oil over medium-high heat and cook the tofu for about 4-5

minutes or until browned completely, stirring occasionally.

2. Transfer the tofu into a bowl
3. In the same skillet, heat the remaining oil over medium heat and sauté the onion for about 3-4 minutes.
4. Add the ginger and garlic and sauté for about 1 minute.
5. Add the tomatoes and cook for about 4-5 minutes, crushing with the back of spoon.
6. Stir in all peas and cook for about 2-3 minutes.
7. Stir in the soy sauce and tofu and cook for about 1-2 minutes.
8. Serve hot with the garnishing of cilantro

Nutrition: Calories: 291 Fat: 11.9g Carbohydrates: 31.6g Dietary Fiber: 10.8g Sugar: 11.5g Protein: 19g

385. Artichoke Hearts with Garlic Aioli

Preparation Time: 15 minutes
Cooking Time: 8 minutes
Serving: 6
Ingredients:
Artichoke hearts:
- 14 water-packed artichoke hearts
- 1/2 cup almond flour
- 1/4 teaspoon baking powder
- 1 pinch salt
- 8 tablespoons water
- 6 tablespoons almond meal
- 1/4 teaspoon dried basil
- 1/4 teaspoon dried oregano
- 1/4 teaspoon paprika
- 1/4 teaspoon granulated garlic
- Spritz canola oil

Lemon garlic aioli:
- 3/4 cup mayonnaise
- 1 garlic clove minced
- 1 teaspoon lemon juice
- 1/8 teaspoon granulated onion
- Pinch salt

Directions:
1. Drain the artichokes and toss with the rest of the ingredients in a bowl.
2. Spread the artichokes in the Air Fryer basket.
3. Return the basket to the Air Fryer.

4. Air fry them for 8 minutes and flip once cooked halfway through.
5. Mix all the garlic aioli ingredients in a bowl.
6. Serve the artichokes with garlic aioli.

Nutrition: Calories 343; Fat 14.5g; Cholesterol 8mg; Carbohydrate 49g; Sugars 5.9g; Protein 14.5g

386. Mushroom Skewers

Preparation Time: 10 minutes
Cooking Time: 9 minutes
Serving: 4
Ingredients:
- 4 tablespoons unsalted butter
- 3 garlic cloves, minced
- 1 1/2 tablespoons soy sauce
- 36 cremini mushrooms with 2-inch caps
- 2 teaspoons fresh thyme leaves, chopped
- Salt

Directions:
1. Toss mushrooms with soy sauce, butter, garlic, thyme and salt in a bowl.
2. Thread these mushrooms on the wooden skewers.
3. Place the seasoned mushroom skewers in the Air Fryer basket.
4. Return the basket to the Air Fryer.
5. Air fry them for 9 minutes and flip once cooked halfway through. Serve warm.

Nutrition: Calories 290; Fat 11.6g; Cholesterol 31mg; Carbohydrate 28.5g; Sugars 9.1g; Protein 18.7g

387. Sumac Roasted Cauliflower

Preparation Time: 10 minutes
Cooking Time: 13 minutes
Serving: 2
Ingredients:
- 4 cups medium-sized cauliflower florets
- 1 teaspoon canola oil
- Pinch salt
- 2 teaspoon lemon juice
- 1/8 teaspoon sumac

Directions:
1. At 400 degrees F, preheat your Air Fryer.

2.   Toss cauliflower with lemon and the rest of the ingredients in a bowl.
3.   Spread the cauliflower in the Air Fryer basket.
4.   Return the Air Fryer basket to the Air Fryer.
5.   Air fry the cauliflower for 13 minutes.
6.   Shake them once cooked halfway through. Serve.
Nutrition: Calories 62; Fat 2.4g; Cholesterol 0mg; Carbohydrate 8.1g; Sugars 2.1g; Protein 2g

388.   Fried Green Tomatoes

Preparation Time: 10 minutes
Cooking Time: 10 minutes
Serving: 2
Ingredients:
• 1/2 cup almond meal
• 3 tablespoons xanthan gum
• 1/4 cup mayonnaise
• 1/2 teaspoon dried basil
• 1/2 teaspoon dried oregano
• 1/2 teaspoon granulated onion
• Salt and black pepper, to taste
• 1 medium-sized green tomato, sliced
• Spritz oil spray
Directions:
1.   Mix mayonnaise, basil, oregano, onion, black pepper, salt, and xanthan gum in a bowl.
2.   Di the green tomatoes slice in the mayo mixture.
3.   Coat them with almond meal.
4.   Place these slices in the Air Fryer basket.
5.   Return the basket to the Air Fryer.
6.   Air fry them for 10 minutes and flip once cooked halfway through.
7.   Serve warm.
Nutrition: Calories 267; Fat 21.9g; Cholesterol 8mg; Carbohydrate 15.5g; Sugars 5.4g; Protein 6.1g

389.   Mushroom Pepper Kabobs

Preparation Time: 10 minutes
Cooking Time: 10 minutes
Serving: 4
Ingredients:

• 1-pint whole mushrooms, portabella
• 1 green pepper, deseeded and diced
• 1 yellow pepper, deseeded and diced
• 1 onion, cut into 2-inch pieces
• 1-pint grape tomatoes
Marinade:
• 1/4 cup olive oil
• 2 garlic cloves, minced
• Juice of 1 lemon
• 1/2 teaspoon dried oregano
• 1/2 teaspoon salt
Directions:
1.   At 400 degrees F, preheat your Air Fryer.
2.   Toss mushrooms with bell pepper and the rest of the ingredients in a bowl.
3.   Thread these mushrooms and veggies on the wooden skewers.
4.   Place the vegetable skewers in the Air Fryer basket.
5.   Return the basket to the Air Fryer.
6.   Air fry them for 10 minutes and flip once cooked halfway through.
7.   Serve warm.
Nutrition: Calories 164; Fat 13.1g; Cholesterol 0mg; Carbohydrate 12.2g; Sugars 4.9g; Protein 3g

390.   Buffalo Cauliflower Steaks

Preparation Time: 10 minutes
Cooking Time: 10 minutes
Serving: 4
Ingredients:
• 1 large cauliflower head, cut into steaks
• Salt and black pepper, to taste
Dry ingredients:
• 1 1/2 cups almond flour
• 1/3 cup xanthan gum
• 1 tablespoon garlic powder
• 1 tablespoon onion powder
• 1 tablespoon salt
• 1 tablespoon paprika
• 2 teaspoon cayenne
Wet ingredients:
• 1 cup soymilk
• 2 teaspoon apple cider vinegar
• 2 tablespoons vegan egg powder
• 1/2 cup ice-cold water
• 2 tablespoons bourbon

- 1 tablespoon hot sauce

Directions:

1. Mix soy milk with all the wet and dry ingredients in a bowl.
2. Dip the cauliflower in the flour batter
3. At 400 degrees F, preheat your Air Fryer.
4. Spread the cauliflower in the Air Fryer basket.
5. Return the Air Fryer basket to the Air Fryer.
6. Air fry the cauliflower for 10 minutes.
7. Shake them once cooked halfway through. Serve.

Nutrition: Calories 230; Fat 5.4g; Cholesterol 38mg; Carbohydrate 39.6g; Sugars 13.4g; Protein 15g

391. Tofu Buddha Bowl

Preparation Time: 10 minutes
Cooking Time: 10 minutes
Serving: 4
Ingredients:
- 14 oz. tofu
- 2 tablespoons sesame oil
- 1/4 cup soy sauce
- ¼ cup edamame beans
- 3 tablespoons maple syrup
- 2 tablespoons lime juice
- 1 tablespoon Sriracha
- 1 lb. fresh broccoli florets only
- 3 medium carrots peeled and sliced
- 1 red bell pepper sliced
- 8 oz. fresh spinach sautéed

Directions:

1. Mix tofu with sesame oil, sriracha, soy sauce and lime juice in a bowl.
2. Spread the tofu in the Air Fryer basket.
3. Air fry them for 10 minutes at 400 degrees F.
4. Toss them once cooked halfway through.
5. Mix broccoli, carrots, edamame beans, bell pepper and spinach in a bowl.
6. Top them with air fried tofu.
7. Enjoy.

Nutrition: Calories 230; Fat 11.5g; Cholesterol 0mg; Carbohydrate 24.2g; Sugars 11.6g; Protein 13.3g

392. Roasted Broccoli Cauliflower

Preparation Time: 10 minutes
Cooking Time: 12 minutes
Serving: 4
Ingredients:
- 3 cups broccoli florets
- 3 cups cauliflower florets
- 2 tablespoons olive oil
- ½ teaspoon garlic powder
- ¼ teaspoon salt
- ¼ teaspoon paprika
- 1/8 teaspoon ground black pepper

Directions:

1. At 400 degrees F, preheat your Air Fryer.
2. Toss cauliflower with broccoli and the rest of the ingredients in a bowl.
3. Spread the cauliflower mixture in the Air Fryer basket.
4. Return the Air Fryer basket to the Air Fryer.
5. Air fry the cauliflower for 12 minutes.
6. Shake them once cooked halfway through.
7. Serve.

Nutrition: Calories 207; Fat 14.6g; Cholesterol 0mg; Carbohydrate 17.7g; Sugars 6.1g; Protein 7g

393. Air Fried Fajitas

Preparation Time: 10 minutes
Cooking Time: 15 minutes
Serving: 4
Ingredients:
- 1 cup mushrooms, sliced
- 1 red bell pepper sliced into ½ inch slices
- 1 yellow bell pepper sliced into ½ inch slices
- 1 green bell pepper sliced into ½ inch slices
- 1 red onion sliced into wedges
- 3 tablespoons fajita seasoning
- 1 tablespoon vegetable oil

Directions:

1. At 390 degrees F, preheat your Air Fryer.
2. Toss mushrooms with peppers, onion fajita seasoning and oil in a bowl.
3. Spread the fajita mixture in the Air Fryer basket.
4. Spray them with cooking spray.
5. Return the Air Fryer basket to the Air Fryer.

6. Air fry these veggies for 15 minutes.
7. Serve warm.
Nutrition: Calories 255; Fat 13.8g; Cholesterol 0mg; Carbohydrate 27.2g; Sugars 5.2g; Protein 3.2g

394. Vegetable Kebabs

Preparation Time: 10 minutes
Cooking Time: 10 minutes
Serving: 2
Ingredients:
• 2 bell peppers, diced
• 1 eggplant, diced
• 1 zucchini, diced
• 1/2 onion, diced
• salt and black pepper, to taste
Directions:
1. At 390 degrees F, preheat your Air Fryer.
2. Thread bell peppers, eggplant, zucchini, and onion on wooden skewers, alternately.
3. Spread the skewers in the Air Fryer basket.
4. Spray them with cooking spray and seasoning with black pepper and salt.
5. Return the Air Fryer basket to the Air Fryer.
6. Air fry these skewers for 10 minutes. Serve warm.
Nutrition: Calories 312; Fat 1.9g; Cholesterol 0mg; Carbohydrate 28.3g; Sugars 15.7g; Protein 4.9g

395. Beans & Barley Soup

Preparation Time: 15 minutes
Cooking Time: 40 minutes
Servings: 4
Ingredients:
• 1 tablespoon olive oil
• 1 white onion, chopped
• 2 celery stalks, chopped
• 1 large carrot, peeled and chopped
• 2 tablespoons fresh rosemary, chopped
• 2 garlic cloves, minced
• 1 teaspoon fresh ginger, minced
• 4 cups fresh tomatoes, chopped
• 4 cups vegetable broth
• 1 cup pearl barley
• 2 cups canned white beans, rinsed and drained

• 2 tablespoons fresh lemon juice
• 2 tablespoons fresh parsley leaves, chopped
Direction:
1. In a large soup pan, heat the oil over medium heat and sauté the onion, celery and carrot for about 4-5 minutes.
2. Add the rosemary, garlic and ginger and sauté for about 1 minute.
3. Add in the tomatoes and cook for about 3-4 minutes, crushing with the back of a spoon.
4. Add the barley and broth and bring to a boil.
5. Now, lower the heat to low and simmer, covered for about 20-25 minutes.
6. Stir in the beans and lemon juice and simmer for about 5 minutes more.
7. Garnish with parsley and serve hot
Nutrition: Calories: 407 Fat: 7.2g Carbohydrates: 70.3g Dietary Fiber: 16.9g Sugar: 8.2g Protein: 18.3g

396. Lentil, Quinoa & Veggie Soup

Preparation Time: 15 minutes
Cooking Time: 1 hour
Servings: 4
Ingredients:
• ½ cup red quinoa, rinsed
• 1 cup dry lentils, rinsed
• ½ cup mushrooms, sliced
• ½ cup carrots, peeled and chopped
• 1 cup celery stalk, chopped
• 1 tablespoon ground ginger
• 1 tablespoon ground cumin
• ½ tablespoon chili powder
• 1 teaspoon red pepper flakes, crushed
• 4 cups water
• 2 tablespoons fresh cilantro, chopped
Direction:
1. In a large soup pan, mix together all ingredients except cilantro over high heat and bring to a boil.
2. Now, lower the heat to medium-low and simmer, covered for about 45-60 minutes or until lentils become tender.
3. Serve hot with the garnishing of cilantro.
Nutrition: Calories: 251 Fat: 2g Carbohydrates: 42.6g Dietary Fiber: 17.3g Sugar: 2.3g Protein: 15.5g

397.   Rice Soup

Preparation Time: 15 minutes
Cooking Time: 50 minutes
Servings: 10
Ingredients:
• 2 tablespoons vegetable oil
• 1 large bell pepper, seeded and chopped
• 2 medium white onions, chopped
• 1 jalapeño pepper, chopped finely
• ¼ teaspoon red pepper flakes, crushed
• ½ teaspoon ground cumin
• ½ teaspoon ground coriander
• 8 cups vegetable broth
• 1 (28-ounce) can diced tomatoes with liquid
• ½ cup uncooked rice
• 1 (18-ounce) jar creamy peanut butter
• ¼ cup peanuts, roasted and chopped
Direction:
1.   In a large soup pan, heat oil over medium heat and sauté bell pepper and onion for about 4-5 minutes.
2.   Add jalapeño pepper, red pepper flakes, cumin and coriander and sauté for about 1 minute.
3.   Add broth and tomatoes and bring to a boil.
4.   Now, lower the heat to medium-low and simmer for about 15 minutes.
5.   Stir in rice and lower the heat to low.
6.   Cover and simmer for about 25 minutes.
7.   Stir in peanut butter and simmer for about 3-4 minutes.
8.   Serve hot with the garnishing of peanuts.
Nutrition: Calories: 440 Fat: 31.4g Carbohydrates: 27.7g Dietary Fiber: 5.3g Sugar: 9.2g Protein: 17.8g

398.   Mixed Veggie Stew

Preparation Time: 20 minutes
Cooking Time: 35 minutes
Servings: 8
Ingredients:
• 2 tablespoons coconut oil
• 1 large sweet onion, chopped
• 1 medium parsnip, peeled and chopped
• 3 tablespoons tomato paste
• 2 large garlic cloves, minced
• 1 teaspoon ground cumin
• ½ teaspoon ground cinnamon
• ½ teaspoon ground ginger

• ¼ teaspoon cayenne pepper
• 2 medium carrots, peeled and chopped
• 2 medium purple potatoes, peeled and chopped
• 2 medium sweet potatoes, peeled and chopped
• 4 cups vegetable broth
• 2 tablespoons fresh lemon juice
• 2 cups fresh kale, tough ribs removed and chopped
• ¼ cup fresh cilantro leaves, chopped
Direction:
1.   In a large soup pan, melt the coconut oil over medium-high heat and sauté the onion for about 5 minutes.
2.   Add the parsnip and sauté for 3 minutes.
3.   Stir in the tomato paste, garlic, and spices and sauté for 2 minutes.
4.   Stir in carrots, potatoes, sweet potatoes, and broth and bring to a boil.
5.   Now, lower the heat to medium-low and simmer, covered for about 20 minutes.
6.   Stir in the lemon juice and kale and simmer for 5 minutes.
7.   Serve hot with a topping of cilantro.
Nutrition: Calories: 168 Fat: 4.4g Carbohydrates: 27.9g Dietary Fiber: 4.9g Sugar: 4.2g Protein: 5.3g

399.   Pasta, Beans & Veggie Stew

Preparation Time: 15 minutes
Cooking Time: 35 minutes
Servings: 6
Ingredients:
• 3 tablespoons canola oil
• 1 large onion, chopped
• 4 ounces' fresh shiitake mushrooms, sliced
• 1 potato, scrubbed and cubed
• 1 medium tomato, chopped
• 2 tablespoons garlic, chopped finely
• 2 bay leaves
• 2 tablespoons mixed fresh herbs (rosemary, thyme, basil), chopped
• 1 teaspoon cayenne pepper
• 4 cups vegetable broth
• 2 tablespoons apple cider vinegar
• 1 cup dry fusilli pasta
• 1/3 cup nutritional yeast

- 1/3 cup roasted tomato salsa
- 6 ounces' fresh collard greens
- 1 (15-ounce) can cannellini beans, rinsed and drained
- Salt and ground black pepper, as required

Direction:

1. In a large saucepan, heat oil over medium heat and cook onion, mushrooms, potato and tomato for about 4-5 minutes, stirring frequently.
2. Add garlic, bay leaves, herbs and cayenne pepper and sauté for about 1 minute.
3. Add broth and bring to a boil.
4. Stir in vinegar, pasta, nutritional yeast and tomato salsa and again bring to a boil.
5. Now, lower the heat to medium-low and simmer, covered for about 20 minutes.
6. Uncover and stir in greens and beans and simmer for about 3-5 minutes.
7. Stir in salt and black pepper and remove from heat.
8. Serve hot.

Nutrition: Calories: 346 Fat: 9.7g Carbohydrates: 30.2g Dietary Fiber: 11.9g Sugar: 5.7g Protein: 17.3g

400. Chickpeas & Spinach Stew

Preparation Time: 15 minutes
Cooking Time: 30 minutes
Servings: 4
Ingredients:
- 1 tablespoon olive oil
- 1 medium onion, chopped
- 2 cups carrots, peeled and chopped
- 2 garlic cloves, minced
- 1 teaspoon red pepper flakes
- ½ teaspoon ground cumin
- ½ teaspoon ground coriander
- 2 large tomatoes, peeled, seeded and chopped finely
- 2 cups vegetable broth
- 2 cups canned chickpeas, rinsed and drained
- 2 cups fresh spinach, chopped
- 1 tablespoon fresh lemon juice
- Salt and ground black pepper, as required

Direction:

1. In a large saucepan, heat oil over medium heat and sauté the onion and carrot for about 6 minutes.
2. Stir in the garlic and spices and sauté for about 1 minute.
3. Add the tomatoes and cook for about 2-3 minutes.
4. Add the broth and bring to a boil.
5. Now, lower the heat to low and simmer for about 10 minutes.
6. Stir in the chickpeas and simmer for about 5 minutes.
7. Stir in the spinach and simmer for 3-4 minutes more.
8. Stir in the lemon juice, salt and black pepper and serve hot.

Nutrition: Calories: 216 Fat: 6.6g Carbohydrates: 31.4g Dietary Fiber: 9.5g Sugar: 7.8g Protein: 10.6g

401. Tofu & Bell Pepper Stew

Preparation Time: 15 minutes
Cooking Time: 15 minutes
Servings: 6
Ingredients:
- 2 tablespoons garlic
- 1 jalapeño pepper, seeded and chopped
- 1 (16-ounce) jar roasted red peppers, rinsed, drained and chopped
- 2 cups vegetable broth
- 2 cups water
- 2 medium bell peppers, seeded and sliced thinly
- 1 (16-ounce) package extra-firm tofu, drained and cubed
- 1 (10-ounce) package frozen baby spinach, thawed

Direction:

1. Add the garlic, jalapeño pepper and roasted red peppers in a food processor and pulse until smooth.
2. In a large saucepan, add the puree, broth and water over medium-high heat and cook until boiling.
3. Add the bell peppers and tofu and stir to combine.
4. Now, lower the heat to medium and cook for about 5 minutes.
5. Stir in the spinach and cook for about 5 minutes.
6. Serve hot.

Nutrition: Calories: 130 Fat: 5.3g Carbohydrates: 12.2g Dietary Fiber: 2.9g Sugar: 6.2g Protein: 11.8g

402.   Black Beans Chili

Preparation Time: 15 minutes
Cooking Time: 2 hours 10 minutes
Servings: 5
Ingredients:
- 2 tablespoons olive oil
- 1 onion, chopped
- 1 large bell pepper, seeded and sliced
- 4 garlic cloves, minced
- 2 jalapeño peppers, sliced
- 1 teaspoon ground cumin
- 1 teaspoon cayenne pepper
- 1 tablespoon red chili powder
- 2 cups tomatoes, finely chopped
- 4 cups cooked black beans
- 2 cups vegetable broth
- Salt and ground black pepper, as required

Direction:
1.   In a large saucepan, heat the oil over medium-high heat and sauté the onion and bell peppers for 3-4 minutes.
2.   Add the garlic, jalapeño peppers, and spices and sauté for about 1 minute.
3.   Add the sweet potato and cook for 4-5 minutes.
4.   Add the remaining ingredients except the pita chips and bring to a boil.
5.   Now, lower the heat to medium-low and simmer, covered for about 1½-2 hours.
6.   Season with the salt and black pepper and serve hot.

Nutrition: Calories: 285 Fat: 7.7g Carbohydrates: 43g Dietary Fiber: 15.g Sugar: 6.3g Protein: 16.4g

403.   Beans & Corn Chili

Preparation Time: 15 minutes
Cooking Time: 1 hour
Servings: 6
Ingredients:
- 2 tablespoons olive oil
- 1 green bell pepper, seeded and chopped
- 2 celery stalks, chopped
- 1 scallion, chopped
- 3 garlic cloves, minced

- 1 teaspoon dried oregano, crushed
- 2 tablespoons red chili powder
- 2 teaspoons ground cumin
- 1 teaspoon ground turmeric
- Salt and ground black pepper, as required
- 4½ cups tomatoes, chopped finely
- 4 cups water
- 1 (15-ounce) can red kidney beans, rinsed and drained
- 1 (15-ounce) can cannellini beans, rinsed and drained
- ½ of (15-ounce) can black beans, rinsed and drained
- 6 ounces frozen corn
- 1 jalapeño pepper, seeded and chopped

Direction:
1.   In a large saucepan, heat oil over medium heat and cook the bell peppers, celery, scallion and garlic for about 8-10 minutes, stirring frequently.
2.   Add the oregano, spices, salt, black pepper, tomatoes and water and bring to a boil.
3.   Simmer for about 20 minutes.
4.   Stir in the beans and jalapeño pepper and simmer for about 30 minutes.
5.   Serve hot.

Nutrition: Calories: 342 Fat: 6.2g Carbohydrates: 58g Dietary Fiber: 21.2g Sugar: 6g Protein: 18.3g

404.   Lentil Chili

Preparation Time: 15 minutes
Cooking Time: 2 hours 40 minutes
Servings: 8
Ingredients:
- 2 teaspoons olive oil
- 1 large onion, chopped
- 3 medium carrots, peeled and chopped
- 4 celery stalks, chopped
- 2 garlic cloves, minced
- 1 jalapeño pepper, seeded and chopped
- ½ tablespoon dried thyme, crushed
- 1 tablespoon chipotle chili powder
- ½ tablespoon cayenne pepper
- 1½ tablespoons ground coriander
- 1½ tablespoons ground cumin
- 1 teaspoon ground turmeric
- Salt and ground black pepper, as required
- 1-pound red lentils, rinsed
- 8 cups vegetable broth
- ½ cup scallion, chopped

Direction:
1.   In a large saucepan, heat the oil over medium heat and sauté the onion, carrot, and celery for 5 minutes.
2.   Add the garlic, jalapeño pepper, thyme, and spices and sauté for about 1 minute.
3.   Add the tomato paste, lentils, and broth and bring to a boil.
4.   Now, lower the heat to low and simmer for 2-2½ hours.
5.   Serve hot with a garnishing of scallion.
Nutrition: Calories: 280 Fat: 3.7g Carbohydrates: 41.5g Dietary Fiber: 19.3g Sugar: 4.3g Protein: 20.5g

405.   Chickpeas & Potato Curry

Preparation Time: 10 minutes
Cooking Time: 55 minutes
Servings: 2
Ingredients:
•   1 teaspoon olive oil
•   1 small onion, chopped
•   2 garlic cloves, chopped finely
•   2 cups tomatoes, chopped finely
•   1 teaspoon curry powder
•   ½ teaspoon red chili powder
•   Salt and ground black pepper, as required
•   ½ of small sweet potato, peeled and cubed
•   ½ of potato, peeled and cubed
•   1 (14-ounce) can chickpeas, drained and rinsed
•   6-7 ounces full-fat coconut milk
Direction:
1.   In a saucepan, heat olive oil over medium heat and sauté the onion and garlic for about 4-5 minutes.
2.   Add the tomatoes, spices, salt and black pepper and cook for about 2-3 minutes, crushing the tomatoes with the back of spoon.
3.   Stir in the potatoes and cook for about 1-2 minutes.
4.   Stir in the chickpeas and coconut milk and bring to a boil over high heat.
5.   Now, lower the heat to medium-low and simmer, partially covered for about 35-40 minutes.
6.   Serve hot.
Nutrition: Calories: 522 Fat: 21g Carbohydrates: 71.8g Dietary Fiber: 14g Sugar: 11.5g Protein: 14.6g

406.   Lentils & Veggie Curry

Preparation Time: 15 minutes
Cooking Time: 1½ hours
Servings: 8
Ingredients:
•   8 cups water
•   ½ teaspoon ground turmeric
•   1 cup brown lentils, rinsed
•   1 cup red lentil, rinsed
•   1 tablespoon vegetable oil
•   1 large white onion, chopped
•   3 garlic cloves, minced
•   2 tomatoes, seeded and chopped
•   1½ tablespoons curry powder
•   2 teaspoons ground cumin
•   3 carrots, peeled and chopped
•   3 cups pumpkin, peeled, seeded and cubed into 1-inch size
•   1 granny smith apple, cored and chopped
•   2 cups fresh spinach, chopped
•   Salt and ground black pepper, as required
Direction:
1.   In a large saucepan, add the water, turmeric and lentils over high heat and bring to a boil.
2.   Now, Now, lower the heat to medium-low and simmer, covered for about 30 minutes.
3.   Drain the lentils, reserving 2½ cups of the cooking liquid.
4.   Meanwhile, in another large saucepan, heat the oil over medium heat and sauté the onion for about 2-3 minutes.
5.   Add in the garlic and sauté for about 1 minute.
6.   Add the tomatoes and cook for about 5 minutes.
7.   Stir in the curry powder and spices and cook for about 1 minute.
8.   Add the carrots, potatoes, pumpkin, cooked lentils and reserved cooking liquid and bring to a gentle boil.
9.   Now, lower the heat to medium-low and simmer, covered for about 40-45 minutes or until desired doneness of the vegetables.
10.   Stir in the apple and spinach and simmer for about 15 minutes.
11.   Stir in the salt and black pepper and remove from the heat.
12.   Serve hot.

Nutrition: Calories: 263 Fat: 2.9g Carbohydrates: 47g Dietary Fiber: 20g Sugar: 9.6g Protein: 14.7g

407. Tofu & Mushroom Curry

Preparation Time: 20 minutes
Cooking Time: 25 minutes
Servings: 4
Ingredients:
For Tofu:
• 16 ounces' extra-firm tofu, pressed, drained and cut into ½-inch cubes
• 1 garlic clove, minced
• 3 tablespoons rice vinegar
• 3 tablespoons low-sodium soy sauce
• 3 tablespoons cornstarch
• 2 tablespoons sesame oil
• 1 tablespoon brown sugar
• 1 teaspoon red pepper flakes
• 2 tablespoons coconut oil
For Curry:
• ¼ cup water
• 1 small yellow onion, minced
• 3 large garlic cloves, minced
• 1 teaspoon fresh ginger, grated
• 2 cups fresh mushrooms, sliced
• 3 tablespoons red curry paste
• 13 ounces' light coconut milk
• 1 tablespoon low-sodium soy sauce
• 1 tablespoon sambal oelek
• 2 tablespoons fresh lime juice
• 1 teaspoon lime zest, grated
• 8 fresh basil leaves, chopped
Direction:
1. For tofu: in a resealable bag, place all ingredients. Seal the bag and shake to coat well.
2. Refrigerate to marinate for 2-4 hours.
3. In a large skillet, melt the coconut oil over medium heat and stir fry the tofu cubes for about 4-5 minutes or until golden brown completely.
4. With a slotted spoon, transfer the tofu cubes into a bowl.
5. For curry: in a large saucepan, add the water over medium heat and ring to a simmer.
6. Add the minced onion, garlic and ginger and cook for about 5 minutes.
7. Add the mushrooms and curry paste and stir to combine well.

8. Stir in the remaining ingredients except for basil and simmer for about 10 minutes.
9. Stir in the tofu and simmer for about 5 minutes.
10. Garnish with basil and serve.
Nutrition: Calories: 550 Fat: 45.1g Carbohydrates: 24.8g Dietary Fiber: 4.1g Sugar: 8.5g Protein: 14.6g

408. Lentils with Kale

Preparation Time: 15 minutes
Cooking Time: 20 minutes
Servings: 6
Ingredients:
• 1½ cups red lentils, rinsed
• 1½ cups vegetable broth
• 1½ tablespoons olive oil
• ½ cup onion, chopped
• 1 teaspoon fresh ginger, minced
• 2 garlic cloves, minced
• 1½ cups tomato, chopped
• 6 cups fresh kale, tough ends removed and chopped
• Salt and ground black pepper, as required
Direction:
1. In a saucepan, add the broth and lentils over medium-high heat and bring to a boil.
2. Now, lower the heat to low and simmer, covered for about 20 minutes or until almost all the liquid is absorbed.
3. Meanwhile, in a large skillet, heat oil over medium heat and sauté the onion for about 5-6 minutes.
4. Add the ginger and garlic and sauté for about 1 minute.
5. Add tomatoes and kale and cook for about 4-5 minutes.
6. Stir in the cooked lentils, salt and black pepper and remove from heat.
7. Serve hot.
Nutrition: Calories: 257 Fat: 4.5g Carbohydrates: 39.3g Dietary Fiber: 16.5g Sugar: 2.8g Protein: 16.2g

409. Veggie Ratatouille

Preparation Time: 20 minutes
Cooking Time: 45 minutes
Servings: 4
Ingredients:
- 6 ounces' tomato paste
- 3 tablespoons olive oil, divided
- ½ onion, chopped
- 3 tablespoons garlic, minced
- Salt and ground black pepper, as required
- ¾ cup filtered water
- 1 zucchini, sliced into thin circles
- 1 yellow squash, sliced into circles thinly
- 1 eggplant, sliced into circles thinly
- 1 red bell pepper, seeded and sliced into circles thinly
- 1 yellow bell pepper, seeded and sliced into circles thinly
- 1 tablespoon fresh thyme leaves, minced
- 1 tablespoon fresh lemon juice

Direction:
1. Preheat oven to 375 °F.
2. In a bowl, add the tomato paste, 1 tablespoon of oil, onion, garlic, salt and black pepper and blend nicely.
3. In the bottom of a 10x10-inch baking dish, spread the tomato paste mixture evenly.
4. Arrange alternating vegetable slices, starting at the outer edge of the baking dish and working concentrically towards the center.
5. Drizzle the vegetables with the remaining oil and sprinkle with salt and black pepper, followed by the thyme.
6. Arrange a piece of parchment paper over the vegetables.
7. Bake for approximately 45 minutes.
8. Serve hot.

Nutrition: Calories: 206 Fat: 11.4g Carbohydrates: 54g Dietary Fiber: 26.4g Sugar: 14.1g Protein: 5.4g

410. Shepherd Pie

Preparation Time: 20 minutes
Cooking Time: 1 hour
Servings: 8
Ingredients:
- ¼ cup pearl barley
- ½ cup lentils, rinsed
- 1 teaspoon nutritional yeast
- 2 cups vegetable broth, divided
- 3 potatoes, scrubbed and chopped
- ½ cup walnuts, chopped
- ½ of onion, chopped
- 1 large carrot, peeled and chopped
- ½ teaspoon water
- 1 teaspoon all-purpose flour
- Salt and ground black pepper, as required

Direction:
1. Preheat your oven to 350 °F.
2. In a large saucepan, add barley, lentils, nutritional yeast and 1¼ cups of broth over medium-low heat.
3. Cover and simmer for about 30 minutes or until all the liquid is absorbed. Transfer the barley mixture into a large bowl.
4. Meanwhile, in another saucepan of salted boiling water, add the potatoes and boil for about 15 minutes.
5. Drain the potatoes well and set aside cool slightly.
6. Then with a potato masher, mash the potatoes completely.
7. Meanwhile, in a third saucepan, add walnuts, onion, carrot and remaining broth over medium heat and cook for about 15 minutes.
8. In a bowl, mix together water and flour.
9. Add flour mixture into the pan of carrot mixture, stirring continuously.
10. Cook for about 2-3 minutes or until thickened.
11. Transfer the carrot mixture into the bowl with barley mixture.
12. Add salt and black pepper and stir to combine.
13. Transfer the mixture into a casserole dish and spread in an even layer.
14. Spread the mashed potatoes on top evenly.
15. Bake for approximately 30 minutes or until top becomes golden brown.
16. Serve hot.

Nutrition: Calories: 186 Fat: 5.3g Carbohydrates: 27.6g Dietary Fiber: 7.6g Sugar: 2.2g Protein: 8.5g

411. Rice & Lentil Casserole

Preparation Time: 20 minutes
Cooking Time1 hour
Servings: 6
Ingredients:
- 2½ cups water, divided
- 1 cup red lentils, rinsed
- ½ cup wild rice
- 1 teaspoon olive oil
- 1 small onion, chopped
- 3 garlic cloves, minced
- 1/3 cup zucchini, chopped
- 1/3 cup carrot, peeled and chopped
- 1/3 cup celery stalk, chopped
- 1 fresh tomato, chopped
- 8 ounces' tomato sauce
- 1 teaspoon ground cumin
- 1 teaspoon dried oregano, crushed
- 1 teaspoon dried basil, crushed
- Salt and ground black pepper, as required

Direction:
1. In a saucepan, add 1 cup of the water and rice over medium-high heat and bring to a rolling boil.
2. Now, lower the heat to low and simmer, covered for about 20 minutes.
3. Meanwhile, in another saucepan, add the remaining water and lentils over medium heat and bring to a rolling boil.
4. Now, lower the heat to low and simmer, covered for about 15 minutes.
5. Transfer the cooked rice and lentils into a casserole dish and set aside.
6. Preheat your oven to 350 °F.
7. Heat the oil in a large skillet over medium heat and sauté the onion and garlic for about 4-5 minutes.
8. Add the zucchini, carrot, celery, tomato and tomato paste and cook for about 4-5 minutes.
9. Stir in the cumin, herbs, salt and black pepper and remove from the heat.
10. Transfer the vegetable mixture into the casserole dish with rice and lentils and stir to combine.
11. Bake for approximately 30 minutes.
12. Remove from the heat and set aside for about 5 minutes.
13. Cut into equal-sized 6 pieces and serve.

Nutrition: Calories: 192 Fat: 1.5g Carbohydrates: 34.5g Dietary Fiber: 12g Sugar: 3.9g Protein: 11.3g

412. Lentil, Oats & Veggie Loaf

Preparation Time: 15 minutes
Cooking Time: 50 minutes
Servings: 6
Ingredients:
For Loaf:
- 2 carrots, peeled and chopped
- 2 celery stalks, chopped
- 1¼ cups Cremini mushrooms, chopped
- ½ cup bell pepper, seeded and chopped
- ½ of yellow onion, chopped
- 2 garlic cloves, minced
- 2 cups cooked French lentils
- ½ cup quick oats
- ½ cup breadcrumbs
- 2 tablespoons flax meal
- 2 tablespoons tomato paste
- 1 tablespoon BBQ sauce
- 1 tablespoon dried parsley
- Salt and ground black pepper, as required

For Topping:
- 1/3 cup ketchup
- Pinch of coconut sugar

Direction:
1. Preheat your oven to 350 °F.
2. Line a baking sheet with parchment paper.
3. For loaf: heat a lightly greased non-stick large skillet over medium heat and sauté the carrots, celery, mushrooms, bell pepper, onion and garlic with a pinch of salt and pepper for about 4-5 minutes.
4. Remove the skillet of veggie mixture from the heat and set aside to cool slightly.
5. In a food processor, add the lentils, cooked vegetables and remaining all ingredients and pulse until a chunky dough is formed.
6. Shape the dough into a ball and place on the prepared baking sheet.
7. Then, press the dough into a loaf shape.
8. Bake for approximately 35 minutes.
9. Remove the baking sheet of loaf from oven and spread the ketchup on top of loaf evenly.
10. Sprinkle the loaf with sugar evenly.
11. Bake for approximately 10 minutes more.

12. Remove the baking sheet from the oven and set aside for at least 10 minutes.
13. Cut the loaf into desired sized slices and serve.

Nutrition: Calories: 189 Fat: 2.2g Carbohydrates: 34.7g Dietary Fiber: 8.4g Sugar: 8.2g Protein: 9.9g

413. Wild Rice & Squash Pilaf

Preparation Time: 15 minutes
Cooking Time: 45 minutes
Servings: 8
Ingredients:
• 1 medium butternut squash, peeled and cubed
• 1/3 cup avocado oil
• Salt, as required
• 2 cups wild rice, rinsed
• 6 cups spring water
• 1 medium onion, chopped
• 2 garlic cloves, minced
• ¼ cup fresh lime juice
• ¼ cup fresh orange juice
• 1 teaspoon fresh lime zest, grated
• ½ teaspoon ground cumin
• ¼ teaspoon ground cinnamon
• ½ teaspoon cayenne pepper
• 1 cup fresh cranberries
• ¾ cup walnuts, chopped
• 3 tablespoons fresh parsley, chopped
Direction:
1. Preheat your oven to 400 °F.
2. In a bowl, add the squash cubes, 1 tablespoon of oil and salt and toss to coat well.
3. Divide the squash cubes onto 2 baking sheets and spread in a single layer.
4. Roast for about 20 minutes.
5. Meanwhile, in a medium skillet, heat 1 tablespoon of oil over medium heat and sauté the onion and garlic for about 3-4 minutes.
6. In a bowl, add the remaining oil, lime juice, orange juice, lime zest and spices and beat until well combined.
7. In a medium saucepan, add the water and rice over medium-high heat and bring to a boil.
8. Now, lower the heat to low and simmer, covered for about 40 minutes.

9. Remove the saucepan of rice from heat and drain completely.
10. Transfer the cooked rice into a bowl.
11. Add the cooked onion mixture, squash cubes, cranberries, walnuts, parsley and dressing and gently stir to combine.
12. Serve immediately.

Nutrition: Calories: 299 Fat: 8.7g Carbohydrates: 48.9g Dietary Fiber: 7g Sugar: 5.4g Protein: 10.3g

414. Barley & Veggie Pilaf

Preparation Time: 15 minutes
Cooking Time: 1 hour 5 minutes
Servings: 15
Ingredients:
• ½ cup pearl barley
• 1 cup vegetable broth
• 2 tablespoons vegetable oil, divided
• 2 garlic cloves, minced
• ½ cup white onion, chopped
• ½ cup green olives, sliced
• 1 cup bell pepper, seeded and chopped
• 2 tablespoons fresh cilantro, chopped
• 2 tablespoons fresh mint leaves, chopped
• 1 tablespoon tamari
Direction:
1. In a saucepan, add the barley and broth over medium-high heat and cook until boiling.
2. Immediately lower the heat to low and simmer, covered for about 45 minutes or until all the liquid is evaporated.
3. In a large skillet, heat 1 tablespoon of the oil over medium-high heat and sauté the garlic for about 30 seconds.
4. Stir in the cooked barley and cook for about 3 minutes.
5. Remove from the heat and set aside.
6. In another skillet, heat the remaining oil over medium heat and sauté the onion for about 7 minutes.
7. Add the olives and bell pepper and stir fry for about 3 minutes.
8. Stir in remaining ingredients except and cook for about 3 minutes.
9. Stir in the barley mixture and cook for about 3 minutes.
10. Serve hot with the garnishing of walnuts.

Nutrition: Calories: 204 Fat: 10.1g Carbohydrates: 25.3g Dietary Fiber: 4.9g Sugar: 2.6g Protein: 4.8g

415. Rainbow Shepherd's Pie

Preparation time: 15 minutes
Cooking time: 45 minutes
Serving: 4
Ingredients:
Topping:
- 4 medium sweet potatoes, peeled and diced (about 4 cups)
- ½ teaspoon salt (optional)
- 1 teaspoon garlic powder
- 2 tablespoons nutritional yeast
- ¼ cup unsweetened plant-based milk
Filling:
- 1 (8-ounce / 227-g) package tempeh
- 2 teaspoons extra-virgin olive oil (optional)
- ½ small yellow onion, diced small
- ½ red or yellow bell pepper, diced small
- 1 large carrot, peeled and diced small
- ½ cup frozen corn
- ½ cup frozen peas
- 2 tablespoons whole-wheat flour
- 2 tablespoons tomato paste
- 2 tablespoons low-sodium soy sauce or gluten-free tamari
- 2 cups water
Direction:
1. Preheat the oven to 375°F (190°C).
2. Make the Topping: Put the sweet potatoes in a medium saucepan and cover with enough water to cover completely. Bring to a boil over high heat. Lower the heat to medium and cook until the sweet potatoes are tender, about 15 minutes. Drain and return the potatoes to the saucepan. Add the salt (if using), garlic powder, nutritional yeast, and plant-based milk and, using a potato masher, mash until creamy. Set aside.
3. Make the Filling: While the potatoes are cooking, in a blender or food processor, pulse the tempeh into very small pieces.
4. In a large skillet over medium heat, heat the oil. Add the tempeh and onion and cook, stirring often, until the onion and tempeh are lightly browned, about

10 minutes. Add the bell pepper, carrot, corn, and peas and cook until the peppers are fragrant, about 5 minutes.
5. Add the flour and stir until well combined. Add the tomato paste, soy sauce, and water and bring to a boil. Lower the heat to medium and cook, stirring often, until a thick gravy forms.
6. Assemble the Dish: In an 8-by-8-inch baking dish, spread out the tempeh and veggie mixture. Top with the mashed sweet potatoes, spreading it to the edges. Cover with aluminum foil and bake for 15 minutes, until bubbly.
Nutrition: Calories: 322 | fat: 9g | protein: 17g | carbs: 48g | fiber: 7g

416. Mango-Ginger Chickpea Curry

Preparation time: 5 minutes
Cooking time: 15 minutes
Serving: 6
Ingredients:
- 3 cups cooked chickpeas
- 2 cups mango chunks
- 2 cups plant-based milk
- 2 tablespoons maple syrup (optional)
- 1 tablespoon curry powder
- 1 tablespoon ground ginger
- 1 teaspoon ground coriander
- 1 teaspoon garlic powder
- 1 teaspoon onion powder
- 1/8 teaspoon ground cinnamon
Direction:
1. Heat a large stockpot or Dutch oven over medium heat.
2. In the pot, combine the chickpeas, mango, milk, maple syrup (if desired), curry powder, ginger, coriander, garlic powder, onion powder, and cinnamon. Cover and cook for 10 minutes, stirring after about 5 minutes.
3. Uncover and cook for an additional 5 minutes, stirring every other minute. Serve.
Nutrition: Calories: 219 | fat: 4g | protein: 8g | carbs: 38g | fiber: 9g

417. Baked Taquitos with Fat-Free Refried Beans

Preparation time: 5 minutes
Cooking time: 25 minutes
Serving: 4
Ingredients:
- 2 cups cooked pinto beans
- 1 teaspoon chili powder
- 1 teaspoon ground cumin
- ½ teaspoon garlic powder
- ½ teaspoon onion powder
- ¼ teaspoon red pepper flakes
- 12 corn tortillas

Direction:
1. Preheat the oven to 400°F (205°C). Line a baking sheet with parchment paper.
2. Combine the beans, chili powder, cumin, garlic powder, onion powder, and red pepper flakes in a food processor or blender. Pulse or blend on low for 30 seconds, or until smooth, then set aside.
3. Place the tortillas on the baking sheet, and bake for 1 to 2 minutes. This helps soften the tortillas and makes rolling them much easier.
4. Remove the tortillas from the oven, then add a couple of heaping tablespoons of the refried beans to the bottom half of each corn tortilla. Roll the tortillas tightly, and place them back on the baking sheet, seam-side down.
5. Bake for 20 minutes, turning once after about 10 minutes, and serve.
Nutrition: Calories: 286 | fat: 3g | protein: 12g | carbs: 56g | fiber: 13g

418. Chickpea and Cauliflower Fajitas

Preparation time: 10 minutes
Cooking time: 30 minutes
Serving: 4
Ingredients:
- 1 tablespoon extra-virgin olive oil (optional)
- ½ large head cauliflower, cut into small florets (about 2 cups)
- 1 small yellow onion, thinly sliced
- 1 red bell pepper, seeded and thinly sliced
- 1 (15-ounce / 425-g) can chickpeas, drained and rinsed
- 1 teaspoon chili powder
- ½ teaspoon smoked paprika
- ½ teaspoon garlic powder
- 1 teaspoon salt (optional)
- 12 (6-inch) soft corn tortillas, for serving
- 1 avocado, pitted, peeled, quartered, and thinly sliced, for serving
- ½ bunch cilantro, chopped, for serving

Direction:
1. In a large sauté pan, heat the oil over medium heat. Add the cauliflower and cook until it begins to brown, about 5 minutes. Add the onion and cook, stirring occasionally, for 5 minutes. Add the bell pepper and cook, stirring occasionally, until the cauliflower is fork-tender, about 5 minutes.
2. Add the chickpeas, chili powder, smoked paprika, garlic powder, and salt (if using) and stir until combined. Cook until the spices flavor the mixture, about 5 minutes. Transfer the fajita mixture to a serving bowl.
3. Wipe out the sauté pan with a paper towel and warm the tortillas over medium heat until they are pliable, about 2 minutes per side.
4. Divide the filling among the tortillas, top each one with 2 or 3 slices of avocado and some chopped cilantro, and serve.
Nutrition: Calories: 500 | fat: 18g | protein: 15g | carbs: 73g | fiber: 13g

419. The Best Veggie Burgers

Preparation time: 15 minutes
Cooking time: 30 minutes
Serving: 12 patties
Ingredients:
- 1 yellow onion, coarsely chopped
- 3 garlic cloves, coarsely chopped
- 1 sweet potato, skin on, cubed
- ½ cup walnuts
- 1 cup precooked brown rice
- 2 cups precooked green lentils or brown lentils

- 1 tablespoon paprika
- 1 tablespoon tamari
- 2 tablespoons tomato paste
- ¼ cup water
- 1 tablespoon Dijon mustard or yellow mustard
- ¼ cup ground flaxseed
- ¾ to 1 cup coarse cornmeal

Direction:

1. Preheat the oven to 450°F (235°C). Line a baking sheet with parchment paper.

2. In a food processor, combine the onion, garlic, sweet potato, and walnuts. Process for 1 to 2 minutes, or until the ingredients are combined and have the consistency of rice.

3. Add the brown rice, cooked lentils, paprika, and tamari. Pulse several times to incorporate the ingredients.

4. In a large bowl, stir together the tomato paste, water, mustard, and flaxseed. Add the blended ingredients to the bowl and mix to combine fully.

5. Starting with ¾ cup, stir in the cornmeal, adding more if the mixture looks too wet. The dough should form a ball without sticking to your hands too much. Divide the dough into 12 equal portions, roughly ¼ cup each. Roll the portions into balls and flatten onto the prepared baking sheet.

6. Bake for 15 minutes. Flip the patties and bake for 15 minutes more. The patties should be browned on the outside and firm to the touch. Serve immediately or let cool completely before freezing in an airtight container for up to 3 months.

Nutrition: Calories: 161 | fat: 5g | protein: 6g | carbs: 24g | fiber: 6g

420. Chickpea, Butternut Squash, and Herb Stuffed Peppers

Preparation time: 5 minutes
Cooking time: 40 minutes
Serving: 4
Ingredients:

- 2 teaspoons extra-virgin olive oil (optional)
- ½ small yellow onion, diced small
- 3 garlic cloves, minced

- 1 (15-ounce / 425-g) can chickpeas, drained and rinsed
- 2 cups frozen cubed butternut squash
- 1 teaspoon smoked paprika
- 1 teaspoon maple syrup (optional)
- ¼ cup plus 2 tablespoons water, divided
- 1 teaspoon salt (optional)
- 1 teaspoon Italian seasoning
- 2 tablespoons chopped fresh parsley
- 2 tablespoons chopped fresh mint
- 2 cups finely chopped baby spinach
- Juice of 1 lemon
- 1 cup frozen or cooked brown rice
- 4 large red or yellow bell peppers

Direction:

1. In a large skillet, heat the olive oil over medium heat. Add the onion and garlic and cook, stirring often, until fragrant, about 5 minutes. Add the chickpeas, squash, smoked paprika, maple syrup (if using), and ¼ cup of water and cook, stirring constantly, for 5 minutes.

2. Remove from the heat and add the salt (if using), Italian seasoning, parsley, mint, spinach, and lemon juice. Add the brown rice and mix well.

3. Preheat the oven to 400°F (205°C). 4. Rinse the bell peppers and pat dry with paper towels. Cut about 2 inches off the top of each pepper. Remove and discard the seeds. Spoon equal amounts of the vegetable-rice mixture into the peppers, packing it in tightly. Cover with the pepper tops.

5. Transfer the stuffed peppers into an 8-by-8-inch baking dish. Pour the remaining 2 tablespoons water into the bottom of the baking dish. Cover the dish with aluminum foil and bake for 30 minutes. Serve hot.

Nutrition: Calories: 254 | fat: 5g | protein: 9g | carbs: 49g | fiber: 8g

421. Burrito Bowl with Oil-Free Tortilla Chips

Preparation time: 10 minutes
Cooking time: 10 minutes
Serving: 2
Ingredients:

- 4 corn tortillas
- 1 cup cooked brown rice

- 1 cup cooked black beans
- 1 cup fresh or frozen corn
- 2 teaspoons chili powder
- 1 teaspoon ground cumin
- ½ teaspoon garlic powder
- ½ teaspoon onion powder
- 2 cups shredded lettuce
- 1 avocado, peeled, pitted, and sliced
- ¼ cup salsa

Direction:

1. Preheat the oven to 350°F (180°C). Line a baking sheet with parchment paper.

2. Cut each tortilla into 6 evenly-sized chips, and place the chips on the baking sheet. Bake for 8 to 10 minutes, or until golden brown. The chips will continue to crisp up as they cool.

3. In a large bowl, combine the rice, black beans, corn, chili powder, cumin, garlic powder, and onion powder. If the rice and beans are cold, warm this mixture in the microwave on high for 2 minutes or on the stovetop in a medium saucepan over medium heat for 5 minutes.

4. Divide the warm rice, bean, and corn mixture into two serving bowls, then top each bowl with 1 cup of shredded lettuce and half of the avocado slices and salsa.

5. Serve with the crispy tortilla chips and any other condiment of your choosing.

Nutrition: Calories: 537 | fat: 17g | protein: 18g | carbs: 86g | fiber: 21g

422.   Black Bean Patties with Carrots and Corn

Preparation time: 15 minutes
Cooking time: 15 minutes
Serving: 6
Ingredients:

- 1½ cups fresh bread crumbs
- 2 tablespoons chia seeds
- 2 tablespoons coconut oil, divided (optional)
- 1 cup diced yellow onion
- ½ cup finely diced carrot
- 1 ear of corn, kernels cut from the cob
- ½ teaspoon dried oregano
- 2 teaspoons chili powder

- ¼ teaspoon ground cumin
- 1 teaspoon salt (optional)
- 2 cloves garlic, finely diced
- ¼ cup sunflower seed kernels
- 2 tablespoons raw shelled hempseed
- 6 whole wheat buns
- Condiments and toppings of your choice

Direction:

1. Make your bread crumbs using any leftover bread that you have. I used whole wheat but you could use sourdough and whatever else you prefer. Place bread in a food processor and process until the bread is a finely ground texture. Set aside. If you have any leftover bread crumbs, they can be frozen for 6 months.

2. Mix the chia seeds with 6 tablespoons water and set aside.

3. Heat 1 tablespoon oil (if desired) in a large skillet, add the onion and carrot, and sauté about 10 minutes. Add the corn and cook another 3 minutes. Add the spices and garlic to the onion and cook another minute.

4. Pat the black beans dry. You want to make sure they aren't wet when mashing and adding to the rest of ingredients. In a large bowl, add the black beans and mash with a potato masher or the back of a fork. You could pulse them in a food processor instead, but not too fine. Stir in the chia seed mixture. Mix in the onion mixture, bread crumbs, sunflower seed kernels, and hempseed.

5. Make into six patties. At this point you can freeze the patties, before frying.

6. Fry the patties in 1 tablespoon medium-hot oil (if desired) until browned on each side.

7. Serve on the whole wheat buns with your favorite toppings.

Nutrition: Calories: 310 | fat: 18g | protein: 22g | carbs: 31g | fiber: 7g

423.   Sweet Potato Patties

Preparation time: 15 minutes
Cooking time: 20 minutes
Serving: 5 to 6 patties
Ingredients:

- 1 cup cooked short-grain brown rice, fully cooled

- 1 cup grated sweet potato
- ½ cup diced onion
- Pinch sea salt (optional)
- ¼ cup fresh parsley, finely chopped
- 1 tablespoon dried dill, or 2 tablespoons fresh
- 1 to 2 tablespoons nutritional yeast (optional)
- ½ cup whole-grain flour, or bread crumbs, or gluten-free flour
- 1 teaspoon olive oil (optional)

Direction:

1. Stir together the rice, sweet potato, onion, and salt (if using) in a large bowl. Allow it to sit for a few minutes, so that the salt can draw the moisture out of the potato and onion. Stir in the parsley, dill, and nutritional yeast (if using), then add enough flour to make the batter sticky, adding a spoonful or two of water if necessary.

2. Form the mixture into tight balls, and squish slightly into patties. 3. Heat a large skillet on medium, then add the oil (if using). Cook for 7 to 10 minutes, then flip. Cook another 5 to 7 minutes, and serve.

Nutrition: Calories: 115 | fat: 1g | protein: 3g | carbs: 23g | fiber: 2g

424. Hawaiian-Inspired Pepper Pot with Brown Rice

Preparation time: 15 minutes
Cooking time: 2 to 3 hours
Serving: 4 to 6
Ingredients:

- Nonstick cooking spray (optional)
- 1 medium onion, diced
- 1 medium red bell pepper, diced
- 1 medium green bell pepper, diced
- 1½ cups brown rice
- 3 cups store-bought low-sodium vegetable broth
- 1 (20-ounce / 567-g) can pineapple pieces in juice, undrained
- 2 tablespoons low-sodium soy sauce, tamari, or coconut aminos
- 2 tablespoons date syrup or maple syrup (optional)

- 1 piece (1-inch) fresh ginger, peeled and minced, or 1 teaspoon ground ginger
- 1 teaspoon garlic powder
- Ground black pepper
- Salt (optional)

Direction:

1. Coat the inside of the slow cooker with cooking spray (if using) or line it with a slow cooker liner.

2. Add the onion, red and green bell peppers, rice, broth, pineapple, soy sauce, syrup (if using), ginger, garlic powder, black pepper, and salt (if using). Stir well to combine.

3. Cover and cook on High for 2 to 3 hours or on Low for 5 to 6 hours. Stir occasionally during the last hour of cooking to keep the rice from settling and overcooking.

Nutrition: Calories: 379 | fat: 3g | protein: 9g | carbs: 87g | fiber: 7g

425. Spiced Green Lentil Sandwich

Preparation time: 15 minutes
Cooking time: 30 minutes
Serving: 8
Ingredients:

- 1 cup green lentils
- 1 small potato, to equal about ½ cup mashed potato
- ½ cup chopped onion
- 1 carrot, finely chopped in a processor
- ¾ cup old-fashioned oats
- ½ cup pepitas or sunflower seed kernels
- 1 tablespoon hempseed, toasted in shell
- 1 cup bread crumbs
- 4 tablespoons tamari
- 1 teaspoon ground ginger
- 1½ teaspoons smoked paprika
- ½ teaspoon salt (optional)
- ¼ teaspoon ground black pepper
- 1 tablespoon coconut oil (optional)
- 8 sandwich buns

Direction:

1. Place 2 cups water and the lentils in a large saucepan. Cover and bring to a boil. Turn down to low and cook for 20 minutes. Drain off remaining liquid from the lentils, if any. Set the lentils aside.

2. Pierce the potato a couple of times with a sharp knife. Wrap in a damp paper towel. Set in the microwave and cook on high for 4 minutes or until you can pinch the potato easily. Peel the potato and mash well. Set aside.

3. Heat 2 tablespoons water in a skillet over medium-high heat. Add the onion and sauté for 10 minutes. Remove from the heat.

4. Add the lentils, potato, onion, and the remainder of the ingredients to a large bowl (excluding the oil and the buns). Mix well. Form eight patties to the size of your sandwich buns.

5. Heat the oil (if desired) in a frying pan and fry the lentil patties on each side without crowding.

6. Spread the buns with all your favorite condiments and any other toppings of your choice.

7. You may also freeze extra patties for future meals.

Nutrition: Calories: 337 | fat: 16g | protein: 15g | carbs: 37g | fiber: 7g

426. Cajun-Style Jambalaya

Preparation time: 15 minutes
Cooking time: 3 to 4 hours
Serving: 4 to 6
Ingredients:

- Nonstick cooking spray (optional)
- 1 medium onion, diced
- 1 medium green bell pepper, diced
- 3 celery stalks, diced
- 4 garlic cloves, minced
- 2 cups uncooked brown rice
- 1 (8-ounce / 227-g) can tomato sauce
- 4 cups store-bought low-sodium vegetable broth
- 1 teaspoon dried thyme
- 1 teaspoon dried oregano
- 2 teaspoons paprika
- ½ teaspoon cayenne powder
- Ground black pepper
- Salt (optional)

Direction:

1. Coat the inside of the slow cooker with cooking spray (if using) or line it with a slow cooker liner.

2. Add the onion, bell pepper, celery, garlic, tomatoes, beans, bay leaf, rice, tomato sauce, broth, thyme, oregano, paprika, cayenne, black pepper, and salt (if using).

3. Cover and cook on High for 3 to 4 hours or on Low for 7 to 8 hours, stirring once per hour after the first two hours to avoid sticking. Remove and discard the bay leaf before serving.

Nutrition: Calories: 466 | fat: 4g | protein: 15g | carbs: 102g | fiber: 15g

427. Lentil Sloppy Joes

Preparation time: 10 minutes
Cooking time: 35 minutes
Serving: 4

- 4 cups water, plus 1 tablespoon and more as needed, divided
- 1 cup dried brown lentils
- 1 tablespoon paprika
- 1 teaspoon onion powder
- 1 teaspoon garlic powder
- 1 teaspoon dried parsley
- 8 ounces (227 g) button mushrooms, chopped
- 1 onion, diced
- 1 red bell pepper, diced
- 1 carrot, diced
- 4 ounces (113 g) tomato paste
- 1 tablespoon tamari
- 1 tablespoon pure maple syrup (optional)
- 1 teaspoon apple cider vinegar
- Multigrain bread, pita, whole wheat buns, or romaine lettuce leaves, for serving

Direction:

1. In an 8-quart pot over high heat, bring 3 cups of water to a boil. Reduce the heat to maintain a simmer and add the lentils. Cover the pot and cook for 20 minutes, or until tender. Transfer the cooked lentils to a bowl.

2. In small bowl, stir together the paprika, onion powder, garlic powder, and parsley. Set aside.

3. Heat a pot over medium-high heat. Add the mushrooms and cook for 3 minutes to remove their moisture. Add the onion, red bell pepper, and carrot. Cook for 3 minutes more, or until the onion becomes translucent. Add water, 1 tablespoon at a time, to prevent burning.

4. Stir in the tomato paste and cook for 30 seconds.

5. Stir in the tamari, maple syrup (if using), and vinegar to combine. Stir in the spice mixture. Add the remaining 1 cup of water and stir to combine.

6. Stir in the cooked lentils, adding more water to thin, as desired. The mixture should be fairly thick. Serve on your choice of bread or wrapped in leafy greens.

Nutrition: Calories: 236 | fat: 2g | protein: 15g | carbs: 46g | fiber: 11g

428. Broccoli and Mushroom Stir-Fry

Preparation time: 10 minutes
Cooking time: 25 minutes
Serving: 4
Ingredients:
- ¼ cup soy sauce
- ¼ cup water, plus 5 tablespoons, divided
- 2 tablespoons seasoned rice vinegar
- ½ teaspoon garlic powder
- ¼ teaspoon ground ginger
- ¼ to ½ teaspoon red pepper flakes
- 2 teaspoons cornstarch
- 3 scallions, green and white parts, thinly sliced (about ½ cup)
- 1 cup sliced (¼-inch-thick) carrots
- 3 cups (1-inch) broccoli florets
- 4 to 6 cups cooked brown rice
- Sesame seeds, for garnish

Direction:
1. In a small bowl, whisk together the soy sauce, ¼ cup of water, the vinegar, garlic powder, ginger, red pepper flakes, and cornstarch.

2. In a large sauté pan or skillet, combine the mushrooms, scallions, and 1 tablespoon of water. Sauté over high heat, stirring occasionally, for about 10 minutes, or until the mushrooms have browned and most of the liquid has evaporated. Transfer to a dish.

3. Return the pan to the stove. Still over high heat, add the carrots and 2 tablespoons of water. Cook, stirring occasionally, for 3 minutes, or until slightly softened.

4. Stir in the broccoli and remaining 2 tablespoons of water. Cook (adding a tablespoon of water as necessary to prevent burning) for about 6 minutes, or until the broccoli is bright green and crisp-tender and the liquid has evaporated.

5. Return the mushrooms with their liquid to the pan.

6. Stir in the soy sauce mixture, and cook for 1 to 2 minutes, or until the sauce thickens. Remove from the heat.

7. Serve the stir-fry over the brown rice, and garnish with sesame seeds.

Nutrition: Calories: 364 | fat: 3g | protein: 11g | carbs: 73g | fiber: 5g

429. Green Pepper, Potato, and Mushroom Scallopini Sandwiches

Preparation time: 15 minutes
Cooking time: 2 to 3 hours
Serving: 6 to 8 sandwiches
Ingredients:
- 1 medium onion, diced
- 4 garlic cloves, minced
- 2 medium green bell peppers, cut into 1½-inch pieces
- 1 pound (454 g) white button or cremini mushrooms, halved
- 6 red or yellow potatoes (about 2 pounds / 907 g), unpeeled and cut into 1½-inch pieces
- 1 tablespoon Italian seasoning
- ¼ teaspoon red pepper flakes (optional)
- Ground black pepper
- Salt (optional)
- 10 fresh basil leaves, torn, divided (optional)
- 6 to 8 (6-inch) whole-grain sub rolls, for serving

Direction:
1. Put the onion, garlic, bell peppers, mushrooms, potatoes, and tomatoes in the slow cooker. Swirl the red wine inside the empty tomato can and pour everything into the slow cooker. Add the Italian seasoning, red pepper flakes (if using), black pepper, and salt (if using). Stir to combine.

2. Cover and cook on High for 2 to 3 hours or on Low for 5 to 6 hours. Stir occasionally and add more water as needed while cooking to avoid sticking.

3. Before serving, stir in 6 torn basil leaves (if using). Portion about ½ cup of scallopini onto each roll, then top with the remaining 4 torn basil leaves.

Nutrition: Calories: 370 | fat: 2g | protein: 16g | carbs: 70g | fiber: 13g

430. Roasted Golden Beet Curry

Preparation time: 15 minutes
Cooking time: 1 hour
Serving: 4
Ingredients:
- 1 large golden beet, peeled and chopped into 1-inch pieces (about 4 cups)
- 1 onion, coarsely chopped
- 3 garlic cloves, peeled and stemmed
- 4 cups no-sodium vegetable broth
- 1 tablespoon coconut aminos or tamari
- 1 tablespoon grated peeled fresh ginger, or 1 teaspoon ground ginger
- 2 teaspoons yellow curry powder
- ½ teaspoon ground turmeric
- ¼ teaspoon cayenne pepper

Direction:
1. Preheat the oven to 400°F (205°C). Line a baking sheet with parchment paper.
2. On the prepared baking sheet, spread the beet pieces in an even layer and top with the onion pieces and garlic cloves.
3. Bake for 45 minutes, until lightly browned and fork-tender. Transfer to a large pot and place it over medium heat.
4. Add the vegetable broth, tofu, coconut aminos, ginger, curry powder, turmeric, and cayenne pepper to the pot. Bring to a simmer. Cover the pot and cook for 15 minutes.
5. Add the coconut milk. Using an immersion blender, purée until smooth. Or transfer the soup to a blender, working in batches as needed, and blend until smooth.
6. Serve with rice or a grain and add a variety of cooked root vegetables and greens, as desired.
Nutrition: Calories: 259 | fat: 20g | protein: 7g | carbs: 18g | fiber: 3g

431. Falafel Burgers

Preparation time: 15 minutes
Cooking time: 30 minutes
Serving: 8
Ingredients:
- 3 cups cooked chickpeas
- ¼ cup vegetable broth
- ¼ cup chopped fresh parsley
- 2 teaspoons garlic powder
- 2 teaspoons onion powder
- 1½ teaspoons ground cumin
- 1 teaspoon ground coriander
- ¼ teaspoon freshly ground black pepper
- Whole-wheat buns
- Lettuce, tomato, and onion, for topping (optional)

Direction:
1. Preheat the oven to 425°F (220°C). Line a baking sheet with parchment paper.
2. In a food processor or blender, combine the chickpeas, rice, broth, parsley, lemon juice, garlic powder, onion powder, cumin, coriander, and pepper. Process on low for 30 to 45 seconds, or until the mixture can easily be formed into patties but isn't so well mixed that you create hummus. You may need to stop the processor and scrape down the sides once or twice.
3. Scoop out ½ cup of the chickpea mixture, and form it into a patty. Place the patty on the baking sheet. Repeat until all of the chickpea mixture is used.
4. Bake for 15 minutes. Flip the patties, cook for 12 to 15 minutes more, and serve on buns with your preferred toppings.
Nutrition: Calories: 230 | fat: 3g | protein: 10g | carbs: 44g | fiber: 8g

432. Broccoli Spinach Stuffed Baguette

Preparation time: 25 minutes
Cooking time: 25 minutes
Serving: 2
Ingredients:
Vegetables:
- 2 cups broccoli florets
- 1 tablespoon extra-virgin olive oil (optional)
- 2 cloves garlic, finely diced
Cashew Cheese:
- ½ cup raw cashews, soaked 1 hour and drained
- 1 cup water
- 1½ tablespoons nutritional yeast
- 4 tablespoons tapioca starch

- ½ teaspoon salt (optional)
- ½ teaspoon garlic powder

Assemble:
- 1 baguette
- 1 ounce (28 g) grape tomatoes, sliced thin
- 2 tablespoons raw shelled hempseed

Direction:

Make Vegetables:

1. Add water to a medium saucepan with a steamer insert and bring to a boil. Add the broccoli to the insert and steam over boiling water for 10 minutes. Remove from steamer and set aside.

2. Heat the oil (if desired) in a large skillet over medium-high heat. Use a skillet that has a lid. Add the garlic and cook for 1 minute. Add the spinach, toss, and cook for 1 minute. Cover and let sit for 2 minutes.

4. Pour into a small saucepan and bring heat up to medium high. Keep cooking and stirring until it goes through its thickening process and becomes a gooey, cheesy sauce. This takes 5 to 10 minutes.

6. Add to the bowl with the broccoli mixture. Stir well. Assemble:

7. Cut off the top of the baguette and scoop out some of the bread from the center using a spoon. Make sure you leave an edge of bread in the shell to help hold the filling.

8. Spoon the broccoli-cheese mixture down the center of the baguette. Top with sliced grape tomatoes and sprinkle with hempseed. Cut in half. You could also cut into slices and serve as an appetizer.

Nutrition: Calories: 365 | fat: 14g | protein: 32g | carbs: 48g | fiber: 6g

433.   Acadian Black Beans and Rice

Preparation time: 15 minutes
Cooking time: 40 minutes
Serving: 6
Ingredients:
- 1½ cups brown rice
- 3½ cups low sodium vegetable broth
- 1 tablespoon extra-virgin olive oil (optional)
- ½ chopped yellow onion
- 1 chopped green bell pepper
- 1 clove garlic, finely chopped

- ¼ cup diced tomatoes
- 1 teaspoon parsley
- 1 teaspoon garlic powder
- 1 teaspoon onion powder
- 1 teaspoon thyme
- ½ teaspoon cayenne pepper
- ¼ teaspoon ground black pepper
- 1 teaspoon salt (optional)

Direction:

1. Cook the rice with vegetable broth for this recipe.

2. In a large skillet, heat the oil (if desired) to medium and then add the onion and bell pepper. Sauté until the onion becomes transparent, about 10 minutes. Add all the remaining ingredients (except the rice) to the large skillet with the onion and bell pepper. Cook for 10 minutes. Add the rice and heat through.

Nutrition: Calories: 291 | fat: 6g | protein: 16g | carbs: 52g | fiber: 7g

434.   Sweet Potato Chickpea Bowl

Preparation Time: 10 minutes
Cooking Time: 35 minutes
Servings: 4
Ingredients:
Veggies:
- 3 tbsp olive oil
- ½ red onion, sliced
- 2 sweet potatoes, halved
- 1 bundle broccoli stems removed and chopped
- 2 handfuls kale, stems removed
- ¼ tsp salt
- ¼ tsp black pepper

Chickpeas:
- 15-ounce chickpeas, drained, rinsed, and patted dry
- 1 tsp cumin
- ¾ tsp chili powder
- ¾ tsp garlic powder
- ¼ tsp salt
- ¼ tsp pepper
- ½ tsp oregano, optional
- ¼ tsp turmeric, optional

Direction:

1.   Preheat your oven to 400 degrees F.

2. Place the sweet potatoes and onions on a baking sheet.

3. Next, drizzle with one tablespoon of oil, making sure that everything is properly coated. Flip the sweet potatoes skin side facing down and bake for 10 minutes.

4. Once ready, remove from the oven and add broccoli. Drizzle with 1 teaspoon of oil and season with salt and pepper. Return to the oven and bake for 10 more minutes and then remove.

5. Add kale and drizzle with a touch of oil. Bake for another 5 minutes then set aside.

6. Next, heat a skillet over medium heat and start mixing the chickpeas with seasonings.

7. Once the skillet starts smoking, add 1 tbsp of oil and toss in the chickpeas. Sauté for 10 minutes until brown, ensuring you stir frequently.

8. Slice the sweet potatoes into bite size pieces and serve with the chickpeas on top.

Nutrition: Calories 488 Kcal, Protein 14 g, Carbs 50g, Fat 24g.

435. Skinny Pasta Primavera

Preparation Time: 10 minutes
Cooking Time: 15 minutes
Servings: 3
Ingredients:
- 4 ounces' spaghetti noodles, broken in half
- 1 leek, sliced
- ¼ lb. asparagus
- ¼ lb. broccoli florets
- ½ cup brown mushrooms, stemmed and sliced
- 2 garlic cloves, peeled and minced
- 1 ½ cups almond milk, unsweetened
- ¼ cup vegetable broth
- ¼ tsp red pepper flakes
- 1 tsp kosher salt
- 3 fresh thyme sprigs, stems removed
- 1 tbsp olive oil
- 6 kale sprouts, ends trimmed and leaves separated
- ¼ cup English peas
- ¼ lemon, juiced and zested
- ½ cup parmesan cheese, grated and more for garnishing
- ¼ cup dill leaves, roughly chopped

Direction:
1. On a Dutch oven, pour the almond milk, vegetable broth, broken spaghetti noodles, asparagus, leek, broccoli, garlic, mushrooms, red pepper flakes, salt, and thyme leaves.

2. Bring to a boil on high heat and then reduce the heat to simmer for 8 minutes, stirring to prevent the pasta from sticking together.

3. Once the time elapse, add the kale sprouts and peas and continue to cook for another 3 minutes.

4. Add in the lemon juice, cheese and dill, and remove from the stove.

5. Allow to cool and serve, not forgetting to garnish with dill leaves.

Nutrition: Calories 240 Kcal, Protein 12g, Carbs 27g, Fat 9g.

436. Grilled Vegetable Sandwich

Preparation Time: 10 minutes
Cooking Time: 25 minutes
Servings: 2
Ingredients:
- 1 cup vegan cashew ricotta cheese
- 1 tbsp parsley, basil, and chives, chopped
- 1 garlic clove, minced
- 1 tbsp extra virgin olive oil, plus more for drizzling
- Kosher salt and freshly ground black pepper to taste
- 1 large Portobello mushroom
- 1 zucchini, sliced lengthwise
- 1 yellow squash, sliced lengthwise
- ½ eggplant, sliced
- ½ red onion, sliced into rounds
- ½ red bell pepper, seeded and sliced in quarters
- 2 tsp oregano, dried
- 1 loaf ciabatta bread, sliced into 6-inch sections
- ½ cup arugula leaves
- Balsamic glaze

Direction:
1. In a small mixing bowl, mix the ricotta, garlic clove, fresh herbs, 1 tbsp olive oil, salt, and black pepper until smooth. Set aside.

2. Oil your grill grates with olive oil and preheat the grill for 15 minutes on high.

3.   Drizzle the veggies with extra virgin olive oil and season with salt, pepper, and dried oregano.

4.   Next, grease the cut side of the ciabatta with some olive oil.

5.   Place your vegetables on the grill and cook for 6 minutes. Once they start to soften, gently flip them using a spatula and cook the underside for another 5 minutes.

6.   Toast the two sides of ciabatta and transfer them along with the vegetables to a platter.

7.   Apply the herbed ricotta mixture on the toasted ciabatta bread and lay the grilled vegetables and arugula sides on top.

8.   Drizzle with the balsamic glaze and serve warm.

Nutrition: Calories 196 Kcal, Protein 9g, Carbs 27g, Fat 12g.

437.   Vegetarian Pancit Bihon

Preparation Time: 10 minutes
Cooking Time: 20 minutes
Servings: 4
Ingredients:
•   2 cups vegetable stock
•   4 oz Bihon noodles
•   2 tbsp canola oil
•   1 medium onion, finely diced
•   3 cloves garlic, crushed
•   ½ lb. mushrooms, sliced into small pieces
•   3 oz firm tofu drained, dried, and sliced (optional)
•   2 tbsp soy sauce
•   Ground pepper to taste
•   ½ cabbage, sliced
•   1 carrot, cut
•   2 celery stalks, sliced on bias
•   ½ cup snow peas
•   Cilantro and lemon wedges for garnish
Direction:
1.   Add the vegetable to a large pot and bring to boil. Toss in your noodles and cook for 4 minutes. Drain and set both the stock and noodles aside.

2.   In a large wok, add the oil and heat over medium-low heat for 3 minutes.

3.   Next, add the onions and garlic and sauté for 8 minutes until transparent. Add tofu, mushrooms, soy sauce, salt, and pepper. Cook for 5 minutes and

add the vegetables, stirring. To prevent your food from sticking, add a little oil or some of the reserved stock.

4.   Once the vegetables are crisp, pour in the noodles and the stock.

5.   Stir well until well incorporated and sprinkle with cilantro and lemon wedges.

6.   Serve immediately.

Nutrition: Calories 200 Kcal, Protein 7g, Carbs 30g, Fat 3g.

438.   Easy Vegetable Lasagna

Preparation Time: 20 minutes
Cooking Time: 1 hour 20 minutes
Servings: 4
Ingredients:
•   7 lasagna noodles, plus 2 more for filling in the holes
•   1 medium zucchini, sliced into ½-inch pieces
•   1 medium yellow squash, sliced into ½-inch pieces
•   6 ounces red peppers, roasted and cut into ½-inch pieces
•   ½ can tomatoes, crushed
•   A generous handful of basil leaves, freshly chopped
•   6 ounces' vegan cashew ricotta cheese
•   1 tbsp extra-virgin olive oil
•   ½ cup onion, chopped
•   ½ tbsp garlic, minced
•   1/8 tsp red pepper flakes, crushed
•   Salt and fresh ground black pepper, to taste
Direction:
For the Noodles:
1.   Add water and salt in a medium cooking pot and bring to boil. Cook your lasagna noodles according to directions indicated on the packaging.

2.   Once ready, drain and lay on a flat aluminum foil sheet.

3.   For the Vegetable Sauce:

4.   Start by preheating your oven to 350 F degrees.

5.   Lightly oil a 13x 9-inch baking dish.

6.   Next, heat the olive oil in a large skillet pan over medium heat and add the onion. Cook for 8 minutes until translucent and add the zucchini, squash, garlic, red pepper flakes, and a pinch of salt.

7. Continue cooking for 8 minutes until softened, stirring. Add in the roasted peppers and crushed tomatoes.

8. Lower the heat and simmer for 5 minutes until the liquid has thickened.

9. Sprinkle the basil on top and adjust the seasoning with additional salt and pepper.

For the Cheese Filling:

1. vegan cashew ricotta cheese

2. Assembling the Lasagna:

3. Spoon enough vegetable mixture into your baking dish and arrange four noodles lengthwise and side by side, ensuring that the bottom is covered.

4. Spread half of your ricotta cheese on top of the noodles. Finish it off with a third of the vegetable mixture.

5. Repeat the process until all your ingredients are done and loosely cover the baking dish with aluminum foil. Bake for 20 minutes, remove the cover and continue baking for 15 minutes.

6. Once ready, remove from the oven and let cool for 20 minutes.

7. Slice and serve.

Nutrition: Calories 450 Kcal, Protein 27g, Carbs 36g, Fat 20g.

439. Completely Stuffed Up Bell Pepper

Preparation Time: 10 minutes
Cooking Time: 10 minutes
Serving: 2
Ingredients:
- 4 bell peppers, halved and hollowed
- ½ cup quinoa, cooked
- 12 black olives, halved
- 1/3 cup tomatoes, sun-dried
- ½ cup baby spinach
- 2 garlic cloves, minced
- Salt and pepper to taste

Direction:

1. Preheat your oven to 400 degrees Fahrenheit

2. Take a bowl and add listed ingredients (except bell pepper), mix well

3. Bake for 10 minutes

4. Once done, stuff pepper with the quinoa mixture

5. Serve and enjoy!

Nutrition: Calories: 126 Fat: 5g Carbohydrates: 19g Protein: 3g

440. Onion and Zucchini Platter

Preparation Time: 15 minutes
Cooking Time: 45 minutes
Serving: 4
Ingredients:
- 3 large zucchinis, julienned
- 1 cup cherry tomatoes, halved
- ½ cup basil
- 2 red onions, thinly sliced
- ¼ teaspoon salt
- 1 teaspoon cayenne pepper
- 2 tablespoons lemon juice

Direction:

1. Create zucchini Zoodles by using a vegetable peeler and shaving the zucchini with a peeler lengthwise, until you get to the core and seeds

2. Turn zucchini and repeat until you have long strips

3. Discard seeds

4. Lay strips on a cutting board and slice lengthwise to your desired thickness

5. Mix Zoodles in a bowl alongside onion, basil, tomatoes, and toss

6. Sprinkle salt and cayenne pepper on top

7. Drizzle lemon juice

8. Serve and enjoy!

Nutrition: Calories: 156 Fat: 8g Carbohydrates: 6g Protein: 7g

441. Interesting Cauliflower Cakes

Preparation Time: 10 minutes
Cooking Time: 10 minutes
Serving: 4
Ingredients:
- 4 cups cauliflower, cut into florets
- 1 cup cashew cheese
- 2 eggs, lightly beaten
- 1 teaspoon paprika
- 1 teaspoon chili powder
- Salt and pepper to taste

- ½ cup fresh parsley, chopped
- 1 tablespoon olive oil

Direction:
1. Add cauliflower, cheese, paprika, eggs, chili, salt, pepper and parsley into a large-sized bowl
2. Mix well
3. Drizzle olive oil into frying pan and place over medium-high heat
4. Shape cauliflower mixture into 12 even patties
5. Once the oil is hot, fry cakes until both sides are golden brown
6. Serve hot and enjoy!

Nutrition: Calories: 180 Fat: 8g Carbohydrates: 6g Protein: 8g

442.   Creamed Leeks

Preparation Time: 10 minutes
Cooking Time: 25 minutes
Serving: 6
Ingredients:
- 1 ½ pound leeks, trimmed and chopped into 4-inch pieces
- 2 ounces' almond butter
- 1 cup coconut cream
- 3 ½ ounces cashew cheese
- Salt and pepper to taste

Direction:
1. Preheat your oven to 400 degrees Fahrenheit
2. Take a skillet and place it over medium heat, add butter and let it heat up
3. Add leeks and sauté for 5 minutes
4. Spread leeks in a greased baking dish
5. Boil cream in a saucepan and lower heat to low
6. Stir in cheese, salt, and pepper
7. Pour sauce over leeks
8. Bake for 15-20 minutes and serve warm
9. Enjoy!

Nutrition: Calories: 204 Fat: 15g Carbohydrates: 9g Protein: 7g

443.   Spiced Up Coconut Cauliflower Rice

Preparation Time: 20 minutes
Cooking Time: 20 minutes

Serving: 4
Ingredients:
- 3 cups cauliflower, riced
- 2/3 cups full-fat coconut milk
- 1-2 teaspoons sriracha paste
- ¼-½ teaspoon onion powder
- Salt as needed
- Fresh basil for garnish

Direction:
1. Take a pan and place it over medium-low heat
2. Add all of the ingredients and stir them until fully combined
3. Cook for about 5-10 minutes, making sure that the lid is on
4. Remove the lid and keep cooking until any excess liquid goes away
5. Once the rice is soft and creamy, enjoy it!

Nutrition: Calories: 95 Fat: 7g Carbohydrates: 4g Protein: 1g

444.   Goodnight, Tomato Platter

Preparation Time: 10 minutes + Chill time
Cooking Time: 0 minute
Serving: 8
Ingredients:
- 1/3 cup olive oil
- 1 teaspoon salt
- 2 tablespoons onion, chopped
- ¼ teaspoon pepper
- ½ a garlic, minced
- 1 tablespoon fresh parsley, minced
- 3 large fresh tomatoes, sliced
- 1 teaspoon dried basil
- ¼ cup red wine vinegar

Direction:
1. Take a shallow dish and arrange tomatoes in the dish
2. Add the rest of the ingredients in a mason jar, cover the jar and shake it well
3. Pour mix over tomato slices
4. Let it chill for 2-3 hours
5. Serve!

Nutrition: Calories: 350 Fat: 28g Carbohydrates: 10g Protein: 14g

445. Full Southern Salad

Preparation Time: 10 minutes
Cooking Time: 0 minute
Serving: 2
Ingredients:
- 5 cups of Romaine lettuce
- ½ cup of sprouted black beans
- 1 cup cherry tomatoes, halved
- 1 avocado, diced
- ¼ cup almonds, chopped
- ½ cup of fresh cilantro
- ½ cup of Salsa Fresca

Direction:
1. Take a large-sized bowl and add lettuce, tomatoes, beans, almonds, cilantro, avocado, Salsa Fresco
2. Toss everything well and mix them
3. Divide the salad into serving bowls and serve!
4. Enjoy!
Nutrition: Calories: 211 Fat: 16g Carbohydrates: 6g Protein: 10g

446. Light Mushroom Sauté

Preparation Time: 4 minutes
Cooking Time: 9 minutes
Serving: 4
Ingredients:
- 2 tablespoons almond butter
- 1 tablespoon olive oil
- 1 1/2 pounds' gourmet mushrooms
- 4 garlic cloves, diced
- 1/3 cup white wine vinegar
- Salt as needed

Direction:
1. Take a heavy pan and place it over medium heat
2. Add olive oil and half the butter
3. When the oil and butter is smoking, add mushrooms and keep stirring until browned
4. Add the remaining butter and garlic
5. Stir everything well
6. Add white wine vinegar and cook until the liquid is absorbed

7. Season with salt and enjoy!
Nutrition: Calories: 256 Fat: 18g Carbohydrates: 16g Protein: 14g

447. Bread Pudding with Raisins

Preparation time: 5 minutes
Cooking time: 60 minutes
Servings: 4
Ingredients:
- 4 cups day-old bread, cubed
- 1 cup brown sugar
- 4 cups coconut milk
- 1/2 teaspoon vanilla extract
- 1 teaspoon ground cinnamon
- 2 tablespoons rum
- 1/2 cup raisins

Directions:
1. Start by preheating your oven to 360ºF. Lightly oil a casserole dish with a nonstick cooking spray.
2. Place the cubed bread in the prepared casserole dish.
3. In a mixing bowl, thoroughly combine the sugar, milk, vanilla, cinnamon, rum and raisins. Pour the custard evenly over the bread cubes.
4. Let it soak for about 15 minutes.
5. Bake in the preheated oven for about 45 minutes or until the top is golden and set. "Bon appétit!"
Nutrition: Calories: 474 Fat: 12.2g Carbs: 72g Protein: 14.4g

448. Vanilla Hot Chocolate

Preparation time: 5 minutes
Cooking time: 10 minutes
Servings: 4
Ingredients:
- 1/4 cup of cocoa powder
- 1/8 teaspoon salt
- 1/2 teaspoon vanilla extract, unsweetened
- 1/4 cup of coconut sugar
- 3 cups almond milk, unsweetened

Directions:

1. Take a medium saucepan, add salt, sugar, vanilla extract and cocoa powder in it, whisk until combined and then whisk in milk.

2. Place the pan over medium-high heat and then bring the milk mixture to a simmer and turn hot, continue whisking.

3. Divide the hot chocolate evenly into four mugs and then serve.

Nutrition: Calories: 137 Fat: 3g Protein: 6g Carbs: 21g Fiber: 2g

449. Vanilla Cupcakes

Preparation time: 10 minutes
Cooking time: 20 minutes
Servings: 18
Ingredients:
• 2 cups white whole-wheat flour
• 1 cup of coconut sugar
• ½ teaspoon salt
• 2 teaspoons baking powder
• 1 (¼) teaspoon vanilla extract, unsweetened
• ½ teaspoon baking soda
• 1 tablespoon apple cider vinegar
• ½ cup coconut oil, melted
• 1 (½) cup almond milk, unsweetened
Directions:
1. Switch on the oven, then set it to 350°F and then let it preheat.

2. Meanwhile, take a medium bowl, place vinegar in it, stir in milk and then let it stand for 5 minutes until curdled.

3. Take a large bowl, place flour in it, add salt, baking soda, baking powder and sugar, and then stir until mixed.

4. Take a separate large bowl, pour in curdled milk mixture, add vanilla and coconut oil and then whisk until combined.

5. Whisk almond milk mixture into the flour mixture until smooth and the batter comes together, and then spoon the mixture into two 12-cups muffin pans lined with muffin cups.

6. Bake the muffins for 15 to 20 minutes until firm and the top turn golden brown, and then let them cool on the wire rack completely.

7. Serve straight away.

Nutrition: Calories: 152.4 Fat: 6.4g Protein: 1.5g Carbs: 22.6g Fiber: 0.5g

450. Hydration Station

Preparation time: 5 minutes
Cooking time: 0 minutes
Servings: 4
Ingredients:
• 1 banana
• 1 orange, peeled and sectioned, or 1 cup pure orange juice
• 1 cup strawberries (frozen or fresh)
• 1 cup chopped cucumber
• ½ cup coconut water
• 1 cup water
• ½ cup ice
Directions:
1. Purée everything in a blender until smooth, adding more water if needed.

2. Add bonus boosters, as desired, and purée until blended.

Nutrition: Calories: 320 Fat: 3g Carbs: 76g Fiber: 13g Protein: 6g

451. Dad's Aromatic Rice

Preparation time: 5 minutes
Cooking time: 20 minutes
Servings: 4
Ingredients:
• 3 tablespoons olive oil
• 1 teaspoon garlic, minced
• 1 teaspoon dried oregano
• 1 teaspoon dried rosemary
• 1 bay leaf
• 1 (½) cup white rice
• ½ cup vegetable broth
• Sea salt and cayenne pepper to taste
Directions:
1. In a saucepan, heat the olive oil over a moderately high flame. Add in the garlic, oregano, rosemary and bay leaf; sauté for about 1 minute or until aromatic.

2. Add in the rice and broth. Bring to a boil; immediately turn the heat to a gentle simmer.

3. Cook for about 15 minutes or until all the liquid has been absorbed. Fluff the rice with a fork, season with salt and pepper and serve immediately.

Nutrition: Calories: 384 Fat: 11.4g Carbs: 60.4g Protein: 8.3g

452. Everyday Savory Grits

Preparation time: 5 minutes
Cooking time: 35 minutes
Servings: 4
Ingredients:
- 2 tablespoons vegan butter
- 1 sweet onion, chopped
- 1 teaspoon garlic, minced
- 4 cups water
- 1 cup stone-ground grits
- Sea salt and cayenne pepper to taste

Directions:
1. In a saucepan, melt the vegan butter over medium-high heat. Once hot, cook the onion for about 3 minutes or until tender.
2. Add in the garlic and continue to sauté for 30 seconds more or until aromatic, reserve.
3. Bring the water to a boil over moderately high heat. Stir in the grits, salt and pepper. Turn the heat to a simmer, cover and continue to cook, for about 30 minutes or until cooked through.
4. Stir in the sautéed mixture and serve warm. "Bon appétit!"
Nutrition: Calories: 238 Fat: 6.5g Carbs: 38.7g Protein: 3.7g

453. Stir-Fry Noodles

Preparation time: 10 minutes
Cooking time: 8 minutes
Servings: 4
Ingredients:
- 1 cup broccoli, chopped
- 1 cup red bell pepper, chopped
- 1 cup mushrooms, chopped
- 1 large onion, chopped
- 1 batch stir-fry sauce, prepared
- Salt and black pepper to taste
- 2 cups spaghetti, cooked
- 4 garlic cloves, minced
- 2 tablespoons sesame oil

Directions:

1. Heat sesame oil in a pan over medium heat and add garlic, onions, bell pepper, broccoli, mushrooms.
2. Sauté for about 5 minutes and add spaghetti noodles and stir-fry sauce.
3. Mix well and cook for 3 more minutes.
4. Dish out in plates and serve to enjoy.
Nutrition: Calories: 567 Total fats: 48g Total carbs: 6g Fiber: 4g Net Carbs: 2g Sodium: 373mg Protein: 33g

454. Spicy Sweet Chili Veggie Noodles

Preparation time: 10 minutes
Cooking time: 7 minutes
Servings: 2
Ingredients:
- 1 head of broccoli, cut into bite-sized florets
- 1 onion, finely sliced
- 1 tablespoon olive oil
- 1 courgetti, halved
- 2 nests of whole-wheat noodles
- 150 grams' mushrooms, sliced

For sauce:
- 3 tablespoons soy sauce
- ¼ cup sweet chili sauce
- 1 teaspoon Sriracha
- 1 tablespoon peanut butter
- 2 tablespoons boiled water

For topping:
- 2 teaspoons sesame seeds
- 2 teaspoons dried chili flakes

Directions:
1. Heat olive oil on medium heat in a saucepan and add onions.
2. Sauté for about 2 minutes and add broccoli, courgetti and mushrooms.
3. Cook for about 5 minutes, stirring occasionally.
4. Whisk sweet chili sauce, soy sauce, Sriracha, water and peanut butter in a bowl.
5. Cook the noodles according to packet instructions and add to the vegetables.
6. Stir in the sauce and top with dried chili flakes and sesame seeds to serve.
Nutrition: Calories: 351 Total fats: 27g Protein: 25g Total carbs: 2g Fiber: 1g Net carbs: 1g

455. Creamy Vegan Mushroom Pasta

Preparation time: 10 minutes
Cooking time: 30 minutes
Servings: 6
Ingredients:
- 2 cups frozen peas, thawed
- 3 tablespoons flour, unbleached
- 3 cups almond beverage, unsweetened
- 1 tablespoon nutritional yeast
- 1/3 cup fresh parsley, chopped, plus extra for garnish
- 1/4 cup olive oil
- 1-pound pasta of choice
- 4 cloves garlic, minced
- 2/3 cup shallots, chopped
- 8 cups mixed mushrooms, sliced
- Salt and black pepper to taste

Directions:
1. Take a bowl and boil pasta in salted water.
2. Heat olive oil in a pan over medium heat.
3. Add mushrooms, garlic, shallots and ½ teaspoon salt and cook for 15 minutes.
4. Sprinkle flour on the vegetables and stir for a minute while cooking.
5. Add almond beverage, stir constantly.
6. Let it simmer for 5 minutes and add pepper to it.
7. Cook for 3 more minutes and remove from heat.
8. Stir in nutritional yeast.
9. Add peas, salt and pepper.
10. Cook for another minute.
11. Add pasta to this sauce.
12. Garnish and serve!

Nutrition: Calories: 364 Total fats: 28g Protein: 24g Total carbs: 4g Fiber: 2g Net carbs: 2g

456. Vegan Chinese Noodles

Preparation time: 15 minutes
Cooking time: 8 minutes
Servings: 4
Ingredients:

- 300 grams mixed oriental mushrooms, such as oyster, shiitake and enoki, cleaned and sliced
- 200 grams' thin rice noodles, cooked according to packet instructions and drained
- 2 garlic cloves, minced
- 1 fresh red chili
- 200 grams courgettes, sliced
- 6 spring onions, reserving the green part
- 1 teaspoon corn flour
- 1 tablespoon agave syrup
- 1 teaspoon sesame oil
- 100 grams' baby spinach, chopped
- Hot chili sauce to serve
- 2 (1-inch) pieces of ginger
- ½ bunch fresh coriander, chopped
- 4 tablespoons vegetable oil
- 2 tablespoons low-salt soy sauce
- ½ tablespoon rice wine
- 2 limes to serve
- 2 tablespoons water

Directions:
1. Heat sesame oil over high heat in a large wok and add the mushrooms.
2. Sauté for about 4 minutes and add garlic, chili, ginger, courgettes, coriander stalks and the white part of the spring onions.
3. Sauté for about 3 minutes until softened and lightly golden.
4. Meanwhile, combine the cornflour and 2 tablespoons of water in a bowl.
5. Add soy sauce, agave syrup, sesame oil and rice wine to the cornflour mixture.
6. Put this mixture in the pan to the veggie mixture and cook for about 3 minutes until thickened.
7. Add the spinach and noodles and mix well.
8. Stir in the coriander leaves and top with lime wedges, hot chili sauce and reserved spring onions to serve.

Nutrition: Calories: 314 Total fats: 22g Protein: 26g Total carbs: 3g Fiber: 0.3g Net carbs: 2.7g

457. Vegetable Penne Pasta

Preparation time: 15 minutes
Cooking time: 20 minutes
Servings: 6
Ingredients:
- ½ large onion, chopped

- 2 celery sticks, chopped
- ½ tablespoon ginger paste
- ½ cup green bell pepper
- 1 (½) tablespoon soy sauce
- ½ teaspoon parsley
- Salt and black pepper to taste
- ½ pound penne pasta, cooked
- 2 large carrots, diced
- ½ small leek, chopped
- 1 tablespoon olive oil
- ½ teaspoon garlic paste
- ½ tablespoon Worcester sauce
- ½ teaspoon coriander
- 1 cup water

Directions:
1. Heat olive oil in a wok on medium heat and add onions, garlic and ginger paste.
2. Sauté for about 3 minutes and stir in all bell pepper, celery sticks, carrots and leek.
3. Sauté for about 5 minutes and add the remaining ingredients except for pasta.
4. Cover the lid and cook for about 12 minutes.
5. Stir in the cooked pasta and dish out to serve warm.

Nutrition: Calories: 385 Total fats: 29g Protein: 26g Total carbs: 5g Fiber: 1g Net carbs: 4g

458.   Spaghetti in Spicy Tomato Sauce

Preparation time: 15 minutes
Cooking time: 40 minutes
Servings: 4
Ingredients:
- 1-pound dried spaghetti
- 1 red bell pepper, diced
- 4 garlic cloves, minced
- 1 teaspoon red pepper flakes, crushed
- 2 (14 ounces) cans of diced tomatoes
- 1 (6 ounces) can tomato paste
- 2 teaspoons vegan sugar, granulated
- 2 tablespoons olive oil
- 1 medium onion, diced
- 1 cup dry red wine
- 1 teaspoon dried thyme
- ½ teaspoon fennel seed, crushed
- 1 (½) cup coconut milk, full-fat
- Salt and black pepper to taste

Directions:

1. Boil water in a large pot and add pasta.
2. Cook according to the package directions and drain the pasta into a colander.
3. Dish out the pasta in a large serving bowl and add a dash of olive oil to prevent sticking.
4. Heat 2 tablespoons of olive oil over medium heat in a large pot and add garlic, onion and bell pepper.
5. Sauté for about 5 minutes and stir in the wine, thyme, fennel and red pepper flakes.
6. Allow simmering on high heat for about 5 minutes until the liquid is reduced by about half.
7. Add diced tomatoes and tomato paste and allow to simmer for about 20 minutes, stirring occasionally.
8. Stir in the coconut milk and sugar and simmer for about 10 more minutes.
9. Season with salt and black pepper and pour the sauce over the pasta.
10. Toss to coat well and dish out in plates to serve.

Nutrition: Calories: 313 Total fats: 25g Protein: 21g Total carbs: 1g Fiber: 0g Net carbs: 1g

459.   20 Minutes Vegetarian Pasta

Preparation time: 5 minutes
Cooking time: 16 minutes
Servings: 4
Ingredients:
- 3 shallots, chopped
- ¼ teaspoon red pepper flakes
- ¼ cup vegan parmesan cheese
- 2 tablespoons olive oil
- 2 garlic cloves, minced
- 8 ounces' spinach leaves
- 8 ounces' linguine pasta
- 1 pinch salt
- 1 pinch black pepper

Directions:
1. Boil salted water in a large pot and add pasta.
2. Cook for about 6 minutes and drain the pasta in a colander.
3. Heat olive oil over medium heat in a large skillet and add the shallots.
4. Cook for about 5 minutes until soft and caramelized and stir in the spinach, garlic, red pepper flakes, salt and black pepper.

5. Cook for about 5 minutes and add pasta and 2 ladles of pasta water.
6. Stir in the parmesan cheese and dish out in a bowl to serve.
Nutrition: Calories: 284 Total fats: 18g Protein: 29g Total carbs: 1.5g Fiber: 0g Net carbs: 1.5g

460. Creamy Vegan Pumpkin Pasta

Preparation time: 15 minutes
Cooking time: 5 minutes
Servings: 6
Ingredients:
• 1 tablespoon olive oil
• 1 cup raw cashews, soaked in water 4-8 hours, drained and rinsed
• 12 ounces dried penne pasta
• 1 cup pumpkin puree, canned
• 1 cup almond milk, plus more as needed
• 3 garlic cloves
• ¼ teaspoon ground nutmeg
• Fresh parsley for garnish
• 1 tablespoon lemon juice
• ¾ teaspoon salt
• 1 tablespoon fresh sage, chopped
Directions:
1. Boil salted water in a large pot and add pasta.
2. Cook according to the package directions and drain the pasta into a colander.
3. Dish out the pasta in a large serving bowl and add a dash of olive oil to prevent sticking.
4. Put the pumpkin, cashews, milk, lemon juice, garlic, salt and nutmeg into the food processor and blend until smooth.
5. Stir in the sauce and sage over the pasta and toss to coat well.
6. Garnish with fresh parsley and dish out to serve hot.
Nutrition: Calories: 431 Total fats: 31g Protein: 35g Total carbs: 3g Fiber: 0.5g Net carbs: 2.5g

461. Loaded Creamy Vegan Pesto Pasta

Preparation time: 15 minutes
Cooking time: 10 minutes

Servings: 6
Ingredients:
• ¼ onion, finely chopped
• 8 romaine lettuce leaves
• 1 celery stalk, thinly sliced
• ½ cup blue cheese, crumbled
• 1 tablespoon olive oil, plus a dash
• 1 cup almond milk, unflavored and unsweetened
• ½ cup vegan pesto
• 1 cup chickpeas, cooked
• 1 cup fresh arugula, packed
• 2 tablespoons lemon juice
• Salt and black pepper to taste
• 6 ounces' orecchiette pasta, dried
• 1 cup full-fat coconut milk
• 2 tablespoons whole wheat flour
• 1 (½) cup cherry tomato halved
• ½ cup Kalamata olives halved
• Red pepper flakes to taste
Directions:
1. Boil salted water in a large pot and add pasta.
2. Cook according to the package directions and drain the pasta into a colander.
3. Dish out the pasta in a large serving bowl and add a dash of olive oil to prevent sticking.
4. Put olive oil over medium heat in a large pot and whisk in the flour.
5. Cook for about 4 minutes, until the mixture begins to smell nutty and stir in the coconut milk and almond milk.
6. Let the sauce simmer for about 1 minute and add the chickpeas, olives and arugula.
7. Stir well and season with lemon juice, red pepper flakes, salt and black pepper.
8. Dish out onto plates and serve hot.
Nutrition: Calories: 220 Total fats: 10g Protein: 31g Total carbs: 1.5g Fiber: 0.5g Net carbs: 1g

462. Creamy Vegan Spinach Pasta

Preparation time: 20 minutes
Cooking time: 5 minutes
Servings: 4
Ingredients:
• 1 cup raw cashews, soaked in water for 8 hours
• 2 tablespoons lemon juice

- 1 tablespoon olive oil
- 1 (½) cup vegetable broth
- 2 tablespoons fresh dill, chopped
- Red pepper flakes to taste
- 10 ounces dried fusilli
- ½ cup almond milk, unflavored and unsweetened
- 2 tablespoons white miso paste
- 4 garlic cloves, divided
- 8 ounces' fresh spinach, finely chopped
- ¼ cup scallions, chopped
- Salt and black pepper to taste

Directions:

1. Boil salted water in a large pot and add pasta.
2. Cook according to the package directions and drain the pasta into a colander.
3. Dish out the pasta in a large serving bowl and add a dash of olive oil to prevent sticking.
4. Put the cashews, milk, miso, lemon juice and 1 garlic clove into the food processor and blend until smooth.
5. Put olive oil over medium heat in a large pot and add the remaining 3 cloves of garlic.
6. Sauté for about 1 minute and stir in the spinach and broth.
7. Raise the heat and allow to simmer for about 4 minutes until the spinach is bright green and wilted.
8. Stir in the pasta and cashew mixture and season with salt and black pepper.
9. Top with scallions and dill, and dish out onto plates to serve.

Nutrition: Calories: 94 Total fats: 10g Protein: 0g Total carbs: 1g Fiber: 0.3g Net carbs: 0.7g

463. Mom's Millet Muffins

Preparation time: 5 minutes
Cooking time: 20 minutes.
Servings: 8
Ingredients:
- 2 cups whole-wheat flour
- 1/2 cup millet
- 2 teaspoons baking powder
- 1/2 teaspoon salt
- 1 cup coconut milk
- 1/2 cup coconut oil, melted
- 1/2 cup agave nectar
- 1/2 teaspoon ground cinnamon

- 1/4 teaspoon ground cloves
- A pinch of grated nutmeg
- 1/2 cup dried apricots, chopped

Directions:

1. Begin by preheating your oven to 400°F. Lightly oil a muffin tin with nonstick oil.
2. In a mixing bowl, mix all dry ingredients. In a separate bowl, mix the wet ingredients. Stir the milk mixture into the flour mixture; mix just until evenly moist and do not over-mix your batter.
3. Fold in the apricots and scrape the batter into the prepared muffin cups.
4. Bake the muffins in the preheated oven for about 15 minutes, or until a tester inserted in the center of your muffin comes out dry and clean.
5. Let it stand for 10 minutes on a wire rack before unfolding and serving. Enjoy!

Nutrition: Calories: 367 Fat: 15.9g Carbs: 53.7g Protein: 6.5g

464. Mango Chickpea Wrap

Preparation time: 15 minutes
Cooking time: 0 minutes
Servings: 3
Ingredients:
- Three tablespoons tahini
- Zest and juice of 1 lime
- One tablespoon curry powder
- ¼ teaspoon of sea salt
- 3 to 4 tablespoons of water
- One can of chickpeas, washed and drained, or 1½ cups cooked
- 1 cup diced mango
- One red bell pepper, seeded and diced small
- ½ cup fresh cilantro, chopped
- Three large whole-grain wraps
- 1 to 2 cups shredded green leaf lettuce

Direction:

1. In a medium bowl, whisk together the tahini, lime zest and juice, curry powder, and salt until creamy and thick.
2. Pour 3-4 tablespoons of water to dilute slightly. Or you can process all of this in a blender. The flavor must be strong and salty, to flavor the whole salad.
3. Toss the chickpeas, mango, pepper, and cilantro with the tahini dressing.

4. Pour the salad into the center of the rolls, garnish with chopped lettuce, then roll up and enjoy.
Nutrition: Calories: 437 Total fats: 8g Carbs: 79g Fiber: 12g Protein: 15g

465.   Black Bean Pizza

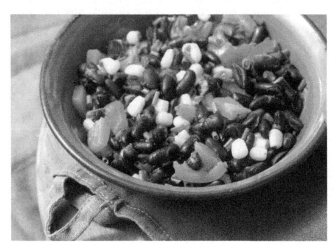

Preparation time: 10 minutes
Cooking time: 10 minutes
Servings: 2

Ingredients:
*   Two prebaked pizza crusts
*   ½ cup Spicy Black Bean Dip
*   One tomato, thinly sliced
*   Pinch freshly ground black pepper
*   One carrot, grated
*   Pinch sea salt
*   One red onion, thinly sliced
*   One avocado, sliced

Direction:
1. Preheat the oven to 400 ° F.
2. Arrange the two crusts on a large baking sheet. Spread half of the spicy black bean sauce over each pizza crust. Then lay the tomato slices with a pinch of pepper if you like.
3. Sprinkle the grated carrot with sea salt and massage it lightly with your hands. Spread the carrot over the tomato and then add the onion.
4. Put the pizzas in the oven for 10-20 minutes or until they are ready according to your taste.
5. Top the cooked pizzas with sliced avocado and another sprinkle of pepper.
Nutrition: Calories: 379 Total fats: 13g Carbs: 59g Fiber: 15g Protein: 13g

Chapter 12. Vegetables

466. Thai Tofu Broth

Preparation time: 5 minutes
Cooking time: 15 minutes
Servings: 4 servings
Ingredients:
• 1 cup rice noodles
• ½ sliced onion
• 6 oz. drained, pressed and cubed tofu
• ¼ cup sliced scallions
• ½ cup water
• ½ cup chestnuts
• ½ cup rice almond milk
• 1 tbsp. lime juice
• 1 tbsp. coconut oil
• ½ finely sliced chili
• 1 cup snow peas
Directions:
1.   Heat the oil in a wok on a high heat and then sauté the tofu until brown on each side.
2.   Add the onion and sauté for 2-3 minutes.
3.   Add the rice almond milk and water to the wok until bubbling.
4.   Lower to medium heat and add the noodles, chili and water chestnuts.
5.   Allow to simmer for 10-15 minutes and then add the sugar snap peas for 5 minutes.
6.   Serve with a sprinkle of scallions.
Nutrition: Calories: 304 kcal; Total Fat: 13 g; Saturated Fat: 0 g; Cholesterol: 0 mg; Sodium: 36 mg; Total Carbs: 38 g; Fiber: 0 g; Sugar: 0 g; Protein: 9 g

467. Delicious Vegetarian Lasagne

Preparation time: 10 minutes
Cooking time: 1 hour
Servings: 4 servings
Ingredients:
• 1 tsp. basil
• 1 tbsp. olive oil
• ½ sliced red pepper
• 3 lasagna sheets
• ½ diced red onion
• ¼ tsp. black pepper
• 1 cup rice almond milk
• 1 minced garlic clove
• 1 cup sliced eggplant
• ½ sliced zucchini
• ½ pack soft tofu
• 1 tsp. oregano
Directions:
1.   Preheat oven to 325°F/Gas Mark 3.
2.   Slice zucchini, eggplant and pepper into vertical strips.
3.   Add the rice almond milk and tofu to a food processor and blitz until smooth. Set aside.
4.   Heat the oil in a skillet over medium heat and add the onions and garlic for 3-4 minutes or until soft.
5.   Sprinkle in the herbs and pepper and allow to stir through for 5-6 minutes until hot.
6.   Into a lasagne or suitable oven dish, layer 1 lasagna sheet, then 1/3 the eggplant, followed by 1/3 zucchini, then 1/3 pepper before pouring over 1/3 of tofu white sauce.
7.   Repeat for the next 2 layers, finishing with the white sauce.
8.   Add to the oven for 40-50 minutes or until veg is soft and easily be sliced into servings.
Nutrition: Calories: 235 kcal; Total Fat: 9 g; Saturated Fat: 0 g; Cholesterol: 0 mg; Sodium: 35 mg; Total Carbs: 10 g; Fiber: 0 g; Sugar: 0 g; Protein: 5 g

468. Chili Tofu Noodles

Preparation time: 5 minutes
Cooking Time: 15 minutes
Servings: 4 servings
Ingredients:
• ½ diced red chili
• 2 cups rice noodles
• ½ juiced lime
• 6 oz. pressed and cubed silken firm tofu
• 1 tsp. grated fresh ginger
• 1 tbsp. coconut oil
• 1 cup green beans
• 1 minced garlic clove
Directions:
1.   Steam the green beans for 10-12 minutes or according to package directions and drain.
2.   Cook the noodles in a pot of boiling water for 10-15 minutes or according to package directions.
3.   Meanwhile, heat a wok or skillet on a high heat and add coconut oil.

4.   Now add the tofu, chili flakes, garlic and ginger and sauté for 5-10 minutes.
5.   Drain the noodles and add to the wok along with the green beans and lime juice.
6.   Toss to coat.
7.   Serve hot!
Nutrition: Calories: 246 kcal; Total Fat: 12 g; Saturated Fat: 0 g; Cholesterol: 0 mg; Sodium: 25 mg; Total Carbs: 28 g; Fiber: 0 g; Sugar: 0 g; Protein: 10 g

469.   Curried Cauliflower

Preparation time: 5 minutes
Cooking time: 20 minutes
Servings: 4 servings
Ingredients:
*   1 tsp. turmeric
*   1 diced onion
*   1 tbsp. chopped fresh cilantro
*   1 tsp. cumin
*   ½ diced chili
*   ½ cup water
*   1 minced garlic clove
*   1 tbsp. coconut oil
*   1 tsp. garam masala
*   2 cups cauliflower florets
Directions:
1.   Add the oil to a skillet on medium heat.
2.   Sauté the onion and garlic for 5 minutes until soft.
3.   Add the cumin, turmeric and garam masala and stir to release the aromas.
4.   Now add the chili to the pan along with the cauliflower.
5.   Stir to coat.
6.   Pour in the water and reduce the heat to a simmer for 15 minutes.
7.   Garnish with cilantro to serve.
Nutrition: Calories: 108 kcal; Total Fat: 7 g; Saturated Fat: 0 g; Cholesterol: 0 mg; Sodium: 35 mg; Total Carbs: 11 g; Fiber: 0 g; Sugar: 0 g; Protein: 2 g

470.   Chinese Tempeh Stir Fry

Preparation time: 5 minutes
Cooking time: 15 minutes
Servings: 2 servings
Ingredients:
*   2 oz. sliced tempeh
*   1 cup cooked rice
*   1 minced garlic clove
*   ½ cup green onions
*   1 tsp. minced fresh ginger
*   1 tbsp. coconut oil
*   ½ cup corn
Directions:
1.   Heat the oil in a skillet or wok on a high heat and add the garlic and ginger.
2.   Sauté for 1 minute.
3.   Now add the tempeh and cook for 5-6 minutes before adding the corn for a further 10 minutes.
4.   Now add the green onions and serve over rice.
Nutrition: Calories: 304 kcal; Total Fat: 4 g; Saturated Fat: 0 g; Cholesterol: 0 mg; Sodium: 91 mg; Total Carbs: 35 g; Fiber: 0 g; Sugar: 0 g; Protein: 10 g

471.   Egg White Frittata with Penne

Preparation time: 15 minutes
Cooking time: 30 minutes
Servings: 4 servings
Ingredients:
*   Egg whites- 6
*   Rice almond milk – ¼ cup
*   Chopped fresh parsley – 1 tbsp.
*   Chopped fresh thyme – 1 tsp
*   Chopped fresh chives – 1 tsp
*   Ground black pepper
*   Olive oil – 2 tsp.
*   Small sweet onion – ¼, chopped
*   Minced garlic – 1 tsp
*   Boiled and chopped red bell pepper – ½ cup
*   Cooked penne – 2 cups
Directions:
1.   Preheat the oven to 350f.

2. In a bowl, whisk together the egg whites, rice almond milk, parsley, thyme, chives, and pepper.

3. Heat the oil in a skillet.

4. Sauté the onion, garlic, red pepper for 4 minutes or until they are softened.

5. Add the cooked penne to the skillet.

6. Pour the egg mixture over the pasta and shake the pan to coat the pasta.

7. Leave the skillet on the heat for 1 minute to set the frittata's bottom and then transfer the skillet to the oven.

8. Bake the frittata for 25 minutes, or until it is set and golden brown.

9. Serve.

Nutrition: Calories: 170 kcal; Total Fat: 3 g; Saturated Fat: 0 g; Cholesterol: 0 mg; Sodium: 90 mg; Total Carbs: 25 g; Fiber: 0 g; Sugar: 0 g; Protein: 10 g

472. Vegetable Fried Rice

Preparation time: 20 minutes
Cooking time: 20 minutes
Servings: 6 servings
Ingredients:
- Olive oil – 1 tbsp.
- Sweet onion – ½, chopped
- Grated fresh ginger – 1 tbsp.
- Minced garlic - 2 tsp
- Sliced carrots – 1 cup
- Chopped eggplant – ½ cup
- Peas – ½ cup
- Green beans – ½ cup, cut into 1-inch pieces
- Chopped fresh cilantro – 2 tbsp.
- Cooked rice – 3 cups

Directions:
1. Heat the olive oil in a skillet.

2. Sauté the ginger, onion, and garlic for 3 minutes or until softened.

3. Stir in carrot, eggplant, green beans, and peas and sauté for 3 minutes more.

4. Add cilantro and rice.

5. Sauté, constantly stirring, for about 10 minutes or until the rice is heated through.

6. Serve.

Nutrition: Calories: 189 kcal; Total Fat: 7 g; Saturated Fat: 0 g; Cholesterol: 0 mg; Sodium: 13 mg; Total Carbs: 28 g; Fiber: 0 g; Sugar: 0 g; Protein: 6 g

473. Couscous Burgers

Preparation time: 20 minutes
Cooking time: 10 minutes
Servings: 4 servings
Ingredients:
- chickpeas – ½ cup
- Chopped fresh cilantro – 2 tbsp.
- Chopped fresh parsley
- Lemon juice - 1 tbsp.
- Lemon zest – 2 tsp
- Minced garlic – 1 tsp
- Cooked couscous – 2 ½ cups
- Eggs – 2, lightly beaten
- Olive oil – 2 tbsp.

Directions:
1. Put the cilantro, chickpeas, parsley, lemon juice, lemon zest, and garlic in a food processor and pulse until a paste form.

2. Transfer the chickpea mixture to a bowl, and add the eggs and couscous. Mix well.

3. Chill the mixture in the refrigerator for 1 hour.

4. Form the couscous mixture into 4 patties.

5. Heat olive oil in a skillet.

6. Place the patties in the skillet, 2 at a time, gently pressing them down with the fork of a spatula.

7. Cook for 5 minutes or until golden, and flip the patties over.

8. Cook the other side for 5 minutes and transfer the cooked burgers to a plate covered with a paper towel.

9. Repeat with the remaining 2 burgers.

Nutrition: Calories: 242 kcal; Total Fat: 10 g; Saturated Fat: 0 g; Cholesterol: 0 mg; Sodium: 43 mg; Total Carbs: 29 g; Fiber: 0 g; Sugar: 0 g; Protein: 9 g

474. Marinated Tofu Stir-Fry

Preparation time: 20 minutes
Cooking time: 20 minutes
Servings: 4 servings
Ingredients:
- For the tofu:
- Lemon juice – 1 tbsp.
- Minced garlic – 1 tsp
- Grated fresh ginger – 1 tsp

- Pinch red pepper flakes
- Extra-firm tofu- 5 ounces, pressed well and cubed
- For the stir-fry:
- Olive oil – 1 tbsp.
- Cauliflower florets – ½ cup
- Thinly sliced carrots – ½ cup
- Julienned red pepper – ½ cup
- Fresh green beans – ½ cup
- Cooked white rice – 2 cups

Directions:

1. In a bowl, mix the lemon juice, garlic, ginger, and red pepper flakes.
2. Add the tofu and toss to coat.
3. Place the bowl in the refrigerator and marinate for 2 hours.
4. To make the stir-fry, heat the oil in a skillet.
5. Sauté the tofu for 8 minutes or until it is lightly browned and heated through.
6. Add the carrots, and cauliflower and sauté for 5 minutes. Stirring and tossing constantly.
7. Add the red pepper and green beans, sauté for 3 minutes more.
8. Serve over white rice.

Nutrition: Calories: 190 kcal; Total Fat: 6 g; Saturated Fat: 0 g; Cholesterol: 0 mg; Sodium: 22 mg; Total Carbs: 30 g; Fiber: 0 g; Sugar: 0 g; Protein: 6 g

475. Curried Veggie Stir-Fry

Preparation Time: 20 minutes
Cooking Time: 10 minutes
Servings: 6
Ingredients:
- 2 tablespoons of extra-virgin olive oil
- 1 onion, chopped
- 4 garlic cloves, minced
- 4 cups of frozen stir-fry vegetables
- 1 cup unsweetened full-fat coconut almond milk
- 1 cup of water
- 2 tablespoons of green curry paste

Directions:

1. In a wok or non-stick, heat the olive oil over medium-high heat. Stir-fry the onion and garlic for 2 to 3 minutes, until fragrant.

2. Add the frozen stir-fry vegetables and continue to cook for 3 to 4 minutes longer, or until the vegetables are hot.
3. Meanwhile, in a small bowl, combine coconut almond milk, water, and curry paste. Stir until the paste dissolves.
4. Add the broth mixture to the wok and cook for another 2 to 3 minutes, or until the sauce has reduced slightly and all the vegetables are crisp-tender.
5. Serve over couscous or hot cooked rice.

Nutrition: Calories: 293 Total fat: 18g Saturated fat: 10g Sodium: 247mg Phosphorus: 138mg Potassium: 531mg Carbohydrates: 28g Fiber: 7g Protein: 7g Sugar: 4g

476. Chilaquiles

Preparation Time: 20 minutes
Cooking Time: 20 minutes
Servings: 4
Ingredients:
- 3 (8-inch) corn tortillas, cut into strips
- 2 tablespoons of extra-virgin olive oil
- 12 tomatillos, papery covering removed, chopped
- 3 tablespoons for freshly squeezed lime juice
- 1/8 teaspoon of salt
- 1/8 teaspoon of freshly ground black pepper
- 4 large egg whites
- 2 large eggs
- 2 tablespoons of water
- 1 cup of shredded pepper jack cheese

Directions:

1. In a dry nonstick skillet, toast the tortilla strips over medium heat until they are crisp, tossing the pan and stirring occasionally. This should take 4 to 6 minutes. Remove the strips from the pan and set aside.
2. In the same skillet, heat the olive oil over medium heat and add the tomatillos, lime juice, salt, and pepper. Cook and frequently stir for about 8 to 10 minutes until the tomatillos break down and form a sauce. Transfer the sauce to a bowl and set aside.
3. In a small bowl, beat the egg whites, eggs, and water and add to the skillet. Cook the eggs for 3 to 4 minutes, stirring occasionally until they are set and cooked to 160°F.
4. Preheat the oven to 400°F.

5. Toss the tortilla strips in the tomatillo sauce and place in a casserole dish. Top with the scrambled eggs and cheese.

6. Bake for 10 to 15 minutes, or until the cheese starts to brown. Serve.

Nutrition: Calories: 312 Total fat: 20g Saturated fat: 8g Sodium: 345mg Phosphorus: 280mg Potassium: 453mg Carbohydrates: 19g Fiber: 3g Protein: 15g Sugar: 5g

477. Roasted Veggie Sandwiches

Preparation Time: 20 minutes
Cooking Time: 35 minutes
Servings: 6
Ingredients:
• 3 bell peppers, assorted colors, sliced
• 1 cup of sliced yellow summer squash
• 1 red onion, sliced
• 2 tablespoons of extra-virgin olive oil
• 2 tablespoons of balsamic vinegar
• 1/8 teaspoon of salt
• 1/8 teaspoon of freshly ground black pepper
• 3 large whole-wheat pita breads, halved
Directions:
1. Preheat the oven to 400°F.
2. Prepare a parchment paper and line it in a rimmed baking sheet.
3. Spread the bell peppers, squash, and onion on the prepared baking sheet. Sprinkle with the olive oil, vinegar, salt, and pepper.
4. Roast for 30 to 40 minutes, turning the vegetables with a spatula once during cooking, until they are tender and light golden brown.
5. Pile the vegetables into the pita breads and serve.

Nutrition: Calories: 182 Total fat: 5g Saturated fat: 1g Sodium: 234mg Phosphorus: 106mg Potassium: 289mg Carbohydrates: 31g Fiber: 4g Protein: 5g Sugar: 6g

478. Grilled squash

Preparation time: 10 minutes
Cooking time: 6 minutes
Servings: 8

Ingredients
• 4 zucchinis, rinsed, drained and sliced
• 4 crookneck squash, rinsed, drained and sliced
• Cooking spray
• 1/4 teaspoon garlic powder
• 1/4 teaspoon black pepper
Directions
1. Arrange squash on a baking sheet.
2. Spray with oil.
3. Season with garlic powder and pepper.
4. Grill for 3 minutes per side or until tender but not too soft.

Nutrition: calories 17 protein 1 g carbohydrates 3 g fat 0 g cholesterol 0 mg sodium 6 mg potassium 262 mg phosphorus 39 mg calcium 16 mg fiber 1.1 g

479. Pasta Fagioli

Preparation Time: 25 minutes
Cooking Time: 25 minutes
Servings: 6
Ingredients:
• 1 (15-ounce) can low-sodium great northern beans, drained and rinsed, divided
• 2 cups frozen peppers and onions, thawed, divided
• 5 cups low-sodium vegetable broth
• 1/8 teaspoon salt
• 1/8 teaspoon freshly ground black pepper
• 1 cup whole-grain orecchiette pasta
• 2 tablespoons extra-virgin olive oil
• 1/3 cup grated Parmesan cheese
Directions:
1. In a large saucepan, place the beans and cover with water. Bring to a boil over high heat and boil for 10 minutes. Drain the beans.
2. In a food processor or blender, combine 1/3 cup of beans and 1/3 cup of thawed peppers and onions. Process until smooth.
3. In the same saucepan, combine the pureed mixture, the remaining 12/3 cups of peppers and onions, the remaining beans, the broth, and the salt and pepper and bring to a simmer.
4. Add the pasta to the saucepan. Make sure to stir it and bring it to boil, reduce the heat to low, and simmer for 8 to 10 minutes, or until the pasta is tender.

5. Serve drizzled with olive oil and topped with Parmesan cheese.

Nutrition: Calories: 245 Total fat: 7g Saturated fat: 2g Sodium: 269mg Phosphorus: 188mg Potassium: 592mg Carbohydrates: 36g Fiber: 7g Protein: 12g Sugar: 4g

480. Roasted Peach Open-Face Sandwich

Preparation Time: 5 minutes
Cooking Time: 15 minutes
Servings: 4
Ingredients:
• 2 fresh peaches, peeled and sliced
• 1 tablespoon of extra-virgin olive oil
• 1 tablespoon of freshly squeezed lemon juice
• 1/8 teaspoon of salt
• 1/8 teaspoon of freshly ground black pepper
• 4 ounces of cream cheese, at room temperature
• 2 teaspoons of fresh thyme leaves
• 4 bread slices

Directions:
1. Preheat the oven to 400°F.
2. Arrange the peaches on a rimmed baking sheet. Brush them with olive oil on both sides.
3. Roast the peaches for 10 to 15 minutes, until they are lightly golden brown around the edges. Sprinkle with lemon juice, salt, and pepper.
4. In a small bowl, combine the cream cheese and thyme and mix well.
5. Toast the bread. Get the toasted bread and spread it with the cream cheese mixture. Top with the peaches and serve.

Nutrition: Calories: 250 Total fat: 13g Saturated fat: 6g Sodium: 376mg Phosphorus: 163mg Potassium: 260mg Carbohydrates: 28g Fiber: 3g Protein: 6g Sugar: 8g

481. Spicy Corn and Rice Burritos

Preparation Time: 10 minutes
Cooking Time: 20 minutes

Servings: 4
Ingredients:
• 3 tablespoons of extra-virgin olive oil, divided
• 1 (10-ounce) package of frozen cooked rice
• 1½ cups of frozen yellow corn
• 1 tablespoon of chili powder
• 1 cup of shredded pepper jack cheese
• 4 large or 6 small corn tortillas

Directions:
1. Put the skillet in over medium heat and put 2 tablespoons of olive oil. Add the rice, corn, and chili powder and cook for 4 to 6 minutes, or until the ingredients are hot.
2. Transfer the ingredients from the pan into a medium bowl. Let cool for 15 minutes.
3. Stir the cheese into the rice mixture.
4. Heat the tortillas using the directions from the package to make them pliable. Fill the corn tortillas with the rice mixture, then roll them up.
5. At this point, you can serve them as is, or you can fry them first. Heat the remaining tablespoon of olive oil in a large skillet. Fry the burritos, seam-side down at first, turning once, until they are brown and crisp, about 4 to 6 minutes per side, then serve.

Nutrition: Calories: 386 Total fat: 21g Saturated fat: 7g Sodium: 510mg Phosphorus: 304mg Potassium: 282mg Carbohydrates: 41g Fiber: 4g Protein: 11g Sugar: 2g

482. Crust less Cabbage Quiche

Preparation Time: 10 minutes
Cooking Time: 40 minutes
Servings: 6
Ingredients:
• Olive oil cooking spray
• 2 tablespoons of extra-virgin olive oil
• 3 cups of coleslaw blend with carrots
• 3 large eggs, beaten
• 3 large egg whites, beaten
• ½ cup of half-and-half
• 1 teaspoon of dried dill weed
• 1/8 teaspoon of salt
• 1/8 teaspoon of freshly ground black pepper
• 1 cup of grated Swiss cheese

Directions:

1.   Preheat the oven to 350°F. Spray pie plate (9-inch) with cooking spray and set aside.
2.   In a skillet, put an oil and put it in medium heat. Add the coleslaw mix and cook for 4 to 6 minutes, stirring, until the cabbage is tender. Transfer the vegetables from the pan to a medium bowl to cool.
3.   Meanwhile, in another medium bowl, combine the eggs and egg whites, half-and-half, dill, salt, and pepper and beat to combine.
4.   Stir the cabbage mixture into the egg mixture and pour into the prepared pie plate.
5.   Sprinkle with the cheese.
6.   Bake for 30 to 35 minutes, or until the mixture is puffed, set, and light golden brown. Let stand for 5 minutes, then slice to serve.
Nutrition: Calories: 203 Total fat: 16g Saturated fat: 6g Sodium: 321mg Phosphorus: 169mg Potassium: 155mg Carbohydrates: 5g Fiber: 1g Protein: 11g Sugar: 4g

483.   Vegetable Confetti

Preparation Time: 25 minutes
Cooking Time: 15 minutes
Servings: 1
Ingredients:
- ½ red bell pepper
- ½ green pepper, boiled and chopped
- 4 scallions, thinly sliced
- ½ tsp. of ground cumin
- 3 tbsp. of vegetable oil
- 1 ½ tbsp. of white wine vinegar
- Black pepper to taste
Directions:
1.   Join all fixings and blend well.
2.   Chill in the fridge.
3.   You can include a large portion of slashed jalapeno pepper for an increasingly fiery blend
Nutrition: Calories: 230 Fat: 25 Fiber: 3g Carbs: 24 Protein: 43g

484.   Creamy Veggie Casserole

Preparation Time: 25 minutes
Cooking Time: 35 minutes

Servings: 4
Ingredients:
- 1/3 cup extra-virgin olive oil, divided
- 1 onion, chopped
- 2 tablespoons flour
- 3 cups low-sodium vegetable broth
- 3 cups frozen California blend vegetables
- 1 cup crushed crisp rice cereal
Directions:
1.   Preheat the oven to 375°F.
2.   Next is heat 2 tablespoons of olive oil in a large skillet over medium heat. Add the onion and cook for 3 to 4 minutes, stirring, until the onion is tender.
3.   Add the flour and stir for 2 minutes.
4.   Add the broth to the saucepan, stirring for 3 to 4 minutes, or until the sauce starts to thicken.
5.   Add the vegetables to the saucepan. Simmer and cook until vegetables are tender (for six to eight minutes).
6.   When the vegetables are done, pour the mixture into a 3-quart casserole dish.
7.   Sprinkle the vegetables with the crushed cereal.
8.   Bake for 20 to 25 minutes or until the cereal is golden brown and the filling is bubbling. Let cool for 5 minutes and serve.
Nutrition: Calories: 234 Total fat: 18g Saturated fat: 3 Sodium: 139mg Phosphorus: 21mg Potassium: 210mg Carbohydrates: 16g Fiber: 3g Protein: 3g Sugar: 5g

485.   Vegetable Green Curry

Preparation Time: 20 minutes
Cooking Time: 20 minutes
Servings: 6
Ingredients:
- 2 tablespoons extra-virgin olive oil
- 1 head broccoli, cut into florets
- 1 bunch asparagus, cut into 2-inch lengths
- 3 tablespoons water
- 2 tablespoons green curry paste
- 1 medium eggplant
- 1/8 teaspoon salt
- 1/8 teaspoon freshly ground black pepper
- 2/3 cup plain whole-almond milk yogurt
Directions:

1. Put olive oil in a large saucepan in a medium heat. Add the broccoli and stir-fry for 5 minutes. Add the asparagus and stir-fry for another 3 minutes.
2. Meanwhile, in a small bowl, combine the water with the green curry paste.
3. Add the eggplant, curry-water mixture, salt, and pepper. Stir-fry or until vegetables are all tender.
4. Add the yogurt. Heat through but avoid simmering. Serve.

Nutrition: Calories: 113 Total fat: 6g Saturated fat: 1gSodium: 174mg Phosphorus: 117mg Potassium: 569mg Carbohydrates: 13g Fiber: 6g Protein: 5g Sugar: 7g

486. Zucchini Bowl

Preparation Time: 10 minutes
Cooking Time: 20 minutes
Servings: 4

Ingredients:
- 1 onion, chopped
- 3 zucchini, cut into medium chunks
- 2 tablespoons coconut almond milk
- 2 garlic cloves, minced
- 4 cups chicken stock
- 2 tablespoons coconut oil
- Pinch of salt
- Black pepper to taste

Directions:
1. Take a pot and place it over medium heat
2. Add oil and let it heat up
3. Add zucchini, garlic, onion, and stir
4. Cook for 5 minutes
5. Add stock, salt, pepper, and stir
6. Bring to a boil and lower down the heat
7. Simmer for 20 minutes.
8. Remove heat and add coconut almond milk

9. Use an immersion blender until smooth
10. Ladle into soup bowls and serve
11. Enjoy!

Nutrition: Calories: 160 Fat: 2g Carbohydrates: 4g Protein: 7g

487. Nice Coconut Haddock

Preparation Time: 10 minutes
Cooking Time: 12 minutes
Servings: 3

Ingredients:
- 4 haddock fillets, 5 ounces each, boneless
- 2 tablespoons coconut oil, melted
- 1 cup coconut, shredded and unsweetened
- ¼ cup hazelnuts, ground
- Salt to taste

Directions:
1. Preheat your oven to 400 °F
2. Line a baking sheet with parchment paper
3. Keep it on the side
4. Pat fish fillets with a paper towel and season with salt
5. Take a bowl and stir in hazelnuts and shredded coconut
6. Drag fish fillets through the coconut mix until both sides are coated well
7. Transfer to a baking dish
8. Brush with coconut oil
9. Bake for about 12 minutes until flaky
10. Serve and enjoy!

Nutrition: Calories: 299 Fat: 24g Carbohydrates: 1g Protein: 20g

Chapter 13. Soups & Stews

488.   Bean and Cabbage Soup

Preparation Time: 20 minutes
Cooking Time: 2 hours
Servings: 4
Ingredients:
- 200 grams of cabbage leaves
- 150 grams of beans already soaked
- 1 carrot
- 1 shallot
- 100 grams of tomato pulp
- 4 bay leaves
- 1 1/2 liters of vegetable broth
- Olive oil to taste
- Salt and pepper to taste

Directions:
1. Add broth to the saucepan and add the beans.
2. Bring to a boil and continue cooking for another 20 minutes.
3. Meanwhile, wash the cabbage leaves, dry them, and cut them into strips.
4. Peel off the carrot, wash it, and then cut it into cubes.
5. Peel and wash the shallot and then chop it.
6. Wash and dry the bay leaves.
7. Add the cabbage to the beans after 20 minutes.
8. Stir and, after 5 minutes, add the carrot, shallot, bay leaves, and tomato pulp.
9. Put salt and pepper, stir, and continue cooking for another 30 minutes.
10. After 30 minutes, turn off and remove the bay leaves.
11. Put the soup on plates, season with oil and pepper, and serve.

Nutrition: Calories: 164 Fat: 4g Carbohydrates: 30g Protein: 11g

489.   Soup with Red Onion

Preparation Time: 20 minutes
Cooking Time: 40 minutes
Servings: 4
Ingredients:
- 200 grams of cabbage
- 2 carrots
- 1 potato
- 2 sticks of celery
- 1 red onion
- 100 grams of beans already boiled
- 100 grams of tomato pulp
- 2 liters of vegetable broth
- Salt and pepper to taste
- Olive oil to taste

Directions:
1. Wash and dry the cabbage leaves. Keep only the tenderest leaves and then cut them into strips.
2. Clean and peel the carrot and then cut it into cubes.
3. Peel the potato, wash it well under running water, and then cut it into cubes.
4. Remove the celery stalk and the side filaments. Wash it and chop it.
5. Peel the onion, wash it, and then slice it.
6. Add vegetable broth in a saucepan, and as soon as it starts to boil, add the potato, cabbage, carrots, and celery.
7. Stir, cook for more minutes, and then add the tomato pulp.
8. Season with salt, pepper, and cook for 30 minutes.
9. Now add the beans, stir, and continue cooking for another 10 minutes.
10. Turn off once cooked and put the soup on serving plates.
11. Season with a drizzle of oil, sprinkle with onion, and serve.

Nutrition: Calories: 80 Fat: 3g Carbohydrates: 12g Protein: 2g

490.   Basil Soup

Preparation Time: 15 minutes
Cooking Time: 40 minutes
Servings: 4
Ingredients:
- 2 carrots
- 1 onion
- 1 potato
- 2 liters of hot vegetable broth
- 8 basil leaves
- Olive oil to taste
- Salt and pepper to taste

Directions:
1. Wash and peel off the carrots, then cut them into slices.
2. Peel and wash the potato and then cut it into cubes.
3. Peel and wash the onion and then cut it into thin slices.
4. Pour two tablespoons of olive oil into a saucepan and as soon as it is hot, add the onion.
5. Sauté for 2 minutes and then add the carrots and potato.
6. Season with salt and pepper, stir and then add the broth.
7. Put a cover and cook for 30 minutes over medium heat.
8. Meanwhile, wash and dry the basil leaves and then cut them into small pieces.
9. After the cooking time, turn off and put the soup on the plates.
10. Season with a drizzle of oil, sprinkle with basil, and serve.

Nutrition: Calories: 210 Fat: 10g Carbohydrates: 14g Protein: 2g

491.   Potato and Carrot Soup

Preparation Time: 20 minutes
Cooking Time: 20 minutes
Servings: 4
Ingredients:
400 grams of potatoes
- 300 grams of carrots
- 1 onion
- 1 1/2 liters of vegetable broth
- 40 grams of soy butter
- 2 sprigs of chopped parsley
- Salt and pepper to taste

Directions:
1. Peel off and wash the potatoes. Then cut them into cubes.
2. Peel off and wash the carrots. Then cut them into slices.
3. Peel and wash the onion and then chop it.
4. Put the vegetable broth in a saucepan and bring to a boil.
5. Put the carrots, potatoes, onion, and season with salt and pepper.
6. Cook for 20 minutes over medium heat.
7. After 20 minutes, turn off and blend everything with an immersion blender.
8. Put the butter cut into chunks and stir until melted.
9. Also, add the parsley and mix.
10. Now put the soup on the serving plates and serve.

Nutrition: Calories: 147 Fat: 4g Carbohydrates: 16g Protein: 0g

492.   Chickpea, Leek, and Rosemary Soup

Preparation Time: 15 minutes+2 hours to rest
Cooking Time: 1 hour and 15 minutes
Servings: 4
Ingredients:
- 200 grams of chickpeas
- 3 leeks
- 2 sprigs of rosemary
- The grated rind of one lemon
- 2 tablespoon Olive oil
- Salt and pepper to taste

Directions:
1. Start by putting the chickpeas in a bowl with cold water. Let it sit for 2 hours.
2. Remove the root and the green part of the leeks, wash them, and cut them into thin slices.
3. Put oil in a saucepan, and as soon as it is hot, put the leeks to dry.
4. Cook them for about 10 minutes and then add the chickpeas. Mix and season with salt and pepper.
5. Now add 1 liter of water and bring to a boil.

6. Wash the rosemary, put it in the pot with the chickpeas, and continue cooking for another 60 minutes.
7. When cooked, remove the rosemary, and take half of the soup.
8. Put it in the blender glass and blend until thick and creamy.
9. Put it back in the pot with the rest of the chickpeas and add the grated lemon zest.
10. Stir to flavor well. Put the soup on the plates and serve.
Nutrition: Calories: 225 Fat: 7g Carbohydrates: 53g Protein: 11g

493. Zucchini and Spinach Soup

Preparation Time: 10 minutes
Cooking Time: 30 minutes
Servings: 4
Ingredients:
- 600 grams of zucchini
- 500 grams of spinach
- 2 tomatoes
- 1 carrot
- 1 onion
- 8 basil leaves
- Olive oil to taste
- Salt and pepper to taste
Directions:
1. Wash the zucchinis and then cut them into thin slices.
2. Wash and dry the spinach and then cut them into thin strips.
3. Peel and wash the onion and carrot and then chop them.
4. Wash and dry the basil leaves.
5. Clean the tomatoes and then cut into cubes.
6. Pour a liter of water into a saucepan and put onion, carrots, tomatoes, spinach, and zucchini inside.
7. Let it boil and season with salt and pepper. Continue cooking for another 25 minutes.
8. After 25 minutes, drain some of the vegetables and put them in the glass of the blender together with the basil leaves. Blend well to get a smooth and homogeneous mixture.
9. Put the vegetable smoothie in the pot and bring it to a boil again.

10. At this point, turn off, put the soup on the plates, season with a drizzle of oil, and serve.
Nutrition: Calories: 133 Fat: 4g Carbohydrates: 21g Protein: 6g

494. Quinoa and Spinach Soup

Preparation Time: 30 minutes
Cooking Time: 50 minutes
Servings: 4
Ingredients:
- 150 grams of quinoa
- 8 mushrooms
- 1 clove of garlic
- 100 grams of spinach
- 2 liters of vegetable broth
- 2 teaspoons of grated ginger
- 1 onion
- 1 carrot
- 150 grams of tofu
- Salt and pepper to taste
- Olive oil
Directions:
1. Wash and dry the mushrooms and then cut them into slices.
2. Bring the vegetable broth to a boil and then add the mushrooms and ginger.
3. Cook for 20 minutes and then remove the mushrooms and turn them off.
4. Peel the onion and carrots and then chop them.
5. Wash the spinach thoroughly and then pat dry.
6. Warm tablespoon of olive oil in a saucepan. Then put the onion and carrots to fry for 10 minutes.
7. Now add the vegetable broth, and when it starts to boil, add the quinoa.
8. Cook over medium heat for 20 minutes.
9. Once the quinoa is cooked, put in the spinach, season with salt and pepper, then mix well. Let it sit for a minute once done.
10. Meanwhile, pat the tofu with absorbent paper and then cut it into cubes.
Nutrition: Calories: 110 Fat: 3.5g Carbohydrates: 17g Protein: 2g

495. Board Beans Cream

Preparation Time: 15 minutes
Cooking Time: 30 minutes
Servings: 4
Ingredients:
- 600 grams of fresh broad beans
- 800 ml of vegetable broth
- 1 shallot
- A tablespoon of cumin seeds
- 2 tablespoons Olive oil
- Salt and pepper to taste

Directions:
1. Shell the beans, remove the skin and then wash them.
2. Peel and wash the shallot and then chop it.
3. Heat olive oil in a saucepan.
4. .As soon as it is hot, brown the shallot for a couple of minutes.
5. .Add the broad beans and cumin and sauté them for 10 minutes, stirring often.
6. Now add the vegetable broth and continue cooking for another 15 minutes.
7. Lower the heat and blend everything with an immersion blender.
8. Cook for another 2 minutes, stirring constantly.
9. Turn off, put the cream on the plates, season with olive oil, and serve.
Nutrition: Calories: 159 Fat: 3.8g Carbohydrates: 23g Protein: 8g

496. Peas Cream

Preparation Time: 15 minutes
Cooking Time: 25 minutes
Servings: 4
Ingredients:
- 300 grams of peas
- 1 onion
- 5 mint leaves
- Salt and pepper to taste
- 1 tablespoon Olive oil

Directions:
1. Peel and wash the onion, then chop it.
2. Wash the peas under running water and then let them drain.

3. Put some olive oil in a saucepan, and once hot, put the onion to fry for a couple of minutes.
4. Now add the peas, mix, and season with salt and pepper.
5. Now add 300 ml of water and cook for 20 minutes.
6. After 20 minutes, take half of the peas and set them aside.
7. Blend the rest with an immersion blender until you get a smooth and creamy mixture.
8. Wash and dry the mint leaves and then chop them.
9. Put the whole peas back into the pot with the mint.
10. Stir, leave to flavor for 2 minutes, and then turn off.
11. Put the cream on the plates, season it with a drizzle of olive oil and serve.
Nutrition: Calories: 236 Fat: 18g Carbohydrates: 13g Protein: 7g

497. Spinach and Kale Soup

Preparation Time: 5 minutes
Cooking Time: 5 minutes
Servings: 2
Ingredients:
- 3 oz. Plant-based butter
- 1 cup fresh spinach, chopped coarsely
- 1 cup fresh kale, chopped coarsely
- 1 large avocado
- 3 tbsp. chopped fresh mint leaves
- 3 1/2 cups coconut cream
- 1 cup vegetable broth
- Salt and black pepper to taste
- 1 lime, juiced

Directions:
1. Liquefy butter in a pot over medium heat and sauté the kale and spinach until wilted, 3 minutes. Turn the heat off.
2. Stir in the remaining ingredients, and using an immersion blender, puree the soup until smooth.
3. Dish the soup and serve warm.
Nutrition: Calories: 743 Proteins: 27g Carbohydrates: 28g Fat: 62g

498.   Coconut and Grilled Vegetable Soup

Preparation Time: 10 minutes
Cooking Time: 45 minutes
Servings: 4
Ingredients:
- 2 small red onions cut into wedges
- 2 garlic cloves
- 10 oz. butternut squash, peeled and chopped
- 10 oz. pumpkins, peeled and chopped
- 4 tbsp. melted butter
- Salt and black pepper to taste
- 1 cup of water
- 1 cup unsweetened coconut milk
- 1 lime juiced
- 3/4 cup plant-based mayonnaise
- Toasted pumpkin seeds for garnishing

Directions:
1.   Preheat the oven to 400 F.
2.   On a baking sheet, spread the onions, garlic, butternut squash, and pumpkins and drizzle half of the butter on top. Season with salt, black pepper, and rub the seasoning well onto the vegetables. Roast in the oven for 45 minutes or until the vegetables are golden brown and softened.
3.   Transfer the vegetables to a pot; add the remaining ingredients except for the pumpkin seeds.
4.   Use a blender to puree the ingredients until smooth.
5.   Dish the soup, garnish with the pumpkin seeds, and serve warm.

Nutrition: Calories: 672 Proteins: 15g Carbohydrates: 12g Fat: 182g

499.   Celery Dill Soup

Preparation Time: 5 minutes
Cooking Time: 25 minutes
Servings: 4
Ingredients:
- 2 tbsp. coconut oil
- 1/2 lb. celery root, trimmed
- 1 garlic clove
- 1 medium white onion
- 1/4 cup fresh dill, roughly chopped
- 1 tsp cumin powder
- 1/4 tsp nutmeg powder
- 1 small head cauliflower, cut into florets
- 31/2 cups seasoned vegetable stock
- 5 oz. Plant-based butter
- Juice from 1 lemon
- 1/4 cup coconut cream
- Salt and black pepper to taste

Directions:
1.   Get a large pot and melt coconut oil. Sauté the celery root, garlic, and onion until softened and fragrant, 5 minutes.
2.   Stir in the dill, cumin, and nutmeg, and stir-fry for 1 minute.
3.   Mix in the cauliflower and vegetable stock.
4.   Let it boil for 15 minutes and turn the heat off.
5.   Add the butter and lemon juice, and puree the soup using an immersion blender.
6.   Stir in the coconut cream, salt, black pepper, and dish the soup. Serve warm.

Nutrition: Calories: 205 Proteins: 3g Carbohydrates: 12g Fat: 232g

500.   Broccoli Fennel Soup

Preparation Time: 15 minutes
Cooking Time: 10 minutes
Servings: 4
Ingredients:
- 1 fennel bulb, white and green parts coarsely chopped
- 10 oz. broccoli, cut into florets
- 3 cups vegetable stock
- Salt and freshly ground black pepper
- 1 garlic clove
- 1 cup dairy-free cream cheese
- 3 oz. Plant-based butter
- 1/2 cup chopped fresh oregano

Directions:
1.   In a medium pot, combine the fennel, broccoli, vegetable stock, salt, and black pepper.
2.   Bring to a boil until the vegetables soften, 10 to 15 minutes.
3.   Stir in the remaining ingredients and simmer the soup for 3 to 5 minutes.
4.   Taste, then adjust the season with salt and black pepper.
5.   Serve warm.

Nutrition: Calories: 690 Proteins: 2g Carbohydrates: 15g Fat: 188g

501. Tofu Goulash Soup

Preparation Time: 35 minutes
Cooking Time: 20 minutes
Servings: 4
Ingredients:
- 4 1/4 oz. Plant-based butter
- 1 white onion, chopped
- 2 garlic cloves, minced
- 1 1/2 cups butternut squash
- 1 red bell pepper, deseeded and chopped
- 1 tbsp. paprika powder
- 1/4 tsp red chili flakes
- 1 tbsp. dried basil
- 1/2 tbsp. crushed cardamom seeds
- Salt and black pepper to taste
- 1 1/2 cups crushed tomatoes
- 3 cups vegetable broth
- 11/2 tsp red wine vinegar
- Chopped parsley to serve

Directions:
1. Put tofu between two paper towels and allow draining of water for 30 minutes. After, crumble the tofu and set it aside.
2. Dissolve butter in a large pot over medium heat and sauté the onion and garlic until the veggies are fragrant and soft, 3 minutes.
3. Stir in the tofu and cook until golden brown, 3 minutes.
4. Add the butternut squash, bell pepper, paprika, red chili flakes, basil, cardamom seeds, salt, and black pepper.
5. Cook for 2 minutes to release some flavor and mix in the tomatoes and 2 cups of vegetable broth.
6. Close the lid, bring the soup to a boil, and then simmer for 10 minutes.
7. Stir in the remaining vegetable broth, the red wine vinegar, and adjust the taste with salt and black pepper.
8. Garnish with the parsley and serve warm.

Nutrition: Calories: 358 Proteins: 4g Carbohydrates: 8g Fat: 36g

502. Vegetable Broth

Preparation Time: 10 minutes
Cooking Time: 60 minutes
Servings: 2
Ingredients:
- 8 cups Water
- 1 Onion, chopped
- 4 Garlic cloves, crushed
- 2 Celery Stalks, chopped
- Pinch of Salt
- 1 Carrot, chopped
- Dash of Pepper
- 1 Potato, medium and chopped
- 1 tbsp. Soy Sauce
- 3 Bay Leaves

Directions:
1. To make the vegetable broth, you need to place all of the ingredients in a deep saucepan.
2. Heat the pan over medium-high heat. Bring the vegetable mixture to a boil.
3. Lower the heat to medium-low once it starts boiling. Allow it to simmer for at least an hour or so. Then, cover it with a lid.
4. When the time is up, pass it through a filter and strain the vegetables, garlic, and bay leaves.
5. Allow the stock to cool completely and store in an air-tight container.

Nutrition: Calories: 40 Protein: 1 g Carbohydrates: 9g Fat: 0g

503. Cucumber Dill Gazpacho

Preparation Time: 10 minutes
Cooking Time: 2 hours
Servings: 4
Ingredients:
- 4 large cucumbers, peeled, deseeded, and chopped
- 1/8 tsp salt
- 1 tsp chopped fresh dill + more for garnishing
- 2 tbsp. freshly squeezed lemon juice
- 1 1/2 cups green grape, seeds removed
- 3 tbsp. extra virgin olive oil
- 1 garlic clove, minced

Directions:

1.   Prepare food processor and put all ingredients. Blend until smooth.
2.   Pour the soup into serving bowls and chill for 1 to 2 hours.
3.   Garnish with dill and serve chilled.
Nutrition: Calories: 118cal Proteins: 2g Carbohydrates: 17g Fat: 5g

504.   Red Lentil Soup

Preparation Time: 5 minutes
Cooking Time: 25 minutes
Servings: 6
Ingredients:
- 2 tbsp. Nutritional Yeast
- 1 cup Red Lentil, washed
- 1/2 tbsp. Garlic, minced
- 4 cups Vegetable Stock
- 1 tsp. Salt
- 2 cups kale, shredded
- 3 cups Mixed Vegetables

Directions:
1.   To start with, place all ingredients needed to make the soup in a large pot.
2.   Heat the pot over medium-high heat and bring the mixture to a boil.
3.   Once it starts boiling, lower the heat to low. Allow the soup to simmer.
4.   Simmer it for 1o to 15 minutes or until cooked.
5.   Serve and enjoy.
Nutrition: Calories: 406 Proteins: 11.8g Carbohydrates: 77.3g Fat: 0.6g

505.   Pesto Pea Soup

Preparation Time: 10 minutes
Cooking Time: 20 minutes
Servings: 4
Ingredients:
- 2 cups Water
- 8 oz. Tortellini
- 1/4 cup Pesto
- 1 Onion, small and finely chopped
- 1 lb. Peas, frozen
- 1 Carrot, medium and finely chopped
- 1 3/4 cup Vegetable Broth, less sodium
- 1 Celery Rib, medium and finely chopped

Directions:

1.   To start with, boil the water in a large pot over medium-high heat.
2.   Stir in the tortellini to the pot and cook it following the Directions given in the packet.
3.   In the meantime, cook the onion, celery, and carrot in a deep saucepan along with the water and broth.
4.   Cook the celery-onion mixture for 6 minutes or until softened.
5.   Now, spoon in the peas and allow it to simmer while keeping it uncovered.
6.   Cook the peas for few minutes or until they are bright green and soft.
7.   Then, spoon in the pesto to the peas mixture. Combine well.
8.   Place mixture into a high-speed blender and blend for 2 to 3 minutes or until you get a rich, smooth soup.
9.   Return the soup to the pan. Spoon in the cooked tortellini.
10.   Finally, pour into a serving bowl and top with more cooked peas if desired.
Nutrition: Calories: 396 Protein: 16.7g Carbohydrates: 51g Fat: 14.3g

506.   Tofu and Mushroom Soup

Preparation Time: 15 minutes
Cooking Time: 10 minutes
Servings: 4
Ingredients:
- 2 tbsp. olive oil
- 1 garlic clove, minced
- 1 large yellow onion, finely chopped
- 1 tsp freshly grated ginger
- 1 cup vegetable stock
- 2 small potatoes, peeled and chopped
- 1/4 tsp salt
- 1/4 tsp black pepper
- 2 (14 oz.) silken tofu, drained and rinsed
- 2/3 cup baby Bella mushrooms, sliced
- 1 tbsp. chopped fresh oregano
- 2 tbsp. chopped fresh parsley to garnish

Directions:
1.   Heat olive oil in a medium pot. Sauté the garlic, onion, and ginger until soft and fragrant.

2. Pour in the vegetable stock, potatoes, salt, and black pepper. Cook until the potatoes soften, 12 minutes.

3. Stir in the tofu, and using an immersion blender, puree the ingredients until smooth.

4. Mix in the mushrooms and simmer with the pot covered until the mushrooms warm up while occasionally stirring to ensure that the tofu doesn't curdle 7 minutes.

5. Stir oregano and dish the soup.

6. Garnish with the parsley and serve warm.

Nutrition: Calories: 325cal Proteins: 33g Carbohydrates: 41g Fat: 27g

507. Beet Soup

Preparation time: 10 minutes
Cooking time: 5 minutes
Serving: 2
Ingredients:
• 2 cups coconut yogurt
• 4 teaspoons fresh lemon juice
• 2 cups beets, trimmed, peeled and chopped
• 2 tablespoons fresh dill
• Salt, as required
Direction:
1. In a high-speed blender, add all ingredients and pulse until smooth.

2. Transfer the soup into a pan over medium heat and cook for about 3-5 minutes or until heated through.

3. Serve immediately.

Meal Prep Tip:
1. Transfer the blended soup into 2 containers.

2. Cover and store in refrigerator for up to 1-2 days.

3. Reheat soup before serving.

Nutrition: Calories: 255, Fats: 11.5g, Carbs: 29.9g, Fiber: 3.9g, Sugar: 21.7g, Proteins: 15.6g, Sodium: 277mg

508. Carrot Soup

Preparation time: 15 minutes
Cooking time: 5 minutes
Serving: 2
Ingredients:
• 2½ cups organic coconut water
• 4 medium carrots, peeled and chopped

• 1 teaspoon fresh ginger, chopped
• ¼ cup raw cashews, chopped
• 1 teaspoon curry powder
• Salt and ground black pepper, as required
• 1 tablespoon fresh cilantro, chopped
Direction:
1. In a high-speed blender, add all ingredients and pulse until smooth.

2. Transfer the soup into a pan over medium heat and cook for about 3-5 minutes or until heated through.

3. Serve immediately.

Meal Prep Tip:
1. Transfer the blended soup into 2 containers.

2. Cover and store in refrigerator for up to 1-2 days.

3. Reheat soup before serving.

Nutrition: Calories: 211, Fats: 8.1g, Carbs: 32.6g, Fiber: 4g, Sugar: 20.7g, Proteins: 3.8g, Sodium: 265mg

509. Broccoli Soup

Preparation time: 15 minutes
Cooking time: 45 minutes
Serving: 4
Ingredients:
• 1 tablespoon olive oil
• 1 white onion, chopped
• 2 garlic cloves, minced
• ¼ teaspoon dried thyme, crushed
• ¼ teaspoon ground cumin
• ¼ teaspoon paprika
• 2 broccoli heads, chopped
• 4 cups homemade hot vegetable broth
• 1 medium avocado, peeled, pitted and chopped
• Salt and ground black pepper, as required
• 2 tablespoons fresh cilantro, chopped
Direction:
1. In a large soup pan, heat the oil over medium heat and sauté the onion for about 4-5 minutes.

2. Add the garlic, thyme, cumin and paprika and sauté for about 1 minute more.

3. Add the broccoli and cook for about 4-5 minutes.

4. Add the broth and bring to a boil over high heat.

5. Reduce the heat to medium-low and simmer, covered for about 25-30 minutes.

6. Stir in salt and black pepper and immediately remove from heat.

7. Set aside to cool it slightly.

8. Transfer the mixture in a high-speed blender with avocado in batches and pulse until smooth.

9. Return the soup to pan over medium heat. Cook for about 3-4 minutes or until heated completely.

10. Garnish with cilantro leaves and serve immediately.

Meal Prep Tip:

1. Transfer the soup into a large bowl and set aside to cool.

2. Divide the soup into 4 airtight containers.

3. Cover and refrigerate for 1-2 days.

4. Reheat in the microwave before serving.

Nutrition: Calories: 199, Fats: 12.3g, Carbs: 15.7g, Fiber: 6.4g, Sugar: 4.3g, Proteins: 9.6g, Sodium: 848mg

510. Yellow Squash Soup

Preparation time: 15 minutes
Cooking time: 3 minutes
Serving: 6
Ingredients:
- 2 tablespoons olive oil
- 2 yellow onions, chopped
- 6 garlic cloves, minced
- 6 cups yellow squash, seeded and cubed
- 4 fresh thyme sprigs
- 4 cups homemade vegetable broth
- Salt and ground black pepper, as required
- 2 tablespoons fresh lemon juice
- 2 teaspoons fresh lemon peel, grated finely

Direction:

1. In a large soup pan, heat the oil over medium heat and sauté the onions for about 5-6 minutes.

2. Add the garlic and sauté for about 1 minute.

3. Add the yellow squash cubes and cook for about 5 minutes.

4. Stir in the thyme, broth, salt and black pepper and bring to a boil.

5. Reduce the heat to low and cook, covered for about 15-20 minutes.

6. Remove from the heat and discard the thyme sprigs.

7. Set the pan aside to cool slightly.

8. In a large blender, add the soup in batches and pulse until smooth.

9. Return the soup into the same pan over medium heat.

10. Stir in the lemon juice and cook for about 2-3 minutes or until heated completely.

11. Serve hot with the garnishing of lemon peel.

Meal Prep Tip:

1. Transfer the soup into a large bowl and set aside to cool.

2. Divide the soup into 6 airtight containers.

3. Cover and refrigerate for 1-2 days.

4. Reheat in the microwave before serving.

Nutrition: Calories: 90, Fats: 5g, Carbs: 10.7g, Fiber: 2.9g, Sugar: 6g, Proteins: 2.1g, Sodium: 395mg

511. Tomato Soup

Preparation Time: 10 minutes
Cooking Time: 10 minutes
Serving: 2 bowls
Ingredients:
- 56 ounces stewed tomatoes
- ¼ teaspoon salt
- ¼ teaspoon ground black pepper
- 1 medium red bell pepper, cored, diced
- ¼ teaspoon dried thyme
- 6 leaves of basil, chopped
- ¼ teaspoon dried oregano
- 1 teaspoon olive oil

Directions:

1. Take a medium pot, place it over medium heat, add oil, and when hot, add bell pepper and then cook for 4 minutes.

2. Add remaining ingredients into the pot, stir until mixed, switch heat to medium-high heat, and bring the mixture to simmer.

3. Remove pot from the heat and then puree the soup until smooth.

4. Taste to adjust seasoning, ladle soup into bowls and then serve.

Nutrition: Calories: 170 Cal; Fat: 1.1 g; Protein: 3.5 g; Carbs: 36 g; Fiber: 2.6 g;

512. Cauliflower Soup

Preparation time: 15 minutes
Cooking time: 26 minutes
Serving: 4
Ingredients:
- 2 tablespoons olive oil
- 1 onion, chopped
- 2 celery stalks, chopped
- 2 carrots, peeled and chopped
- 2 garlic cloves, minced
- ½ teaspoon ground coriander
- ½ teaspoons ground cumin
- ½ teaspoon ground turmeric
- 1 head cauliflower, chopped
- 4 cups homemade vegetable broth
- 1 cup coconut milk
- Salt and ground black pepper, as required

Direction:
1. In a large soup pan, heat the oil over medium heat and sauté onion, celery and carrot for about 4-5 minutes.
2. Add the garlic and spices and sauté for about 1 minute.
3. Add the cauliflower and cook for about 5 minutes, stirring occasionally.
4. Add the broth and coconut milk and bring to a boil over medium-high heat.
5. Reduce the heat to low and simmer for about 15 minutes or until desired doneness of vegetables.
6. Season the soup with salt and black pepper and remove from heat.
7. Serve hot.

Meal Prep Tip:
1. Transfer the soup into a large bowl and set aside to cool.
2. Divide the soup into 4 airtight containers.
3. Cover and refrigerate for 1-2 days.
4. Reheat in the microwave before serving.

Nutrition: Calories: 259, Fats: 21.5g, Carbs: 16.5g, Fiber: 5.6g, Sugar: 8.4g, Proteins: 3.5g, Sodium: 672mg

513. Navy Bean Chili

Preparation time: 15 minutes
Cooking time: 35 minutes
Serving: 6
Ingredients:
- 1 large green pepper, deseeded and diced
- 1 large yellow onion, peeled and diced
- 3 jalapeño peppers, deseeded and minced
- 6 cloves garlic, peeled and minced
- 2 tablespoons ground cumin seeds, toasted
- 4 cups cooked navy beans, drained and rinsed
- 1 (28-ounce / 794-g) can diced tomatoes
- 3 cups low-sodium vegetable broth
- Zest of 1 lime and juice of 2 limes
- 1 cup finely chopped cilantro
- Salt, to taste (optional)

Direction:
1. Put the green pepper, onion, and jalapeño peppers in a large saucepan and sauté over medium cook for 8 minutes.
2. Add the garlic and cumin and cook for 2 minutes. Add the beans, tomatoes, and vegetable broth and bring to a boil over high heat.
3. Reduce the heat to medium and cook, covered, for 25 minutes. Add the lime zest and juice and cilantro and season with salt, if desired.
4. Serve immediately.

Nutrition: Calories: 373 | fat: 8.9g | carbs: 61.1g | protein: 15.4g | fiber: 20.1g

514. Spicy Lentil Chili

Preparation time: 15 minutes
Cooking time: 30 to 35 minutes
Serving: 6 to 8
Ingredients:
- 1-pound (454 g) lentils
- 8 cups water or low-sodium vegetable broth, plus more as needed
- 2 cups diced onion
- 1 cup crushed tomatoes
- ¼ cup tomato paste
- 2 tablespoons chopped garlic
- 2 tablespoons balsamic vinegar
- 2 tablespoons fresh lime juice
- 1 tablespoon ground cumin
- 2 tablespoons chili powder

- 1 teaspoon cayenne (use less if you don't like your chili spicy)

Direction:

1. In a large pot, add all the ingredients and bring to a boil over high heat.
2. Reduce the heat to medium-low and let simmer covered for 30 to 35 minutes, or until the lentils are softened, adding more water or broth if needed for desired chili consistency.
3. Remove from the heat and serve.

Nutrition: Calories: 145 | fat: 1.0g | carbs: 26.7g | protein: 7.3g | fiber: 3.4g

515.   Three Bean Chili

Preparation time: 25 minutes
Cooking time: 2 hours 10 minutes
Serving: 12
Ingredients:

- 1 cup black beans
- 1 cup pinto beans
- 1 cup kidney beans
- 6½ cups water, divided
- 1 red bell pepper, chopped
- 1 green bell pepper, chopped
- 1 cup chopped celery
- 1 cup chopped onion
- 3 cloves garlic, minced
- ½ tablespoon ground cumin
- ¼ cup chili powder
- ¼ teaspoon crushed red pepper flakes
- 1 teaspoon ground oregano
- 1 (4-ounce/ 113-g) can chopped green chilies
- 1 (28-ounce / 794-g) can crushed tomatoes

Direction:

1. Add the beans and 6 cups of the water to a large pot over medium heat and bring to a boil. Allow to boil for 2 minutes and remove from the heat. Cover the pot and let sit for 1 hour.
2. Combine the bell pepper, celery, onion, garlic, and remaining ½ cup of water in another pot. Sauté for about 6 minutes or until the vegetables are tender.
3. Stir in the beans and their water, cumin, chili powder, red pepper, and oregano and bring to a boil. Reduce the heat to low and let simmer covered for 1 hour, stirring occasionally.
4. Add the chilies and tomatoes and stir well. Cook for an additional 1 hour, stirring occasionally.
5. Allow to cool for 5 minutes before ladling into bowls to serve.

Nutrition: Calories: 177 | fat: 2.5g | carbs: 29.4g | protein: 9.3g | fiber: 9.6g

516.   Sumptuous Dal

Preparation time: 20 minutes
Cooking time: 40 minutes
Serving: 4
Ingredients:

- 1 cup red split lentils, rinsed
- 1 cup cherry tomatoes, halved
- 1 cup finely diced carrots
- 1 small yellow onion, finely diced
- 4 cloves garlic, minced
- 2-inch piece of fresh ginger, peeled and minced
- Pinch of dried chili flakes
- 1 teaspoon ground turmeric
- 3½ cups water
- Salt, to taste (optional)
- Ground black or white pepper, to taste
- 2 tablespoons low-sodium vegetables broth
- ½ teaspoon cumin seeds
- ½ teaspoon mustard seeds
- ½ teaspoon coriander seeds
- 1/3 cup chopped fresh cilantro leaves, for garnish
- Lemon wedges, for serving

Direction:

1. Add the lentils, cherry tomatoes, carrots, onion, garlic, ginger, chili flakes, turmeric, and water to a large pot. Stir to mix well.
2. Bring to a boil over medium heat, then simmer for 40 minutes or until the vegetables are tender and the lentils are soft. Stir constantly. Sprinkle with salt (if desired) and pepper.
3. Meanwhile, heat the vegetable broth in a nonstick skillet over medium-high heat. Add the seeds and sauté for 6 minutes until toasted.
4. Pour the cooked soup in a large serving bowl, then pour in the toasted seeds and garnish with cilantro and lemon wedges before serving.

Nutrition: Calories: 219 | fat: 1.6g | carbs: 40.5g | protein: 13.0g | fiber: 7.5g

517. Caramelized Sweet Onion Garlic Soup

Preparation time: 20 minutes
Cooking time: 35 minutes
Serving: 4
Ingredients:
- 2 tablespoons vegan margarine
- 2 tablespoons olive oil
- 4 banana shallots, halved then finely sliced
- 3 large white onions, halved then finely sliced
- 2 red onions, halved then finely sliced
- 3 Teaspoon Sea salt
- Black pepper
- 1 tablespoon fresh thyme leaves, plus extra for serving
- 2 teaspoons dried sage
- 1 tablespoon plain (all-purpose) flour or gluten-free flour
- 240ml (1 cup) vegan-friendly dry white wine
- 35ml (1 shot) brandy
- 1 liter (1¾ pints) hot vegetable stock
- 1 bay leaf
- 1 rosemary sprig
- 4–6 slices of French baguette (day-old bread works best)
- 1 garlic clove
- Grated vegan cheese

Direction:
1. First up, place a large heavy-based saucepan over a low heat, then add the margarine and olive oil.
2. When hot, add the shallots and onions with the salt, pepper, thyme and sage. Allow the onions to sweat down and caramelize, this should take approximately 15–20 minutes. At first, it may look as though there are way too many onions in the pan, but after a little while they will shrink right down. Stir the onions often.
3. When the onions are beautiful and golden, add the flour and stir well to coat the onions. Cook out the flour for a minute or so before deglazing the pan with the white wine and the brandy.
4. Bring the liquid to a boil before adding the hot vegetable stock, bay leaf and rosemary. Place a lid on the pan and let the soup cook away for 15–20 minutes.
5. Preheat your grill (broiler) to high.
6. Toast your slices of baguette. Cut the garlic clove in half and rub the cut side on each side of the slices of toasted bread.
7. Remove the bay leaf and rosemary sprig, then ladle the soup into your serving bowls and float a slice or two of toasted baguette on the surface of the soup in each bowl.
8. Top each slice of baguette with a handful of the grated vegan cheese. Place your bowls onto a flat baking sheet then place each one under the grill (broiler) for 2 minutes.
9. Once the cheese has melted and is nice and golden, sprinkle over a few fresh thyme leaves, grind over some black pepper and serve up.
Nutrition: Calories: 1481 | fat: 111.2g | carbs: 54.71g | protein: 67.44g

518. Nourishing Veggie Soup

Preparation time: 15 minutes
Cooking time: 35 minutes
Serving: 4
Ingredients:
- 2 leeks
- 3 celery sticks
- 2 garlic cloves, minced
- 1 swede (rutabaga)
- 2 medium potatoes
- 2 carrots
- 1 tablespoon olive oil
- 1 teaspoon sea salt
- 2 teaspoons cracked black pepper
- 3 liters (6 pints) vegetable stock
- 1 tablespoon mint sauce
- 1 tablespoon Marmite or miso paste
- 1 x 400-g (14-oz) can butter (lima) beans, drained and rinsed
- large handful of cavolo nero or curly kale, stems removed and cut into bite-sized pieces
- handful of flat-leaf parsley
- Juice of 1 lemon

Direction:
1. Peel and chop all the vegetables into approximately 2cm pieces. Slice the leek, carrot and celery at an angle, for presentation purposes.
2. Place a large saucepan over a low heat and add the oil. When it is hot, add the leek, celery and garlic then sauté for 2–3 minutes before adding the remaining vegetables and the seasoning.
3. Continue to sauté the vegetables for 5 minutes, getting a little color on them, then deglaze

the pan with the vegetable stock, mint sauce and Marmite.

4.	Bring the soup to a simmer and let it bubble away until the swede (rutabaga) is tender. This usually takes 25–30 minutes.

5.	Once the swede (rutabaga) has cooked, add the butter (lima) beans, cavolo nero, parsley and lemon juice and stir.

6.	Add the lemon halves to the pan for extra flavor, if you like. Let the soup simmer for an additional 5 minutes before serving.

Nutrition: Calories: 1070 | fat: 17.15g | carbs: 215.23g | protein: 26.99g

# 519.	Mom's Special Spicy Vegan Pumpkin Soup

Preparation time: 15 minutes
Cooking time: 35 minutes
Serving: 4
Ingredients:
•	1 medium-sized pumpkin, peeled, deseeded and cubed (my pumpkin was 8kg/17lb 10oz)
•	3 tablespoons Cajun spice mix
•	1 tablespoon dried sage
•	Drizzle of olive oil
•	2 onions, roughly chopped
•	3 garlic cloves, roughly chopped
•	480ml (2 cups) non-dairy milk
•	Approx. 720ml (3 cups) hot vegetable stock (you may need more if your pumpkin is large)
•	Squeeze of lemon juice, optional
•	Sea salt and ground pepper
To garnish
•	Handful of pumpkin seeds
•	Drizzle of vegan cream, such as soy or oat
•	Sprinkle of dried chili flakes
Direction:
Toasted bread
1.	Preheat your oven to 180°C (350°F).
2.	Place the pumpkin into a roasting pan with the Cajun spice mix, sage, 2 teaspoons of salt and 1 teaspoon of pepper and a drizzle of oil. Mix it all up using your hands so the pumpkin is well coated.
3.	Roast the pumpkin in your oven for around 45 minutes to 1 hour – or until it is tender.
4.	When the pumpkin is cooked, place a large saucepan over a medium heat and add a drop of oil (or water if you're keeping this recipe oil-free). Add

the chopped onion and garlic and sauté the mix with a pinch of salt for 4 minutes.

5.	Add the roasted pumpkin to the saucepan, followed by the milk and vegetable stock.

6.	Allow the soup to simmer for 10 minutes before blending it until super smooth. Blend the soup a few ladlefuls at a time and if it's too thick added more vegetable stock.

7.	Check the soup is seasoned to your liking. If it needs an extra lift, add a squeeze of lemon juice, before serving with a few pumpkin seeds, a drizzle of vegan cream, a sprinkle of chili flakes and some toasted bread.

8.	This soup can be kept in the fridge for up to 4 days.

Nutrition: Calories: 2201 | fat: 219.04g | carbs:65.2g | protein: 7.17g

# 520.	Spicy Butternut Squash Soup

Preparation Time: 15 minutes
Cooking Time: 60 minutes
Serving: 6 to 8
Ingredients:
•	1 large butternut squash, halved
•	1 medium white onion, diced
•	1 15-ounces can of full-fat coconut milk
•	4 leaves fresh sage
•	1/4 teaspoon of ground nutmeg
•	1/2 teaspoon of apple cider vinegar
•	2 medium jalepeños (or poblano for less spicy)
•	1 shallot, minced
•	5 cloves of garlic
•	2 cups of vegetable broth
Direction:
1.	Preheat the oven to 400 degrees f.
2.	Prepare a baking sheet by spraying it using nonstick cooking spray.
3.	Cut the butternut squash into half hot dog style, and remove the seeds. Place on pan.
4.	Bake squash for about 30 minutes, remove from oven and add jalapeno, onion, garlic, and shallot to the same pan. Use olive oil to drizzle the veggies and then bake for extra 30 minutes.
5.	Remove pan from the oven. Then let cool for 10 to 15 mins.

6. Scoop out the squash flesh. Discard the ring and place it in a large pot with other roasted ingredients from the baking sheet.

7. Add coconut milk, broth, fresh sage, apple cider vinegar, and nutmeg to the pot.

8. Blend all the ingredients together using an emulsifier.

9. Bring soup to a boil. Turn heat to low and let it simmer for about 30 minutes.

10. Serve and enjoy.

Nutrition: Calories: 197cal | Fat: 12g | Protein: 5g | Fiber: 3g | Sodium: 46mg | Sugar: 3g | Carbohydrate: 18g

521. Coconut Thai Curry Soup

Preparation Time: 10 minutes
Cooking Time: 20 minutes
Serving: 6
Ingredients:
- 4 cups, broth (any kind)
- 1 15 ounces can of full-fat coconut milk
- 1/2 tablespoon of sriracha (or more, to taste)
- 2 tablespoons of diced green onion
- 2 tablespoons of chopped cilantro
- 1 lime, juiced
- salt, to taste
- 8 ounces of frozen green peas
- 1.5 tablespoons of coconut oil
- 1 large sweet potato, peeled and chopped
- 4 large carrots, peeled and diced
- 4 cloves garlic, minced
- 1 medium yellow onion, finely diced
- 1 large red pepper, finely stripped
- 5 tablespoons of red curry paste
- salt, to taste

Optional Toppings:
- 1/4 cup of brown rice, cooked (per serving)
- chopped jalapenos
- fresh cilantro, chopped
- green onions, chopped

Direction:
1. In a large pot, heat coconut-oil over medium/high heat.

2. Add the carrots and sweet potatoes. Let cook for about 7 to 10 mins, stirring occasionally.

3. Then, add onion, garlic, and red pepper—Cook for 2 to 3 minutes.

4. Place other ingredients except for the peas into the pot. Bring to a boil.

5. Turn the heat to low. Add peas and let simmer for about 10 to 15 minutes.

6. Remove from heat. Then, serve with green onion, jalapeno, cilantro, and rice.

7. Enjoy!

Nutrition: Calories: 282cal | Fat: 15g | Protein: 11g | Fiber: 6g | Sodium: 3039mg | Sugar: 11g | Carbohydrate: 25g

522. Minestrone Soup

Preparation Time: 5 minutes
Cooking Time: 25 minutes
Serving: 6
Ingredients:
- 5 cloves garlic, minced
- 10 ounces of zucchini (about 1 medium), halved lengthwise and thinly sliced
- 1 (15 ounce) can of no-salt-added cannellini beans, rinsed
- 3 cups of fresh baby kale or chopped kale
- 1 cup of frozen peas, thawed, 1/2 teaspoon of ground pepper
- 3 tablespoons of extra-virgin olive oil, divided, 1 cup of cubed whole-grain rustic bread
- 1 cup of chopped leek, light green and white parts only, rinsed well
- 1 cup of chopped carrots, 3 cups of low-sodium vegetable broth, 3 cups of water
- 3/4 teaspoon of kosher salt, 1 cup of ditalini pasta or other small pasta

Direction:
1. Preheat oven to 350 degrees f.

2. Cook 2 tablespoons of oil and garlic in a medium skillet over medium heat, stirring constantly, for about 4 minutes, until the garlic is softened.

3. Add bread and toss to coat. On a baking sheet, spread the mixture evenly, and bake for about 10 minutes, until toasted.

4. In a large pot, heat remaining 1 tablespoon of oil over medium high heat. Add carrots and leek; cook, for about 5 minutes, stirring occasionally. Add water, broth, and salt.

5. Cover and bring to a boil on a high heat.

6. Add pasta. Reduce the heat to medium-high; stirring often, for about 5 minutes (cooked uncovered).

7. Add zucchini. Cook and stir occasionally for 5 minutes, until the pasta is al dente. Stir in the beans, peas, kale and pepper.
8. Cook and stir occasionally for 2 minutes until the kale is wilted.
9. Ladle the soup evenly into 6 bowls. Then sprinkle with the croutons and enjoy.
Nutrition: Calories: 267cal | Fat: 8.6g | Protein: 9.7g | Fiber: 7.2g | Sugar: 6.7g | Carb: 38.7g

523. Slow-Cooker Mediterranean

Preparation Time: 15 minutes
Cooking Time: 6 hours 30 minutes
Serving: 6
Ingredients:
• 4 cloves garlic, minced
• 1 teaspoon of dried oregano
• 3/4 teaspoon of salt
• 1/2 teaspoon of crushed red pepper
• 1/4 teaspoon of ground pepper
• 1 (15 ounce) can of no-salt-added chickpeas, rinsed, divided
• 1 bunch of lacinato kale, stemmed and chopped (about 8 cups)
• 1 tablespoon of lemon juice
• 2 (14 ounce) cans of no-salt-added fire-roasted diced tomatoes
• 3 cups of low-sodium vegetable broth
• 1 cup of coarsely chopped onion
• 3/4 cup of chopped carrot
• 3 tablespoons of extra-virgin olive oil
• 8 leaves Fresh basil leaves, torn if large
• 6 eaches lemon wedges
Direction:
1. Combine broth, tomatoes, carrot, onion, oregano, garlic, crushed red pepper, salt, and pepper in a 4-quart slow cooker—cover and cook on low for 6 hrs.
2. Measure 1/4 cup of the cooking liquid from the slow cooker inside a small bowl.
3. Add 2 tablespoons of chickpeas; mash until smooth using a fork.
4. Add the kale, mashed chickpeas, lemon juice, and other whole chickpeas to the mixture in the slow cooker. Stir to combine.
5. Cover & cook for about 30 minutes, until the kale is tender, on low.

6. Ladle the stew evenly into 6 bowls. Use oil to drizzle and garnish with basil.
7. Serve with lemon wedges if you want. Enjoy!
Nutrition: Cal: 191cal | Fat: 7.8g | Protein: 5.7g | Fiber: 5.6g | Sodium: 415.5mg | Calcium: 128mg | Sugar: 6.5g | Carb: 22.9g

524. Cabbage Soup

Preparation Time: 5 minutes
Cooking Time: 25 minutes
Serving: 6
Ingredients:
• 6 cups of low-sodium vegetable broth
• 1 (15 ounce) can of no-salt-added diced tomatoes with basil, garlic and oregano
• 1 small head green cabbage (1 1/2 pounds), chopped
• 1 (15 ounce) can of unsalted cannellini beans, rinsed
• 2 teaspoons of sugar
• 1 teaspoon of chopped fresh oregano
• 2 tablespoons of extra-virgin olive oil
• 1 cup of chopped carrots
• 1 cup of sliced fennel, fronds reserved for garnish
• 1/2 cup of chopped onion
• 2 teaspoons of minced garlic
• 1/2 teaspoon of ground coriander
• 1/2 teaspoon of salt
• 1 teaspoon of Lemon zest for garnish
Direction:
1. In a large heavy-pot, heat oil over medium-high heat.
2. Add fennel, carrots, and onion; cook, occasionally stirring, for about 5 minutes, until starting to soften.
3. Add garlic, salt, and coriander, constantly stirring, for about a minute, until fragrant.
4. Add tomatoes & broth; bring to a boil.
5. Add cabbage. Reduce heat to medium.
6. Cook, occasionally stirring, for 20 to 25 mins, until the cabbage is tender.
7. Stir in sugar, beans, and oregano.
8. Cook for about 3 mins, until the beans are heated through.
9. Sprinkle with reserved fennel fronds and lemon zest.
10. Serve immediately.
11. Enjoy!

Nutrition: Cal: 205cal | Fat: 5.5g | Protein: 6.2g | Fiber: 9.6g | Sodium: 426.5mg | Calcium: 153.5mg | Sugar: 14.5g | Carb: 41g

525. Butternut Squash Chili & Black Beans

Preparation Time: 15 minutes
Cooking Time: 35 minutes
Serving: 6
Ingredients:
- 1/4 teaspoon of ground chipotle chili, or to taste, 2 cups of vegetable broth (no-salt-added)
- 3 cups of cubed butternut-squash
- 1 (14 ounces) can of no-salt-added diced tomatoes
- 1 tablespoon plus 1 teaspoon of avocado oil or canola oil
- 4 cloves garlic, minced
- 1 large onion, diced
- 2 cans of black beans (14 ounces), rinsed & drained, 1 (14 ounces) can of no-salt-added crushed tomatoes
- 1/2 teaspoon of salt
- 2 tablespoons of chili powder, 1 tablespoon of ground cumin, 1/4 teaspoon of ground cinnamon, 1/2 cup of Greek yogurt, for serving
- 1/4 cup of chopped fresh cilantro, for serving
- 1/4 cup of minced red onion, for serving

Direction:
1. In an oven, heat oil over medium-high. Add garlic, salt, and onion; cook until starting to brown, often stirring for 5 mins. Add chili powder, cinnamon, cumin, and chipotle, and stir to coat. Cook until the spices are fragrant but not scorched, stirring often.
2. Add squash and broth; increase heat to high. Bring to a simmer, stirring occasionally. Cover and reduce heat to medium-low. Simmer for 20-mins, until the squash is tender.
3. Stir in crushed tomatoes, black beans, and diced tomatoes.
4. Increase heat to medium-high, stirring often, then bring to a simmer. Reduce heat to medium-low, simmer, uncovered, and often stir for 5 mins until the flavors have melded and chili is thickened.

5. Serve the chili topped with yogurt and sprinkled with red onion and cilantro. Enjoy!
Nutrition: Cal: 246cal | Fat: 4.9g | Protein: 10.8g | Fiber: 12.5g | Sugar: 7.5g | Carb: 41g

526. Instant Pot Lentil Soup

Preparation Time: 10 minutes
Cooking Time: 30 minutes
Serving: 6
Ingredients:
- 6 cups of low-sodium vegetable broth
- 2 cups of brown lentils, rinsed
- 3/4 teaspoon of salt
- 5 cups of fresh baby spinach
- 1 1/2 tablespoons of balsamic vinegar
- 2 tablespoons of extra-virgin olive oil, divided
- 1 cup of chopped yellow onion
- 1 cup of chopped carrots
- 1 cup of chopped turnip
- 1 tablespoon of chopped fresh thyme
- 3 eaches radishes, cut into matchsticks
- 1/4 cup of packed fresh flat-leaf parsley leaves

Direction:
1. Select Sauté setting on the instant pot. Select a high-temperature setting. Allow preheating.
2. Add 1 tablespoon of oil into the cooker; heat until shimmering.
3. Add carrots, onion, thyme, and turnip; cook until the onion is tender, for 5 min, stirring occasionally.
4. Stir in lentils, broth, and salt.
5. Press cancel and cover the cooker, then lock the lid in place.
6. Turn the steam release handle to the sealing-position. Select a pressure/manual cook setting.
7. Select high pressure for 10 min.
8. Turn the steam release handle carefully to the venting position when cooking is complete and let the steam fully escape.
9. Toss parsley, radishes with 1 tablespoon of oil in a small bowl.
10. Ladle the soup evenly into 6 bowls.
11. Top with the radish mixture and enjoy.
Nutrition: Calories: 305cal | Fat: 5.5g | Protein: 18g | Fiber: 17.7g | Sugar: 8.8g | Carbohydrate: 47.5g

527. Chickpea and Vegetable Soup

Preparation Time: 15 minutes
Cooking Time: 20 minutes
Serving: 4
Ingredients:
- 1/2 teaspoon of kosher salt
- 1/2 teaspoon of ground pepper
- 2 teaspoons of extra-virgin olive oil
- 1 large carrot, diced
- 1 small onion, diced
- 2 cloves garlic, minced
- 1 (15 ounces) can of no-salt-added chickpeas, rinsed
- 2/3 cup of frozen corn
- 2/3 cup of frozen peas
- 4 cups of low-sodium vegetable broth
- 1/2 cup of packed chopped spinach
- 6 sprigs of Fresh cilantro for garnish

Direction:
1. In a large saucepan, heat oil over medium heat.
2. Add onion, carrot, and garlic; cook for about 4 minutes, until the onion is soft, stirring.
3. Stir in chickpeas, broth, peas, corn, pepper and salt.
4. Bring to a boil over high-heat.
5. Reduce the heat to simmer; then cook, for about 10 minutes, stirring occasionally.
6. Stir in spinach, and cook for about 1 minute, until wilted.
7. Serve the soup topped with cilantro, if you want.
8. Enjoy.

Nutrition: Calories: 175cal | Fat: 3.4g | Protein: 7.1g | Fiber: 6g | Sugar: 5.3g | Carbohydrate: 28.5g

528. Pasta e fagioli Soup

Preparation Time: 5 minutes
Cooking Time: 20 minutes
Serving: 4
Ingredients:
- 1 tablespoon of minced fresh garlic
- 1 bay leaf
- 1 sprig fresh rosemary
- 1/2 teaspoon of salt
- 1/4 teaspoon of crushed red pepper
- 1 Parmesan rind (optional)
- 1 (32 fluid ounces) container of low-sodium vegetable broth
- 1/2 cup of ditalini pasta or mini shells
- 1 tablespoon of olive oil
- 1 cup of diced onion
- 3/4 cup of diced carrot
- 3/4 cup of diced celery
- 1 (14 ounces) can of no-salt-added diced tomatoes
- 1 (15 ounces) can of white beans, rinsed

Direction:
1. Cook pasta according to the package direction. Drain and set it aside.
2. Heat oil in a large pot over medium heat.
3. Add carrot, onion, and celery; cook for about 5 minutes until softened, stirring occasionally.
4. Add bay leaf, garlic, salt, rosemary, Parmesan rind, and crushed red pepper.
5. Cook for about 30 seconds, until fragrant.
6. Stir in tomatoes with their juice and broth; bring to a simmer.
7. Stir in beans. Cook for about 5 minutes, until heated through.
8. Discard the bay leaf, Parmesan rind, rosemary sprig.
9. Stir in the cooked pasta.
10. Serve and enjoy.

Nutrition: Calories: 229cal | Fat: 5g | Protein: 10g | Fiber: 10g | Sodium: 756mg | Sugar: 9g | Carbohydrate: 41g

529. Potato Leek Soup

Preparation Time: 25 minutes
Cooking Time: 30 minutes
Serving: 6
Ingredients:
- 6 cups of no-salt-added vegetable broth
- 2 pounds of russet potatoes, cubed and peeled
- 1 pound of small red potatoes, cubed
- 1/2 teaspoon of ground pepper
- 4 eaches leeks (white parts only), cleaned and thinly sliced (about 4 cups)
- 2 tablespoons of olive oil
- 5 cloves garlic, chopped

- 1 tablespoon of chopped fresh thyme
- 3/4 teaspoon of salt
- 2 tablespoons of chopped fresh chives

Direction:

1. In a large heavy-pot, cook leeks, and oil over medium-high heat, covered and occasionally stirring, for about 5 to 6 minutes, until the leeks are slightly tender.
2. Stir in thyme, garlic, and salt; reduce heat to medium and cook, covered, occasionally stirring, for about 10 mins, until the leeks are very soft.
3. Add russet potatoes, broth, and red potatoes to the leek mixture; bring to simmer on a high heat.
4. Cover & reduce heat to medium; then cook until the soup thickens slightly and russet potatoes start to break down, for about 30 minutes.
5. Stir in pepper and ladle evenly into 6 bowls.
6. Sprinkle with chives.
7. Serve and enjoy.

Nutrition: Calories: 281cal | Fat: 5.1g | Protein: 5.8g | Fiber: 4.5g | Sodium: 534.2mg | Sugar: 8.3g | Carbohydrate: 54.8g

530.   Pumpkin Soup

Preparation time: 15 minutes
Cooking time: 20 minutes
Serving: 6
Ingredients:

- 2 teaspoons olive oil
- 1 yellow onion, chopped
- ½ teaspoon fresh ginger
- 2 tablespoons fresh cilantro, chopped
- 3 cups pumpkin, peeled and cubed
- 1 garlic clove, chopped
- 5½ cups homemade vegetable broth
- Salt and ground black pepper, as required
- ½ cup coconut cream
- 2 tablespoons fresh lime juice

Direction:

1. In a large soup pan, heat the oil over medium heat and sauté the onion, ginger and cilantro for about 2-3 minutes.
2. Add the pumpkin, garlic and broth and bring to a boil
3. Reduce the heat to low and simmer, covered for about 15 minutes.
4. Stir in the salt and black pepper and remove from the heat.

5. Add the coconut cream and lime juice and with an immersion blender, blend until smooth.
6. Serve immediately.

Meal Prep Tip:

1. Transfer the soup into a large bowl and set aside to cool.
2. Divide the soup into 6 airtight containers.
3. Cover and refrigerate for 1-2 days.
4. Reheat in the microwave before serving.

Nutrition: Calories: 166, Fats: 6g, Carbs: 27.8g, Fiber: 5g, Sugar: 19.4g, Proteins: 1.9g, Sodium: 529mg

531.   Sweet Potato Soup

Preparation time: 15 minutes
Cooking time: 30 minutes
Serving: 6
Ingredients:

- 2 tablespoons olive oil
- 1 medium onion, chopped
- 3 large scallions, chopped
- 2 garlic cloves, minced
- 1 teaspoon fresh ginger, minced
- 4 sweet potatoes, peeled and chopped
- 4 cups homemade vegetable broth
- 1½ cups coconut milk
- Salt and ground black pepper, as required
- 2 tablespoons fresh lemon juice

Direction:

1. In a large soup pan, heat the oil over medium heat and sauté onion for about 4-6 minutes.
2. Add the scallions and sauté for about 1-2 minutes.
3. Add the garlic and ginger and sauté for about 1 minute.
4. Add the sweet potato and cook for about 4-5 minutes.
5. Add the broth and bring to a boil over high heat.
6. Reduce the heat to medium-low and simmer for about 10 minutes.
7. Stir in the coconut milk and cook for 5 minutes.
8. Season with salt and black pepper and remove from heat.
9. Set aside to cool slightly.
10. In a blender, add the soup in batches and pulse until smooth.
11. Return the soup in pan and cook for 3-4 minutes.

12.   Stir in the lemon juice and remove from heat.
13.   Serve hot.
Meal Prep Tip:
1.   Transfer the soup into a large bowl and set aside to cool.
2.   Divide the soup into 6 airtight containers.
3.   Cover and refrigerate for 1-2 days.
4.   Reheat in the microwave before serving.
Nutrition: Calories: 31, Fats: 19.2g, Carbs: 34.2, Fiber: 6.6g, Sugar: 5g, Proteins: 3.3g, Sodium: 402mg

532.   Greens Soup

Preparation time: 15 minutes
Cooking time: 35 minutes
Serving: 8
Ingredients:
• 2 cups collard greens, chopped
• 2 cups mustard greens, chopped
• 1 large onion, chopped
• 2 teaspoons fresh ginger, chopped
• 2 tablespoons soy sauce
• 8 cups homemade vegetable broth
• Salt and ground black pepper, as required
Direction:
1.   In a large soup pan, add all the ingredients over high heat and bring to a boil.
2.   Reduce the heat to medium and simmer, covered for about 25-30 minutes.
3.   Remove from heat and set aside to cool slightly.
4.   In a blender, add soup in batches and pulse until smooth.
5.   Return the soup in pan and cook for 3-4 minutes.
6.   Stir in the lemon juice and remove from heat.
7.   Serve hot.
Meal Prep Tip:
1.   Transfer the soup into a large bowl and set aside to cool.
2.   Divide the soup into 8 airtight containers.
3.   Cover and refrigerate for 1-2 days.
4.   Reheat in the microwave before serving.
Nutrition: Calories: 56, Fats: 1.5g, Carbs: 4.6g, Fiber: 1.3g, Sugar: 1.8g, Proteins: 6g, Sodium: 995mg

533.   Squash & Apple Soup

Preparation time: 15 minutes
Cooking time: 40 minutes
Serving: 5
Ingredients:
• 1 tablespoon olive oil
• 1 medium white onion, chopped
• 1½ pounds butternut squash, peeled, seeded and chopped
• 2 apples, peeled, cored and chopped
• 4½ cups homemade vegetable broth
• ½ cup unsweetened coconut milk
• Salt and ground black pepper, as required
Direction:
1.   In a large soup pan, heat the oil over medium heat and sauté the onion for 5-6 minutes.
2.   Add the squash, apples and broth and bring to a boil on high heat.
3.   Reduce the heat to medium-low. Cover and simmer for about 20-25 minutes.
4.   Stir in the coconut milk and simmer for 5 minutes more.
5.   Stir in the salt and black pepper and remove from the heat.
6.   Set aside to cool slightly.
7.   In a blender, add the soup in batches and pulse until smooth.
8.   Return the soup in pan and cook for about 3-4 minutes or until heated completely.
9.   Serve hot.
Meal Prep Tip:
1.   Transfer the soup into a large bowl and set aside to cool.
2.   Divide the soup into 5 airtight containers.
3.   Cover and refrigerate for 1-2 days.
4.   Reheat in the microwave before serving.
Nutrition: Calories: 209, Fats: 8.8g, Carbs: 34.3g, Fiber: 6.8g, Sugar: 15.8g, Proteins: 2.4g, Sodium: 519mg

534.   Mexican-Inspired Soup

Preparation time: 10 minutes
Cooking time: 25 minutes
Serving: 6
Ingredients:
• 3 tablespoons water
• 1½ teaspoons minced garlic
• 1 cup diced red, white, or yellow onion

- 2 carrots, thinly sliced
- 2 ribs celery, thinly sliced
- 2 cups chopped frozen or fresh broccoli
- 1 (15.5-ounce / 439-g) can hominy, drained
- 1 tablespoon lime juice
- 4 cups vegetable broth
- ¼ cup minced cilantro
- Salt and pepper, to taste (optional)

Direction:

1. In a large pot over medium-high heat, heat the water.

2. Add the garlic and onion and sauté until the onion becomes tender and translucent.

3. Add the carrots, celery, broccoli, hominy, and lime juice.

4. Pour in the broth. Bring to a boil, then reduce the heat and simmer for 20 minutes.

5. Stir in the cilantro and add salt (if desired) and pepper.

Nutrition: Calories: 98 | fat: 1g | protein: 3g | carbs: 21g | fiber: 4g

535.   Curried Acorn Squash Soup

Preparation time: 20 minutes
Cooking time: about 1 hour
Serving: 6
Ingredients:

- 1 acorn squash
- 1 yellow onion, chopped
- 2 garlic cloves, chopped
- 2 celery stalks, coarsely chopped
- 1 tablespoon water, plus more as needed
- 2 tablespoons whole wheat flour
- 2 cups no-sodium vegetable broth
- 1 teaspoon curry powder, plus more for seasoning
- ½ teaspoon dill
- 1/8 teaspoon cayenne pepper
- 1 (14-ounce / 397-g) can full-fat coconut milk
- Chopped scallions, green parts only, for serving

Direction:

1. Preheat the oven to 350ºF (180ºC).

2. Halve the acorn squash lengthwise and scoop out the seeds and stringy center. Place the squash halves, cut-side down, in a 9-by-13-inch baking dish and add enough water to come up about 1 inch all around.

3. Bake for 30 to 45 minutes, or until the squash is easily pierced with a fork. Remove the squash from the baking dish and let cool to the touch, about 10 minutes. Scoop out the soft flesh and set aside in a bowl.

5. Sprinkle in the flour and stir to coat the vegetables.

6. Add the vegetable broth, roasted squash, curry powder, dill, and cayenne pepper. Bring the mixture to a boil. Reduce the heat to maintain a simmer, cover the pot, and cook for 10 minutes.

7. Pour in the coconut milk. Using an immersion blender, blend the soup until smooth. Serve immediately or refrigerate in an airtight container for up to 1 week.

8. Top with scallions and a sprinkle of curry powder.

Nutrition: Calories: 169 | fat: 13g | protein: 2g | carbs: 14g | fiber: 2g

536.   Carrot Ginger Soup

Preparation time: 15 minutes
Cooking time: 25 minutes
Serving: 6
Ingredients:

- 3 tablespoons water
- 1 cup diced red, white, or yellow onion
- 1 teaspoon minced garlic
- 2 tablespoons minced ginger
- 3 cups chopped carrots
- 2 cups chopped russet potatoes
- 4 cups vegetable broth
- Salt and pepper, to taste (optional)

Direction:

1. In a large pot, heat the water over medium-high heat.

2. Add the onion, garlic, and ginger and sauté for 2 to 3 minutes or until the onion becomes translucent and tender.

3. Add the carrots, potatoes, and broth, and cook for 20 minutes or until the carrots and potatoes are tender.

4. Remove from the heat. Purée the soup using an immersion blender (or with a regular blender, working in batches). Add salt and pepper.

Nutrition: Calories: 80 | fat: 0g | protein: 2g | carbs: 18g | fiber: 3g

537. Spicy Thai Sweet Potato Stew

Preparation time: 30 minutes
Cooking time: 40 minutes
Serving: 6
Ingredients:
- 2 large yellow onions, peeled and diced
- 2 celery stalks, diced
- 2 medium carrots, peeled and diced
- 2 serrano chiles, seeded and minced
- 4 cloves garlic, peeled and minced
- 2 teaspoons grated ginger
- 1 tablespoon ground coriander
- 3 tablespoons Thai red chili paste
- 6 cups vegetable stock, or low-sodium vegetable broth
- 4 large sweet potatoes, peeled and cut into ½-inch pieces (about 8 cups)
- Zest of 1 lime and juice of 2 limes
- ½ teaspoon cayenne pepper (optional)
- Salt and freshly ground black pepper, to taste
- ½ cup chopped cilantro

Direction:
1. Place the onions, celery, and carrots in a large saucepan and sauté over medium heat for 10 minutes. Add water 1 to 2 tablespoons at a time to keep the vegetables from sticking to the pan.
2. Add the serrano chiles, garlic, ginger, coriander, red chili paste, and ½ cup of water. Whisk to combine well and cook 3 to 4 minutes. Add the vegetable stock and sweet potatoes and bring to a boil over high heat. Reduce the heat to medium and cook, covered, for 25 minutes, or until the potatoes are tender.
3. Stir in the lime zest and juice and cayenne pepper (if using). Season with salt and pepper and serve garnished with cilantro.

Nutrition: Calories: 134 | fat: 0g | protein: 2g | carbs: 30g | fiber: 5g

538. Tex-Mex Quinoa Vegetable Soup

Preparation time: 20 minutes
Cooking time: 3 to 8 hours
Serving: 6
Ingredients:
- 1 cup dried quinoa
- ½ large yellow onion, diced
- 2 garlic cloves, minced
- 2 carrots, cut into coins
- 2 celery stalks, cut into slices
- 1 tablespoon water, plus more as needed
- ¼ cup tomato paste
- 1 zucchini, cut into coins and quartered
- 1 (15-ounce /425-g) can red kidney beans, drained and rinsed
- 2 teaspoons chili powder
- 1 teaspoon ground cumin
- 6 cups no-sodium vegetable broth, plus more as needed

Direction:
1. Place the quinoa in a fine-mesh sieve and rinse under cold water for 2 to 3 minutes, or until the cloudy water becomes clear.
2. On a 5-quart or larger slow cooker, set the temperature to High and let it heat for 5 to 10 minutes.
3. In the preheated slow cooker, combine the onion, garlic, carrots, celery, and 1 tablespoon of water. Cook for 2 to 3 minutes. Stir in the tomato paste to combine.
4. Add the zucchini, corn, tomatoes, black beans, kidney beans, chili powder, cumin, and vegetable broth. Stir well. The tomato paste will fully incorporate as the soup cooks.
5. Turn the heat to low. Cover the slow cooker and cook on Low for 6 to 8 hours or cook on High for 3 to 4 hours. If the soup seems too thick, add more broth or water, ½ cup at a time.
6. Refrigerate leftovers in an airtight container for up to 1 week or freeze for 4 to 6 months.

Nutrition: Calories: 334 | fat: 4g | protein: 16g | carbs: 62g | fiber: 14g

539.   Bloody Caesar Gazpacho

Preparation time: 20 minutes
Cooking time: 0 minutes
Serving: 6
Ingredients:
- 6 cups chopped ripe tomatoes
- 1 small red onion, chopped
- 1 English cucumber, chopped
- 2 stalks celery, chopped
- 2 cloves garlic, chopped
- Fresh chili pepper, chopped, to taste (optional)
- 2 teaspoons celery salt (optional)
- Vegan gluten-free worcestershire sauce or gluten-free tamari soy sauce, to taste
- Hot sauce, to taste
- Freshly ground black pepper, to taste

Garnishes:
- Thinly sliced celery
- Thinly sliced red onion
- Lime wedges
- Pitted green olives
- Additional hot sauce

Direction:
1. In a large bowl, toss together the chopped tomatoes, red onions, cucumber, celery, garlic, chili, if using, and celery salt, if using. Cover the bowl with plastic wrap, and let it sit at room temperature for 1 hour.
2. Uncover the vegetables and transfer them to the bowl of a food processor. Pour all the marinating liquid from the bowl into the food processor as well. Drain the almonds and add them to the food processor. Run the motor on high until the vegetables and almonds are puréed. Reduce the speed to low, and drizzle in the red wine vinegar and olive oil, if using. Stop the machine when you have a smooth mixture.
3. Run the gazpacho through a fine strainer into a large bowl. Season with vegan Worcestershire sauce, hot sauce, and black pepper.
4. Store the gazpacho, covered, in the refrigerator until ready to serve with the garnishes. The gazpacho will keep in the refrigerator for up to 5 days.
Nutrition: Calories: 140 | fat: 10g | protein: 4g | carbs: 12g | fiber: 4g

540.   Roasted Red Pepper and Butternut Squash Soup

Preparation time: 10 minutes
Cooking time: 40 to 50 minutes
Serving: 6 bowls
Ingredients:
- 1 small butternut squash
- 1 tablespoon olive oil (optional)
- 2 red bell peppers
- 1 yellow onion
- 1 head garlic
- Zest and juice of 1 lime
- 1 to 2 tablespoons tahini
- Pinch cayenne pepper
- ½ teaspoon ground coriander
- Toasted squash seeds (optional)

Direction:
1. Preheat the oven to 350°F (180°C).
2. Prepare the squash for roasting by cutting it in half lengthwise, scooping out the seeds, and poking some holes in the flesh with a fork. Reserve the seeds if desired. Rub a small amount of oil over the flesh and skin, then rub with a bit of sea salt and put the halves skin-side down in a large baking dish. Put it in the oven while you prepare the rest of the vegetables.
3. After the squash has cooked for 20 minutes, add the peppers, onion, and garlic, and roast for another 20 minutes. Optionally, you can toast the squash seeds by putting them in the oven in a separate baking dish 10 to 15 minutes before the vegetables are finished. Keep a close eye on them.
4. When the vegetables are cooked, take them out and let them cool before handling them. The squash will be very soft when poked with a fork.
5. Scoop the flesh out of the squash skin into a large pot (if you have an immersion blender) or into a blender. Chop the pepper roughly, remove the onion skin and chop the onion roughly, and squeeze the garlic cloves out of the head, all into the pot or blender. Add the water, the lime zest and juice, and the tahini. Purée the soup, adding more water if you like, to your desired consistency.
7. Season with the salt (if using), cayenne, coriander, and cumin. Serve garnished with toasted squash seeds (if using).

Nutrition: Calories: 58 | fat: 3g | protein: 1g | carbs: 5g | fiber: 0g

541.   Corn Chowder

Preparation time: 25 minutes
Cooking time: 40 minutes
Serving: 6
Ingredients:
- 2 medium yellow onions, peeled and diced small
- 2 red bell peppers, seeded and finely chopped
- 3 ears corn, kernels removed (about 2 cups)
- 3 cloves garlic, peeled and minced
- 2 large russet potatoes, peeled and diced
- 1½ pounds (680 g) tomatoes (4 to 5 medium), diced
- 6 cups vegetable stock, or low-sodium vegetable broth
- ¾ cup finely chopped basil
- Salt and freshly ground black pepper, to taste

Direction:
1. Place the onions and peppers in a large saucepan and sauté over medium heat for 10 minutes. Add water 1 to 2 tablespoons at a time to keep the vegetables from sticking to the pan. Add the corn and garlic, and sauté for 5 more minutes. Add the potatoes, tomatoes, peppers, and vegetable stock. Bring the mixture to a boil over high heat. Reduce the heat to medium and cook, uncovered, for 25 minutes, or until the potatoes are tender.
2. Purée half of the soup in batches in a blender with a tight-fitting lid, covered with a towel. Return the puréed soup to the pot. Add the basil and season with salt and pepper.
Nutrition: Calories: 209 | fat: 0g | protein: 6g | carbs: 48g | fiber: 5g

542.   Kale and White Bean Soup

Preparation time: 10 minutes
Cooking time: 2 to 3 hours
Serving: 4 to 6
Ingredients:
- 2 medium shallots, finely diced
- 3 garlic cloves, minced
- 2 (14½-ounce / 411-g) cans white beans, drained and rinsed
- 1 pound (454 g) fresh Tuscan or curly kale (about 5 large stalks), chopped
- 6 cups store-bought low-sodium vegetable broth
- Ground black pepper
- Salt (optional)
- ½ bunch fresh flat-leaf parsley, chopped

Direction:
1. Put the shallots, garlic, beans, kale, broth, pepper, and salt (if using) in the slow cooker. 2. Cover and cook on High for 2 to 3 hours or on Low for 4 to 5 hours. Stir in the parsley just before serving.
Nutrition: Calories: 233 | fat: 2g | protein: 13g | carbs: 42g | fiber: 12g

543. Zucchini Soup

Preparation time: 10 minutes
Cooking time: 25 minutes
Serving: 2 quarts
Ingredients:

- 2 tablespoons extra-virgin coconut oil (optional)
- 1 medium yellow onion, diced
- 2 large garlic cloves, finely chopped
- 1½ teaspoons fine sea salt, plus more to taste (optional)
- 8 medium-large zucchinis, cut into 1-inch pieces
- 3¼ cups filtered water
- Freshly ground black pepper
- Tamari (optional)

Direction:

1. Warm the oil in a large pot over medium-high heat. Add the onion and cook for 6 to 8 minutes, until beginning to brown. Stir in the garlic and salt, if using, and cook for 3 to 4 minutes, until the garlic is golden and fragrant. Add the zucchini and water, raise the heat, and bring a boil. Cover the pot, reduce the heat to low, and simmer for 8 to 10 minutes, until the zucchini is tender, pressing it down into the liquid a couple of times during cooking to ensure that it cooks evenly. Test by pressing a piece of zucchini against the side of the pot; it should crush easily. Remove from the heat and set aside to cool slightly.

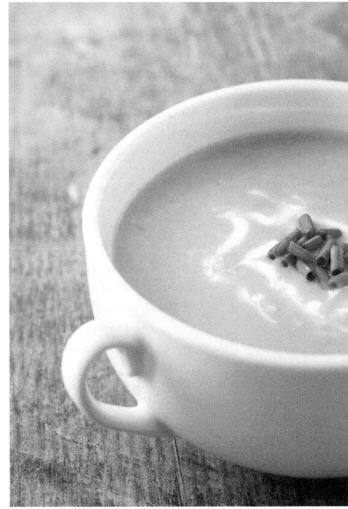

Nutrition: Calories: 153 | fat: 14g | protein: 2g | carbs: 8g | fiber: 2g

Chapter 14. Dessert

544. Raspberry Jelly

Preparation Time: 10 minutes
Cooking Time: 4 minutes
Servings: 4
Ingredients:
• 2 pounds' fresh raspberries
• ¼ cup water
• 1 tablespoon freshly squeezed lemon juice
Direction:
1. In a medium saucepan, add the raspberries and water and cook over low heat for 8-10 minutes or until raspberries become soft, stirring occasionally.
2. Add the lemon juice and cook for 30 minutes.
3. Remove from the heat and place the mixture into a sieve.
4. Strain the mixture into a bowl by pressing with the back of a spoon.
5. Now, transfer the mixture into a blender and pulse until a jelly like texture is formed.
6. Transfer into glass serving bowls and refrigerate for at least 1 hour before serving.
Nutrition: Calories: 119 Fat: 1.5g Carbohydrates: 27.2g Dietary Fiber: 14.8g Sugar: 10.1g Protein: 2.8g

545. Mint Mousse

Preparation Time: 15 minutes
Cooking time: 0 minutes
Servings: 4
Ingredients:
• 1½ cups raw coconut meat, chopped
• 1 tablespoon fresh mint leaves
• 1 tablespoon chia seeds
• 1¼ cups unsweetened almond milk
• 12 drops liquid stevia
• ¼ cup almond butter
• 1 teaspoon organic vanilla extract
• 3 tablespoons fresh raspberries
Direction:
1. In a blender, add all ingredients except the raspberries and pulse until creamy and smooth.
2. Transfer into serving bowls and refrigerate to chill before serving.
3. Garnish with raspberries and serve
Nutrition: Calories: 149 Fat: 12.9g Carbohydrates: 8.1g Dietary Fiber: 5.1g Sugar: 2.3g Protein: 2.4g

546. Chocolate Tofu Mousse

Preparation Time: 15 minutes
Cooking time: 0 minutes
Servings: 6
Ingredients:
• 1-pound firm tofu, drained
• ¼ cup unsweetened almond milk
• 2 tablespoons cacao powder
• 10-15 drops liquid stevia
• 1 tablespoon organic vanilla extract
• ¼ cup fresh strawberries
Direction:
1. In a blender, add all ingredients except the strawberries and pulse until creamy and smooth.
2. Transfer into serving bowls and refrigerate to chill for at least 2 hours.
3. Garnish with strawberries and serve.
Nutrition: Calories: 67 Fat: 3.7g Carbohydrates: 2.9g Dietary Fiber: 3.5g Sugar: 1g Protein: 6.6g

547. Brown Rice Pudding

Preparation Time: 15 minutes
Cooking Time: 1¼ hours
Servings: 3
Ingredients:
• ½ cup brown basmati rice, soaked for 15 minutes and drained
• 1½ cups water
• 2½ cups unsweetened almond milk
• 4 tablespoons cashews
• 2-3 tablespoons maple syrup
• 1/8 teaspoon ground cardamom
• Pinch of salt
• 3 tablespoons golden raisins
Direction:
1. In a saucepan, add the rice and water over medium-high heat and bring to a boil.
2. Lower the heat to medium and cook for about 30 minutes.
3. Meanwhile, in a blender, add the almond milk and cashews and pulse until smooth.

4.   In the pan of rice, slowly add the milk mixture stirring continuously.

5.   Sir in the maple syrup, cardamom and salt and cook for about 15-20 minutes, stirring occasionally.

6.   Stir in the raisins and cook for about 15-20 minutes, stirring occasionally.

7.   Remove from the heat and set aside to cool slightly.

8.   Serve warm.

Nutrition: Calories: 274 Fat: 8.5g Carbohydrates: 46.2g Dietary Fiber: 1.9g Sugar: 13.9g Protein: 5.1g

548.   Tofu & Strawberry Mousse

Preparation Time: 10 minutes
Cooking time: 0 minutes
Servings: 4
Ingredients:
•   2 cups fresh strawberries, hulled and sliced
•   2 cups firm tofu, pressed and drained
•   3 tablespoons maple syrup

Direction:
1.   In a blender, add the strawberries and pulse until just pureed.
2.   Add the tofu and maple syrup and pulse until smooth.
3.   Transfer the mousse into serving bowls and refrigerate to chill before serving.

Nutrition: Calories: 195 Fat: 10.1g Carbohydrates: 14.5g Dietary Fiber: 3g Sugar: 13.3g Protein: 12.7g

549.   No-Bake Cheesecake

Preparation Time: 20 minutes
Cooking time: 0 minutes
Servings: 12
Ingredients:
For Crust:
•   1 cup dates, pitted and chopped
•   1 cup raw almonds
•   2-3 tablespoons unsweetened coconut, shredded
For Filling:
•   3½ cups cashews, soaked overnight
•   ½ cup coconut oil, melted

•   2 tablespoons fresh lemon rind, grated finely
•   ¾ cup freshly squeezed lemon juice
•   ¾ cup maple syrup
•   10 drops liquid stevia
•   1 teaspoon organic vanilla extract
•   Salt, as required

Direction:
1.   For crust: in a food processor, add the dates, almonds, and coconut and pulse until mixture just starts to combine.
2.   Transfer the mixture into a greased spring form pan and, with the back of a spatula, smooth the surface of the crust.
3.   For filling: in the clean food processor, add the cashews and oil and pulse until well combined.
4.   Add the remaining ingredients except lemon slices and pulse until creamy and smooth.
5.   Pour the mixture over crust evenly and with the back of a spatula, smooth the top.
6.   Refrigerate for about 1 hour.
7.   Cut into 12 equal-sized slices and serve.

Nutrition: Calories: 455 Fat: 32.1g Carbohydrates: 39.8g Dietary Fiber: 3.6g Sugar: 23.9g Protein: 8.3g

550.   Coconut Macaroons

Preparation Time: 15 minutes
Cooking Time: 16 minutes
Servings: 12
Ingredients:
•   1¼ cups unsweetened coconut, shredded finely
•   ¼ cup blanched almond flour
•   ¼ cup maple syrup
•   3 tablespoons coconut oil

Direction:
1.   Preheat your oven to 350 °F.
2.   Line a baking sheet with parchment paper.
3.   In a food processor, add all the ingredients and pulse until a thick, sticky mixture forms.
4.   With a scooper, place the balls onto the prepared baking sheet about 1 inch apart.
5.   Bake for approximately 12-16 minutes until golden.
6.   Remove from the oven and immediately transfer the macaroons onto a wire rack to cool completely before serving.

Nutrition: Calories: 90 Fat: 7.3g Carbohydrates: 6.2g Dietary Fiber: 1g Sugar: 4.4g Protein: 0.8g

551. Chocolate Cupcakes

Preparation Time: 15 minutes
Cooking Time: 25 minutes
Servings: 6
Ingredients:
- 1 cup water
- 1 cup dates, pitted
- 1 cup gluten-free oat flour
- 1/3 cup cacao powder
- 1 tablespoon baking powder
- ¼ teaspoon salt
- ¼ cup unsweetened almond milk

Direction:
1. Preheat your oven to 350 °F.
2. Line 6 cups of a muffin tin with paper liners.
3. In a food processor, add water and dates and pulse until smooth.
4. In a large bowl, mix together flour, cacao powder, baking powder, and salt.
5. Add the almond milk and date paste and beat until well combined.
6. Transfer the mixture into paper muffin cups, filling them about ¾ of the way full.
7. Bake for approximately 25 minutes or until a toothpick inserted in the center comes out clean.
8. Remove the muffin tin from oven and place onto a wire rack to cool for about 10 minutes.
9. Carefully invert the cupcakes onto a wire rack to cool completely before serving.
Nutrition: Calories: 159 Fat: 2.2g Carbohydrates: 36.2g Dietary Fiber: 5.3g Sugar: 18.8g Protein: 3.7g

552. Chickpea Fudge

Preparation Time: 15 minutes
Cooking time: 0 minutes
Servings: 12
Ingredients:
- 2 cups cooked chickpeas
- 8 Medjool dates, pitted and chopped
- ½ cup almond butter
- ½ cup unsweetened almond milk
- 1 teaspoon organic vanilla extract
- 2 tablespoons cacao powder

Direction:
1. Line a large baking dish with parchment paper.
2. In a food processor, add all the ingredients except cacao powder and pulse until well combined.
3. Transfer the mixture into a large bowl and stir in the cacao powder.
4. Transfer the mixture into the prepared baking dish, evenly spread. Smooth the surface with the back of a spatula.
5. Refrigerate for about 2 hours or until set completely.
6. Cut into desired sized squares and serve.
Nutrition: Calories: 61 Fat: 1.4g Carbohydrates: 10.8g Dietary Fiber: 2.8g Sugar: 3.9g Protein: 2.5g

553. Beans Brownies

Preparation Time: 15 minutes
Cooking Time: 30 minutes
Servings: 12
Ingredients:
- 2 cups cooked black beans
- 12 Medjool dates, pitted and chopped
- 2 tablespoons almond butter
- 2 tablespoons gluten-free quick rolled oats
- 2 teaspoons organic vanilla extract
- ¼ cup cacao powder
- 1 tablespoon ground cinnamon

Direction:
1. Preheat your oven to 350 °F.
2. Line a large baking dish with parchment paper.
3. In a food processor, add all the ingredients except the cacao powder and cinnamon and pulse until well combined and smooth.
4. Transfer the mixture into a large bowl.
5. Add the cacao powder and cinnamon and stir to combine.
6. Now, transfer the mixture into prepared baking dish evenly and with the back of a spatula, smooth the top surface.
7. Bake for approximately 30 minutes.
8. Remove from oven and place onto a wire rack to cool completely.
9. With a sharp knife, cut into 12 equal-sized brownies and serve.
Nutrition: Calories: 216 Fat: 2.3g Carbohydrates: 2.3g Dietary Fiber: 8g Sugar: 18.9g Protein: 9g

554. Carrot Flaxseed Muffins

Preparation time: 10 minutes
Cooking time: 20 minutes
Servings: 12
Ingredients:

- 2 tablespoons ground flax
- 5 tablespoons water
- ¾ cup almond milk
- ¾ cup applesauce
- ½ cup maple syrup
- 1 teaspoon vanilla extract
- 1½ cups whole wheat flour
- ½ cup rolled oats
- 1 teaspoon baking soda
- 1½ teaspoons baking powder
- ½ teaspoon salt
- 1 teaspoon ground cinnamon
- ¼ teaspoon ground ginger
- 1 cup grated carrot

Direction:
1. Whisk flaxseed with water in a bowl and leave it for 10 minutes
2. Preheat your oven to 350°F.
3. Separately, whisk together the dry ingredients in one bowl and the wet ingredients in another bowl.
4. Beat the two mixtures together until smooth.
5. Fold in flaxseed and carrots, give it a gentle stir.
6. Line a muffin tray with muffin cups and evenly divide the muffin batter among the cups.
7. Bake for 20 minutes and serve.
Nutrition: Calories 172 Total Fat 11.8 g Saturated Fat 4.4 g Cholesterol 62 mg Sodium 871 mg Total Carbs 45.8 g Fiber 0.6 g Sugar 2.3 g Protein 4 g

555. Chocolate Peanut Fat Bombs

Preparation time: 10 minutes
Cooking time: 1 hour 1 minute
Servings: 12
Ingredients:

- ½ cup coconut butter

- 1 cup plus 2 tablespoons peanut butter
- 5 tablespoons cocoa powder
- 2 teaspoons maple syrup

Direction:
1. In a bowl, combine all the ingredients.
2. Melt them in the microwave for 1 minute.
3. Mix well then divide the mixture into silicone molds.
4. Freeze them for 1 hour to set.
5. Serve.
Nutrition: Calories 246 Total Fat 7.4 g Saturated Fat 4.6 g Cholesterol 105 mg Sodium 353 mg Total Carbs 29.4 g Sugar 6.5 g Fiber 2.7 g Protein 7.2 g

556. Protein Fat Bombs

Preparation time: 10 minutes
Cooking time: 1 hour
Servings: 12
Ingredients:

- 1 cup coconut oil
- 1 cup peanut butter, melted
- ½ cup cocoa powder
- ¼ cup plant-based protein powder
- 1 pinch of salt
- 2 cups unsweetened shredded coconut

Direction:
1. In a bowl, add all the ingredients (except coconut shreds).
2. Mix well then make small balls out of this mixture and place them into silicone molds.
3. Freeze for 1 hour to set.
4. Roll the balls in the coconut shreds
5. Serve.
Nutrition: Calories 293 Total Fat 16 g Saturated Fat 2.3 g Cholesterol 75 mg Sodium 386 mg Total Carbs 25.2 g Sugar 2.6 g Fiber 1.9 g Protein 4.2 g

557. Mojito Fat Bombs

Preparation time: 10 minutes
Cooking time: 1 hour 1 minute
Servings: 12
Ingredients:

- ¾ cup hulled hemp seeds
- ½ cup coconut oil
- 1 cup fresh mint

- ½ teaspoon mint extract
- Juice & zest of two limes
- ¼ teaspoon stevia

Direction:
1. In a bowl, combine all the ingredients.
2. Melt in the microwave for 1 minute.
3. Mix well then divide the mixture into silicone molds.
4. Freeze them for 1 hour to set.
5. Serve.

Nutrition: Calories 319 Total Fat 10.6 g Saturated Fat 3.1 g Cholesterol 131 mg Sodium 834 mg Total Carbs 31.4 g Fiber 0.2 g Sugar 0.3 g Protein 4.6 g

558.   Apple Pie Bites

Preparation time: 10 minutes
Cooking time: 1 hour
Servings: 12
Ingredients:
- 1 cup walnuts, chopped
- ½ cup coconut oil
- ¼ cup ground flax seeds
- ½ ounce freeze dried apples
- 1 teaspoon vanilla extract
- 1 teaspoon cinnamon
- Liquid stevia, to taste

Direction:
1. In a bowl add all the ingredients.
2. Mix well then roll the mixture into small balls.
3. Freeze them for 1 hour to set.
4. Serve.

Nutrition: Calories 211 Total Fat 25.5 g Saturated Fat 12.4 g Cholesterol 69 mg Sodium 58 mg Total Carbs 32.4 g Fiber 0.7 g Sugar 0.3 g Protein 1.4 g

559.   Apple Hand Pies

Preparation Time: 15 minutes
Cooking Time: 10 minutes
Serving: 6
Ingredients:
- 14 ounces refrigerated package pie crust (2 crusts)
- 1/2 (21 ounces) can apple pie filling
- 2 tablespoons almond butter
- 3 teaspoon turbinado sugar
- Caramel sauce for dipping

Directions:
1. At 350 degrees F, preheat your air fryer.
2. Spread the pie crusts on the working surface.
3. Cut 5-inch circles out of the crusts using a cookie cutter.
4. Add two slices of apples from the pie filling at the center of each round.
5. Fold the dough circles in half and press edges with a fork to seal the filling.
6. Place the apple hand pies in the air fryer basket.
7. Brush the almond butter over the handpieces and drizzle sugar on top.
8. Cut three slits on top of each hand pie and air fry for 10 minutes.
9. Serve with caramel sauce.

Nutrition: Calories 349; Fat 13.2g; Cholesterol 5mg; Carbohydrate 56.7g; Sugars 26.4g; Protein 4.6g

560.   Air Fryer Beignets

Preparation Time: 10 minutes
Cooking Time: 12 minutes
Serving: 6
Ingredients:
- 1 cup self-rising flour
- 1 cup soy yogurt
- 2 tablespoons sugar
- 1 teaspoon vanilla
- 2 tablespoons melted almond butter
- 1/2 cup powdered sugar

Directions:
1. Mix yogurt, sugar and vanilla in a mixing bowl.
2. Stir in flour and mix until it makes a smooth dough.
3. Knead the dough for 5 minutes, then spread into a 1inch thick rectangle.
4. Cut this dough into 9 equal pieces and dust each piece with some flour.
5. Leave these dough pieces for 15 minutes.
6. At 350 degrees F, preheat your air fryer.
7. Grease the air fryer basket with cooking oil spray.
8. Transfer the prepared dough pieces to the basket and brush them with melted butter.
9. Air fry the beignets for 12 minutes until golden brown.

10. Flip the beignets once cooked halfway through.

11. Dust the beignets with powdered sugar.

12. Serve.

Nutrition: Calories 294; Fat 6.1g; Cholesterol 0mg; Carbohydrate 52.7g; Sugars 25.7g; Protein 7.7g

561. Air Fryer Baked Apples

Preparation Time: 15 minutes
Cooking Time: 15 minutes
Serving: 4
Ingredients:
- 2 apples
- 1 teaspoon almond butter, melted
- ½ teaspoon cinnamon

Topping:
- 1/3 cup old fashioned oats
- 1 tablespoon almond butter, melted
- 1 tablespoon maple syrup
- 1 teaspoon whole meal flour
- ½ teaspoon cinnamon

Directions:
1. At 350 degrees F, preheat your air fryer.
2. Cut the whole apples in half crosswise and remove the core using a knife.
3. Brush the apples with butter and spring cinnamon over them.
4. Mix oats with butter, maple syrup, cinnamon and a whole meal in a bowl.
5. Stuff the apples with the oats mixture and place them in the air fryer basket.
6. Air fry these apples for 15 minutes in the preheated air fryer.
7. Serve once cooled.

Nutrition: Calories 168; Fat 3.5g; Cholesterol 0mg; Carbohydrate 32.5g; Sugars 15.1g; Protein 3.6g

562. Bread Pudding

Preparation Time: 10 minutes
Cooking Time: 10 minutes
Serving: 6
Ingredients:
- 2 cups bread cubed
- 2/3 cup coconut cream
- 1/2 teaspoon vanilla extract
- 1/4 cup sugar
- 1/4 cup chocolate chips

Directions:
1. At 350 degrees F, preheat your air fryer.
2. Grease a baking dish suitable for your air fryer with cooking spray.
3. Spread the bread cubes in the baking dish.
4. Add chocolate chips on top of the bread cubes.
5. Beat cream with vanilla extract and sugar in a bowl.
6. Spread the cream mixture over the bread cubes.
7. Air fry the pudding for 10 minutes in the air fryer.

Nutrition: Calories 154; Fat 8.8g; Cholesterol 2mg; Carbohydrate 17.9g; Sugars 13.4g; Protein 2.4g

563. Berry Hand Pies

Preparation Time: 10 minutes
Cooking Time: 12 minutes
Serving: 8
Ingredients:
- 1 box store-bought pie crust
- 1/2 cup berry jam
- 1/2 cup berries
- ¼ cup almond butter, melted
- 2 tablespoons caster sugar

Directions:
1. At 375 degrees F, preheat your air fryer.
2. Roll out the pie crusts and cut 14 (4 inches) circles out of this dough using a cookie cutter.
3. Knead the leftover dough and roll out again to cut 2 more circles.
4. Add 2 tablespoons of berry jam at the center of 8 dough circles.
5. Place the remaining dough circles on top and press the edges with a fork to seal them.
6. Brush the hand pies with almond butter and drizzle sugar on top.
7. Place the berry hand pies in the air fryer basket and air fry for 12 minutes.
8. Flip the hand pies once cooked halfway through.
9. Serve.

Nutrition: Calories 167; Fat 7.3g; Cholesterol 0mg; Carbohydrate 25.3g; Sugars 13.8g; Protein 1.1g

564. Cheesecake Chimichangas

Preparation Time: 15 minutes
Cooking Time: 10 minutes
Serving: 8
Ingredients:
• 1 (8 ounces) can vegan cream cheese, softened
• 1/4 cup coconut cream
• 1-1/2 tablespoons granulated sugar
• 1 teaspoon vanilla extract
• 8 medium strawberries, quartered
• 1 medium banana, peeled and sliced
• 8 soft flour tortillas
• 8 teaspoons Nutella
• olive oil spray

Directions:
1. Mix sugar, vegan cream cheese, sugar and coconut cream in a bowl.
2. Divide the vegan cream cheese mixture into two bowls.
3. Add strawberries to one bowl and sliced bananas to another bowl.
4. Spread a tortilla on the working surface.
5. Add ¼ of the strawberry mixture to the left of the center of the tortilla.
6. Add a teaspoon of Nutella on the side and roll the tortilla like a burrito.
7. Repeat the same steps with the remaining strawberry and banana filling and tortillas.
8. At 350 degrees F, preheat your air fryer.
9. Place the rolled chimichangas in the air fryer basket.
10. Spray them with cooking oil and the air fryer for 10 minutes.
11. Flip the rolls once cooked halfway through.
12. Serve.

Nutrition: Calories 299; Fat 17g; Cholesterol 0mg; Carbohydrate 32.7g; Sugars 10g; Protein 5g

565. Chocolate Chip Skillet Cookie

Preparation Time: 15 minutes
Cooking Time: 15 minutes
Serving: 6
Ingredients:
• 1 cup 2 tablespoons all-purpose flour
• ½ teaspoon baking soda
• ½ teaspoon salt
• 6 tablespoons almond butter
• 1/3 cup granulated sugar
• ¼ cup light brown sugar
• 2 tablespoons almond milk
• ½ teaspoon vanilla extract
• 1 cup semisweet chocolate chips

Directions:
1. At 350 degrees F, preheat your air fryer.
2. Mix flour with salt and baking soda in a mixing bowl.
3. Stir in vanilla extract, milk, brown sugar, sugar and butter, then mix well.
4. Fold in chocolate chips and mix evenly.
5. Grease a 7 inches round pan with oil.
6. Spread the cookie batter in the pan and place it in the air fryer basket.
7. Air fryer the cookie dough for 15 minutes.
8. Serve.

Nutrition: Calories 333; Fat 15.4g; Cholesterol 0mg; Carbohydrate 46.6g; Sugars 29.3g; Protein 4.3g

566. Air Fryer Peaches

Preparation Time: 15 minutes
Cooking Time: 10 minutes
Serving: 2
Ingredients:
• 2 yellow peaches
• 1/4 cup graham cracker crumbs
• 1/4 cup brown sugar
• 1/4 cup almond butter

Directions:
1. Cut the peaches into wedges.
2. Layer the air fryer basket with a baking or parchment paper.
3. Spread peaches in the prepared basket.
4. At 350 degrees F, preheat your air fryer.
5. Air fry the peaches for 5 minutes.
6. Add butter, sugar and crumbs on top of the peaches.
7. Continue air frying for 5 minutes.
8. Serve.

Nutrition: Calories 187; Fat 2.5g; Cholesterol 0mg; Carbohydrate 40.8g; Sugars 33.7g; Protein 2.5g

567. Cherry Hand Pies

Preparation Time: 15 minutes
Cooking Time: 15 minutes
Serving: 6-8
Ingredients:
- 1 (2-count package) refrigerated pie crusts
- 1 (21-ounce) can cherry pie filling
- 2¼ cups confectioners' sugar
- 1/4 cup almond milk

Directions:
1. At 370 degrees F, preheat your air fryer.
2. Roll out the pie crusts and cut 4-inch circles out of this dough using a cookie cutter.
3. Add a tablespoon of pie at the center of the dough circles.
4. Fold them in half and press the edges with a fork to seal.
5. Brush the hand pies with almond milk and drizzle sugar on top.
6. Place the cherry hand pies in the air fryer basket and air fry for 15 minutes.
7. Flip the hand pies once cooked halfway through.
8. Serve.
Nutrition: Calories 248; Fat 10.5g; Cholesterol 0mg; Carbohydrate 37.2g; Sugars 19.9g; Protein 1.4g

568. Apple Pie Roll

Preparation Time: 10 minutes
Cooking Time: 8 minutes
Serving: 4
Ingredients:
- 21 ounces can apple pie filling
- 1/2 teaspoon lemon juice
- 1/4 teaspoon apple pie spice
- 1/8 teaspoon ground cinnamon
- 1 tablespoon all-purpose flour
- 4 roll wrappers

Directions:
1. Mix apple pie filling with lemon juice, apple pie spice, cinnamon and flour in a bowl.
2. Spread a roll wrapper on the working surface in a diamond shape position.
3. Add ¼ of the apple pie filling on one corner of the wrapper.
4. Fold the top and bottom of the wrapper and roll it neatly.

5. Wet the edges and press to seal the roll.
6. Place the rolls in the air fryer basket and spray with cooking spray.
7. At 400 degrees F, preheat your air fryer.
8. Air fry the apple pie rolls for 8 minutes in the preheated air fryer.
9. Serve.
Nutrition: Calories 156; Fat 0.6g; Cholesterol 0mg; Carbohydrate 34.5g; Sugars 3.6g; Protein 5.2g

569. Hippie Bonbons

Preparation time: 10 minutes
Cooking time: 0 minutes
Serving: 19 bonbons
Ingredients:
- 1½ cups Medjool dates, pitted
- 1 cup mixed raw nuts or seeds
- 1 tablespoon fresh orange juice
- ½ teaspoon orange zest
- 1 teaspoon pure vanilla extract
- ½ teaspoon fine sea salt (optional)
- ½ teaspoon ground cinnamon

Direction:
1. In the bowl of a food processor, combine the pitted dates, nuts or seeds, orange juice, orange zest, vanilla, sea salt, if using, and cinnamon. Pulse the mixture a couple of times to chop everything. Then mix on high speed until the mixture sticks together and the nut pieces are quite small.
2. Scoop out a heaped tablespoon portion of the date and nut mixture, and roll the portion into a ball. Set the bonbon onto a dinner plate. Repeat with the remaining date and nut mixture.
3. The bonbons will keep in a sealed container in the refrigerator for about 1 week.
Nutrition: Calories: 104 | fat: 8g | protein: 3g | carbs: 7g | fiber: 2g

570. Berry Compote

Preparation time: 5 minutes
Cooking time: 5 minutes
Serving: 2 cups
Ingredients:
- 3 to 4 cups fresh or frozen berries,
- ½ cup freshly squeezed orange juice
- 1 teaspoon vanilla extract

- Tiny pinch of fine sea salt (optional)
- 2 teaspoons arrowroot powder
- 1 tablespoon filtered water

Direction:

1. Combine the berries, orange juice, vanilla, and salt, if using, in a medium pot and bring to a boil over high heat. Cover the pan, reduce the heat to low, and simmer for 5 minutes, or until the berries have softened and released their juice. Dissolve the arrowroot in the water in a small cup, then slowly drizzle into the simmering berries, stirring constantly. Once the compote has returned to a simmer and thickened, remove from the heat.

2. Serve warm or at room temperature. Store the cooled compote in a sealed jar in the fridge for up to 5 days.

Nutrition: Calories: 81 | fat: 1g | protein: 1g | carbs: 19g | fiber: 3g

571.   Blueberry-Lime Sorbet

Preparation time: 5 minutes
Cooking time: 0 minutes
Serving: 6
Ingredients:

- 1 cup frozen blueberries
- 1 cup fresh blueberries
- 3 to 6 ice cubes
- ¼ cup unsweetened raisins
- 2 tablespoons lime juice

Direction:

1. In a high-efficiency blender, combine the frozen blueberries, fresh blueberries, ice, raisins, and lime juice. Blend for about 30 seconds, or until smooth. (You may need to use the tamping tool to move frozen ingredients toward the blades.) Serve immediately.

Nutrition: Calories: 116 | fat: 1g | protein: 2g | carbs: 30g | fiber: 4g

572.   Dutch Apple Pie Oatmeal Squares

Preparation time: 10 minutes
Cooking time: 30 minutes

Serving: 4
Ingredients:

- 2¼ cups rolled oats, divided
- 1 cup unsweetened plant-based milk
- 4 tablespoons maple syrup, divided (optional)
- 2 teaspoons ground cinnamon
- 1 apple, peeled, cored, and chopped
- 1 teaspoon vanilla extract
- ¼ cup ground flaxseeds
- 1 cup plus 3 tablespoons water, divided
- ¼ cup macadamia nuts
- ½ cup whole-wheat flour

Direction:

1. Preheat the oven to 375°F (190°C).

2. In an 8-by-8-inch baking dish, mix together 2 cups of oats, the plant-based milk, 2 tablespoons of maple syrup (if using), the cinnamon, apple, vanilla, flaxseeds, and 1 cup of water.

3. In a blender, pulse the macadamia nuts to a meal-like texture.

4. In a medium bowl, mix together the whole-wheat flour, macadamia nuts, the remaining ¼ cup oats, remaining 2 tablespoons maple syrup, and 3 tablespoons water to form a loose dough. Crumble the mixture over the top of the oatmeal mixture.

5. Bake for 35 minutes, or until the top is crispy. Let cool for 10 minutes to set, then cut into 4 squares. Refrigerate for up to 4 days.

Nutrition: Calories: 438 | fat: 14g | protein: 14g | carbs: 69g | fiber: 11g

573.   Zesty Orange-Cranberry Energy Bites

Preparation time: 10 minutes
Cooking time: 0 minutes
Serving: 12 bites
Ingredients:

- 2 tablespoons almond butter, or cashew or sunflower seed butter
- 2 tablespoons maple syrup or brown rice syrup (optional)
- 1 tablespoon chia seeds
- ½ teaspoon almond extract or vanilla extract
- Zest of 1 orange
- 1 tablespoon dried cranberries
- ¼ cup ground almonds

Direction:

1. In a medium bowl, mix together the nut or seed butter and syrup (if using) until smooth and creamy.

2. Stir in the rest of the ingredients, and mix to make sure the consistency is holding together in a ball.

3. Form the mix into 12 balls. Place them on a baking sheet lined with parchment or waxed paper and put in the fridge to set for about 15 minutes.

Nutrition: Calories: 71 | fat: 4g | protein: 2g | carbs: 6g | fiber: 1g

574. Caramel-Coconut Frosted Brownies

Preparation time: 10 minutes
Cooking time: 25 minutes
Serving: 12 brownies
Ingredients:
Brownies:
- 1 (15-ounce / 425-g) can black beans, drained and rinsed
- ½ cup rolled oats
- 6 tablespoons pure maple syrup
- 2 tablespoons unsalted, unsweetened almond butter
- 1 teaspoon vanilla extract
- Pinch ground cinnamon

Frosting:
- 1 cup pitted dates
- 6 tablespoons unsweetened plant-based milk
- 2 tablespoons nutritional yeast
- ¼ teaspoon vanilla extract
- 1/8 teaspoon red miso paste
- ¼ cup chopped pecans
- 3 tablespoons unsweetened coconut flakes

Direction:
Make the Brownies:

1. Preheat the oven to 350°F (180°C). Line a 12-cup cupcake tin with liners.

2. In a food processor, combine the beans, oats, maple syrup, cocoa powder, applesauce, almond butter, vanilla, and cinnamon. Process until smooth.

3. Transfer the mixture to the prepared cupcake tin, about 2 tablespoons per cup to start, then evenly divide the remaining mixture.

4. Bake for 20 to 22 minutes, or until the tops are crispy and a toothpick inserted into the center of a cupcake comes out mostly clean. Remove from the oven. Remove the brownies from the tin, and transfer to a wire rack to cool for about 5 minutes. Make the Frosting:

5. Add 1 heaping tablespoon of the frosting per brownie, and serve.

Nutrition: Calories: 235 | fat: 11g | protein: 10g | carbs: 30g | fiber: 12g

575. Zabaglione Cashew Cream

Preparation time: 5 minutes
Cooking time: 0 minutes
Serving: 4
Ingredients:
- ½ cup raw cashews
- ½ cup apple juice
- ½ cup unsweetened raisins
- 2 teaspoons lemon juice
- Fresh berries or other fruits, for serving

Direction:

1. In a high-efficiency blender, combine the cashews, apple juice, raisins, and lemon juice. Blend until smooth. Transfer to an airtight container, and refrigerate until ready to serve.

2. To serve, put fruit in a bowl or dessert dish, and drizzle with the zabaglione.

Nutrition: Calories: 231 | fat: 8g | protein: 3g | carbs: 40g | fiber: 3g

576. Sweet Red Beans

Preparation time: 10 minutes
Cooking time: 30 minutes
Serving: 6
Ingredients:
- 1 cup adzuki beans, soaked overnight, drained and rinsed
- ¼ teaspoon vanilla bean powder or ½ teaspoon vanilla extract
- 2 cup water
- 3 tablespoons maple syrup (optional)
- 1/8 teaspoon salt (optional)

Direction:

1. Place the beans and vanilla in a medium saucepan. Add the water and bring to a boil. Cover and continue to boil until tender, about 30 minutes. (If your beans are still tough and need more water to cook, add it sparingly; you don't want soupy beans.)

2. Remove from the heat and stir in the sugar and salt, if desired. Let cool before serving.

Nutrition: Calories: 76 | fat: 0g | protein: 3g | carbs: 16g | fiber: 3g

577. Cherry Chocolate Bark

Preparation time: 5 minutes
Cooking time: 0 minutes
Serving: 8
Ingredients:
- 1 cup vegan semisweet chocolate chips
- 1 cup sliced almonds
- 1 cup dried tart cherries, chopped
- ½ teaspoon flaky sea salt, for sprinkling (optional)

Direction:
1. Line a rimmed baking sheet with parchment paper and place in the fridge or freezer to get very cold.

2. In a heatproof glass bowl set over a pan of simmering water, melt the chocolate, stirring occasionally. Be careful not to let water droplets get into the bowl or the chocolate will seize.

3. Pour the melted chocolate onto the chilled prepared pan and use a thin spatula to spread it evenly almost to the edges of the pan. Immediately sprinkle the almonds and cherries evenly over the chocolate, followed by a sprinkling of salt (if using). Refrigerate until firm.

4. Break the bark into pieces and store in an airtight container in the refrigerator for up to 1 week.

Nutrition: Calories: 189 | fat: 12g | protein: 3g | carbs: 17g | fiber: 3g

578. Spinach Sorbet

Preparation Time: 15 minutes
Cooking time: 0 minutes
Servings: 4
Ingredients:
- 3 cups fresh spinach, torn
- 1 tablespoon fresh basil leaves
- ½ of avocado, peeled, pitted and chopped
- ¾ cup almond milk
- 20 drops liquid stevia
- 1 teaspoon almonds, chopped very finely
- 1 teaspoon vanilla extract
- 1 cup ice cubes

Direction:
1.   In a blender, add all the ingredients and pulse until creamy and smooth.

2.   Transfer into an ice cream maker and process according to manufacturer's directions.

3.   Transfer into an airtight container and freeze for at least 4-5 hours before serving.

Nutrition: Calories: 166 Fat: 16g Carbohydrates: 5.7g Dietary Fiber: 3.2g Sugar: 1.9g Protein: 2.3g

579. Raspberry Ice Cream

Preparation Time: 15 minutes
Cooking time: 0 minutes
Servings: 8
Ingredients:
- 2¼ cups fresh raspberries, divided
- 1 small avocado, peeled, pitted and chopped
- 10 dates, pitted and chopped
- ¼ cup cashews, soaked for 30 minutes and drained
- 1¾ cups unsweetened almond milk
- 2/3 cup filtered water
- 1 tablespoon fresh lemon juice
- 1 tablespoon fresh beet juice

Direction:
1.   In a blender, add 2 cups of raspberries and reaming all ingredients and pulse until creamy and smooth.

2.   Transfer into an ice cream maker and process according to manufacturer's directions.

3.   Transfer into an airtight container and freeze for at least 4-5 hours.

4.   Top with the remaining raspberries and serve.

Nutrition: Calories: 187 Fat: 11.5g Carbohydrates: 21.9g Dietary Fiber: 7.1g Sugar: 11.4g Protein: 3g

580. Mixed Berries Granita

Preparation Time: 15 minutes
Cooking time: 0 minutes
Servings: 4
Ingredients:
- ½ cup fresh strawberries, hulled and sliced
- ½ cup fresh raspberries
- ½ cup fresh blueberries
- ½ cup fresh blackberries
- 1 tablespoon maple syrup
- 1 tablespoon fresh lemon juice
- 1 cup ice cubes, crushed

Direction:
1. In a high-powered blender, add the berries, maple syrup, lemon juice, and ice cubes and pulse on high speed until smooth.
2. Transfer the berry mixture into an 8x8-inch baking dish, spread evenly, and freeze for at least 30 minutes.
3. Remove from the freezer and, with a fork, stir the granita completely.
4. Freeze for 2-3 hours, stirring every 30 minutes with a fork.
Nutrition: Calories: 46 Fat: 0.3g Carbohydrates: 11g Dietary Fiber: 2.8g Sugar: 7.3g Protein: 0.7g

581. Blueberry & Tofu Mousse

Preparation Time: 10 minutes
Cooking time: 0 minutes
Servings: 2
Ingredients:
- ¾ cup silken tofu, drained and pressed
- ¾ cup frozen blueberries
- 2 tablespoons fresh lemon juice
- 1½ tablespoons maple syrup
- ¼ teaspoons vanilla extract

Direction:
1. Place tofu in a blender and pulse on high speed until a creamy.
2. Add the remaining ingredients and pulse until well combined.
3. Transfer the mixture into serving bowls and refrigerate to chill for about 1 hour before serving.

Nutrition: Calories: 142 Fat: 4.3g Carbohydrates: 19.9g Dietary Fiber: 2.2g Sugar: 15.3g Protein: 8.3g

582. Chocolaty Beans Mousse

Preparation Time: 10 minutes
Cooking time: 0 minutes
Servings: 2
Ingredients:
- 1 (15-ounce) can black beans, rinsed and drained
- ¼ cup unsweetened cocoa powder
- 3-4 tablespoons maple syrup
- 2 tablespoons vanilla soy milk
- ¼ teaspoon vanilla extract
- 1/8 teaspoon salt
- 2-3 tablespoons fresh blueberries

Direction:
1. In a food processor, add all ingredients except for raspberries and pulse until smooth.
2. Transfer the mixture into a bowl and refrigerate to chill in the fridge for at least 20 minutes.
3. Serve with the garnishing of blueberries.
Nutrition: Calories: 399 Fat: 3g Carbohydrates: 78.7g Dietary Fiber: 22.4g Sugar: 19.6g Protein: 21.5g

583. Raspberry Brownies

Preparation Time: 15 minutes
Cooking Time: 23 minutes
Servings: 10
Ingredients:
- 1 tablespoon flax meal
- 2½ tablespoons water
- ¼ cup plus 2 tablespoons vegan chocolate chips, divided
- 2 tablespoons coconut oil
- ¼ cup rolled oats
- ½ cup unsweetened vegan chocolate protein powder
- ½ cup cacao powder
- 2/3 cup unsweetened chocolate almond milk
- ½ cup unsweetened applesauce
- 1 tablespoon maple syrup
- 1 teaspoon vanilla extract

- ½ cup fresh raspberries, broken up into large pieces

Direction:
1. Preheat your oven to 350 °F.
2. Grease an 8x8-inch baking dish.
3. In a large bowl, add the ground flax and water and mix well.
4. Set aside for about 5 minutes.
5. In a microwave-safe bowl, place ¼ cup of chocolate chips and coconut oil and microwave on High for about 1 minute, stirring after every 20 seconds.
6. Remove from microwave and stir until just smooth.
7. Place oats in blender and pulse until a flour like texture is formed.
8. In a large bowl, add oat flour, protein powder and cacao powder and mix well.
9. In the bowl of flaxseed mixture, add almond milk, applesauce, maple syrup and vanilla extract and whisk until smooth.
10. I the bowl of flaxseed mixture, add the flour mixture and mix until just combined.
11. Add the chocolate chips mixture and gently stir to combine.
12. Place the mixture into prepared baking dish and with the back of a spoon, smooth the top surface.
13. Place the remaining chocolate chips and raspberries on top and with a knife, swirl them in the mixture.
14. Bake for approximately 18-22 minutes.
15. Remove the baking dish from oven and place onto a wire rack to cool completely.
16. With a sharp knife, cut into equal-sized brownies and serve.

Nutrition: Calories: 95 Fat: 5g Carbohydrates: 9.7g Dietary Fiber: 0.8g Sugar: 2.4g Protein: 5.3g

584. Blackberry Crumble

Preparation Time: 10 minutes
Cooking Time: 40 minutes
Servings: 4
Ingredients:
- ¼ cup coconut flour
- ¼ cup arrowroot flour
- ¾ teaspoon baking soda
- 2 tablespoons coconut oil, melted

- ¼ cup banana, peeled and mashed
- ½ tablespoon fresh lemon juice
- 3 tablespoons water
- 1½ cups fresh blackberries

Direction:
1. Preheat your oven to 3oo °F.
2. Lightly grease an 8x8-inch baking dish.
3. In a large bowl, mix together all ingredients except blackberries.
4. Place blackberries in the bottom of prepared baking dish.
5. Spread flour mixture over blackberries evenly.
6. Bake for 35-40 minutes or until top becomes golden brown.
7. Serve warm.

Nutrition: Calories: 99 Fat: 7.3g Carbohydrates: 8.9g Dietary Fiber: 3.5g Sugar: 3.9g Protein: 1.3g

585. Apple Crisp

Preparation Time: 15 minutes
Cooking Time: 20 minutes
Servings: 8
Ingredients:
For Filling:
- 2 large apples, peeled, cored, and chopped
- 2 tablespoons fresh apple juice
- 2 tablespoons water
- ¼ teaspoon ground cinnamon

For Topping:
- ½ cup quick rolled oats
- 2 tablespoons walnuts, chopped
- ¼ cup unsweetened coconut flakes
- ½ teaspoon ground cinnamon
- ¼ cup water

Instructions:
1. Preheat your oven to 300 °F.
2. In a baking dish, add all filling ingredients and gently mix.
3. In a bowl, add all topping ingredients and mix until well combined.
4. Spread the topping over the filling mixture evenly.
5. Bake for approximately 20 minutes or until top becomes golden brown.
6. Serve warm.

Nutrition: Calories: 115 Fat: 3.7g Carbohydrates: 19.4g Dietary Fiber: 2.9g Sugar: 12.2g Protein: 1.8g

586.   Grilled Peaches

Preparation Time: 10 minutes
Cooking Time: 10 minutes
Servings: 4
Ingredients:
• 2 large peaches, halved and pitted
• 1/8 teaspoon ground cinnamon
Direction:
1. Preheat the grill to medium-high heat.
2. Grease the grill grate.
3. Arrange the peach halves on the prepared grill, cut side down and cook for 3-5 minutes per side.
4. Sprinkle with cinnamon and serve.
Nutrition: Calories: 30 Fat: 0.2g Carbohydrates: 7.1g Dietary Fiber: 1.2g Sugar: 7g Protein: 0.7g

587.   Carrot Cake

Preparation time: 15 minutes
Cooking time: 45 minutes
Servings: 4
Ingredients:
For the carrot cake:
• 3 cups of flour
• 2 cups of sugar
• 2 tsp. ground cinnamon
• 2 tsp. baking powder
• 1 tsp. baking soda
• 1 tsp. of salt
• 4 large eggs
• 1 ¼ cups of vegetable oil
• ¾ cup sugar-free and fat-free applesauce
• 1 tsp. vanilla extract
• 2 cups carrots, crumbled
• 1 pineapple, drained and chopped
• 1 cup chopped walnuts
For the cream cheese topping:
• 1 cup unsalted butter, softened
• 1 cup cream cheese, soft
• 1 ½ cups powdered sugar
• 1 cup chopped walnuts
Direction:
1. Preheat oven to 360ºF and grease three 8-inch round cake pans with non-stick spray.

2. In large bowl, beat together flour, sugar, cinnamon, baking powder, baking soda, and salt.
3. In a small bowl, beat the eggs, oil, applesauce, and vanilla.
4. Add the egg mixture into the flour mixture until combined. Fold the carrots, pineapple and walnuts.
5. Evenly distribute the dough between the prepared pans and bake in the oven for about 45 minutes. Let cool.
6. For the Coverage: Place the butter and cream cheese in a bowl and beat on medium low speed until smooth and creamy, about 3 minutes. Gradually add powdered sugar. Whisk over medium until light and fluffy, scraping bowl as needed.
7. Remove the cooled cakes from their cans and place one of the layers, flat side down, on a flat plate or cake stand. Cover with ¾ cup of frosting. Put another layer of cake. Cover with ¾ cup of frosting. Place with the final layer of cake. Using a spatula, cover the cake with the remaining topping. Garnish with chopped walnuts along the bottom edge of the sides. Enjoy!
Nutrition: Calorie: 133.5 Protein: 4.3g Fat: 3.7g Carbohydrates: 23.7g

588.   Carrot and Tofu Cake

Preparation time: 15 minutes
Cooking time: 40 minutes
Servings: 4
Ingredients:
• ½ lb. of raw carrots, peeled and grated
• ½ lb. silky tofu
• ½ cup of sunflower oil
• ½ lb. of flour
• ½ lb. of brown sugar
• 4 tsp (one sachet) of chemical yeast
• 4 eggs
• 1 tsp of baking soda
• 1 tsp of cinnamon
Direction:
1. Crush the carrots together with the oil and reserve. Sift together the dry ingredients (flour, yeast, baking soda, and cinnamon). In a large bowl beat the sugar with the eggs until they are frothy.

2. Add the tofu and continue beating to integrate. Add the carrot, mix, and then dry ingredients twice, mixing well.

3. Pour into a 24 cm mold previously greased and floured. Take to the oven preheated to 360° F for about 40 minutes, to know if the cake is ready click with a toothpick in the center, if it comes out clean it is cooked.

4. Remove from the oven, let cool in the mold and then unmold.

Nutrition: Calorie: 133.5 Protein: 4.3g Fat: 3.7g Carbohydrates: 23.7g

589. Strawberry Cream Cake

Preparation time: 10 minutes
Cooking time: 40 minutes
Servings: 4
Ingredients:
- 4 eggs
- 1 cup of sugar
- ¼ cup oil
- 1 cup of flour
- 1 pinch of salt
- ½ cup boiling water
- ½ tsp. vanilla extract tea
- Powdered tea
- 1 ½ teaspoon of baking soda
- ½ lb. of fresh cream
- 3 ½ oz. condensed milk
- 1 lb. strawberry

Direction:
1. Separate the whites from the yolks and reserve the whites. In a bowl, beat the egg yolks with the sugar and oil. Mix the flour with the salt.

2. Add the water and wheat flour to the yolk mixture and mix. Then add the vanilla essence. Beat the egg whites.

3. Add the yeast mixture and finally the egg whites gently.

4. Grease and flour a mold with a round shape and place the mixture

5. Bake at 3600F for 40 minutes.

6. Mix the cream with condensed milk to form whipped cream.

7. Cut ½ lb. of strawberries in small cubes and add to the mixture of whipped cream Mix with the rest of the whipped cream.

8. Cover the cake with the cream and decorate.
Nutrition: Calorie: 212.5 Protein: 2.3g Fat: 8.3g Carbohydrates: 31.9g

590. Quince Sweet

Preparation time: 40 minutes
Cooking time: 40-50 minutes
Servings: 4
Ingredients:
- Quince pulp 1 lb. (already peeled and cored)
- 1 lb. sugar

Direction:
1. Wash the quinces well, put them in a large pot and cover with water. Once the water starts to boil, lower the heat and cook for 45 minutes.

2. After the time, remove the quinces from the water, let cool until they do not burn, peel them, remove the heart and cut the pulp into pieces.

3. Arrange the pieces in a saucepan next to the sugar and bring to the fire. Little by little the sugar will be integrated into the pulp of the quince; after about 10 minutes you will see that the sugar is completely dissolved: at that moment grind with the mixer and cook for about 40 more minutes.

4. After the time has passed, to shape the homemade quince, we pour the quince jelly onto the container you have chosen and distribute it well; Cover with plastic wrap and take to the fridge overnight.

Nutrition: Calorie: 52 Protein: 0.3g Fat: 0g Carbohydrates: 14g

591. Oat and Banana Cookies

Preparation time: 10 minutes
Cooking time: 15-20 minutes
Servings: 4
Ingredients:
- 3 ripe bananas
- 1 and a half glass of oatmeal
- Chocolate chips (to taste)
- 1 tablespoon brown sugar

Direction:
1. Preheat the oven to 360ºF, heat up and down.

2. Cut the three bananas into slices and arrange them in a bowl, with the handle of a mortar crush the bananas well.

3. Next add the oats, chocolate chips and a tablespoon of brown sugar, knead well until a ball form.

4. Form small balls and crush lightly, put the cookies on a suitable dish for oven and bake for 15 - 20 minutes.

5. After the time, remove the cookies from the oven and let them warm on a rack.

Nutrition: Calorie: 34.1 Protein: 1g Fat: 0.4g Carbohydrates: 7.2g

592. Orange and Chocolate Cake

Preparation time: 1h minutes
Cooking time: 455 minutes
Servings: 2
Ingredients:
For the Cake:
- 3 cups of flour
- 2 cups butter
- 2 tsp. baking powder
- 2 cups of sugar
- a pinch of salt
- 2 ½ tbsp. orange zest
- 1 ½ tbsp. lemon zest
- 5 eggs
- 1 ½ cups orange juice.
For the filling:
- 1 cup of sugar
- 2 ½ tbsp. Of flour
- 1 cup orange juice
- 2 egg yolks
- 2 tbsp. of butter
Direction:
1. Beat the butter, orange zest, lemon and sugar.

2. Add the eggs and gradually integrate the flour, baking powder and salt, alternating with the orange juice.

3. Flour and butter 2 molds of the same size. Distribute the mixture evenly in the two molds and bake for 45 minutes. Unmold and let cool. For the filling, in a saucepan mix the sugar, flour, orange juice and yolks. Heat over low heat and stir until it boils slightly and thickens.

4. Remove from the heat, add the butter and let cool.

5. Put one layer of cake, filling, the other layer of cake and more filling.

Nutrition: Calorie: 168.1 Protein: 3.1g Fat: 11.9g Carbohydrates: 13.8g

593. Vegan Kefir

Preparation time: 15 minutes
Cooking time: 0 minutes
Servings: 4
Ingredients:
- 4 ¼ cup of filtered drinking water
- 5 tbsp of water kefir nodules
- 1 ½ oz. of raisins
- 5 tbsp of muscobo sugar
- 1 apple
Direction:
1. In a liter of drinking water, dissolve 3 tablespoons of sugar; squeeze the juice of half a lemon (cut that half of the squeezed lemon and add it to the water), 5 tablespoons of nodules and 1 handful of raisins. Stir with a wooden spoon (do not use metal). Cover with a canvas and let stand 12 hours at room temperature. At 12 o'clock stir carefully again and cover again. 12 hours later strain the liquid. Wash the nodules and store in the refrigerator.

Nutrition: Calorie: 110 Protein: 11g Fat: 0g Carbohydrates: 12g

594. Azteca Cake

Preparation time: 15 minutes
Cooking time: 30-40 minutes
Servings: 2
Ingredients:
- 5 chilies from heaven
- 2 cloves of garlic
- ¼ onion
- 3 cups. of water
- 8 wheat tortillas
- 1 cup corn kernels
- ½ cup cream
- 2 tbsp. chopped coriander
- 1 ½ cup of mozzarella or cheese of preference
- Salt oil
Direction:

1. Heat the chilies, garlic, and onion with 3 cups of water.
2. Boil 10m. Transfer to a blender and blend with the same cooking juice.
3. Strain and reserve the sauce.
4. Brown the tortillas in oil and reserve. Dip it in the sauce and arrange in the base of an ovenproof dish.
5. Sprinkle some corn kernels, a little of the chili sauce, cream and coriander.
6. Repeat this operation until you finish with all the ingredients.
7. Gratin in the oven at 4000F until the cheese is gratin.
Nutrition: Calorie: 140 Protein: 11g Fat: 12g Carbohydrates: 10g

595. Strawberry Milkshake

Preparation time: 5 minutes
Cooking time: 0 minutes
Servings: 1-2
Ingredients:
- ½ lb. strawberry
- 2 strawberry soy yogurts
- 1 cup of soy milk
- 4 cookies without ingredients of animal origin
- 2 tbsp of sugar

Direction:
1. Clean the strawberries and put them in the blender glass together with the yogurts, sugar and milk. You can use the yogurt cups to measure the milk, filled the same ones and add that amount. When it is well mixed, break the cookies and add them. Continue beating until everything is homogeneous and ready. You can leave it a little in the fridge so that it is very cold.
Nutrition: Calorie: 640 Protein: 12g Fat: 22g Carbohydrates: 101g

596. Potato and Mushroom Cake

Preparation time: 20 minutes
Cooking time: 1hour
Servings: 8

Ingredients:
- 8 medium potatoes
- ½ lb. of mushroom
- ½ lb. of portobello in thin sheets
- 1 cup of grated gruyere
- ½ cup grated Parmesan
- 3 tbsp. parsley
- 1 tbsp. oregano
- ½ cup vegetable broth
- salt, pepper and nutmeg
- 1 tbsp. butter

Direction:
1. Heat the oven to 360ºF and grease a baking dish with the tablespoon of butter
2. Cut the potatoes and mushrooms into very thin sheets
3. In the greased refractory make layers of potatoes, mushrooms, gruyere, seasoning between layers.
4. At the end add the vegetable stock, cover with aluminum and bake for 1h.
5. Uncover, cover with cheese and gratin with Parmesan until golden.
Nutrition: Calorie: 117.5 Protein: 2.9g Fat: 3.2g Carbohydrates: 20.2g

597. Oat Milk

Preparation time: 5 minutes
Cooking time: 15 minutes
Servings: 1-2
Ingredients:
- ½ cup rolled whole oats
- 3 cups of water
- 2 tsp maple syrup
- ½ tsp vanilla extract
- Ta tsp of sea salt

Direction:
1. Mix the oats, water, maple syrup, vanilla, and salt in a blender and mix for 30 seconds.
2. Place the fine mesh strainer over a large bowl and strain the milk without pushing excess pulp through the strainer. This will create a creamier texture that is not gritty or sticky.
3. Add more maple syrup, to taste, if desired. Let cool overnight. but if you want to take it once prepared, put an ice on it. It is much tastier fresh.
Nutrition: Calorie: 120 Protein: 3g Fat: 5g Carbohydrates: 16g

598. Strawberry Biscuit Cake

Preparation time: 15 minutes
Cooking time: 30-40 minutes
Servings: 4
Ingredients:
- 1 can of condensed milk
- ½ cup milk
- 4 egg yolks
- 1 tablet of semi-bitter chocolate
- 1 pot of cream
- ½ lb. of cookies
- 1 cup of whipping cream
- ½ lb. sliced strawberries

Direction:
1. Place the milk, condensed milk and egg yolks over low heat, stirring constantly until thick. Cool for 1 hour.
2. In a bowl, mix the melted chocolate with the cream. Reserve.
3. On a platter, put the condensed milk mixture, a large number of cookies on top, then the chocolate mixture, the second portion of wafers and cover with the whipping cream.
4. Finish the preparation with strawberry slices on top. Arrange in circular shapes.
5. Enjoy it!

Nutrition: Calorie: 90 Protein: 2.3g Fat: 2.7g Carbohydrates: 15.3g

599. Red Fruit Shake

Preparation time: 5 minutes
Cooking time: 0 minutes
Servings: 1-2
Ingredients:
- ½ lb. of strawberries
- ½ lb. raspberries
- ½ lb. of blackberries
- ½ cup of water
- Agave syrup (optional)
- Flax or chia seeds (optional)

Direction:
1. First wash the fruits well. Cut the strawberries too, but if they are not very large, it is not necessary.
2. Put the fruits in the base of the mixer and crush until you have a smooth and homogeneous texture.
3. Raspberries and frozen blackberries give a very creamy texture and also makes the smoothie super cool. If you use them frozen, keep in mind the type of mixer you use, if it is not very powerful; better take them out of the freezer a few minutes before so they are not too hard.
4. You can also add some seeds, flax or chia, crushing them at the same time as the fruits and you will provide extra nutrients.

Nutrition: Calorie: 130 Protein: 1g Fat: 0g Carbohydrates: 31g

600. Oreo Crepes Tower

Preparation time: 25 minutes
Cooking time: 40 minutes
Servings: 8
Ingredients:
- 1 cup flour
- 2 tbsp. cocoa powder
- 4 tbsp. of sugar
- 2 eggs
- 2 tbsp. melted butter
- 1 cup milk
- 1 1/3 cup heavy cream
- ¼ cup sugar
- 1 tsp. vanilla essence
- 7 crushed Oreo cookies

Direction:
1. Mix all the ingredients for the pancakes.
2. Make 15 pancakes.
3. Separate the cream from the Oreo and crush them.
4. Make the pancake tower sandwiching with the whipped cream and the crushed Oreo.
5. Decorate with whipped cream and Mini-Oreos.

Nutrition: Calorie: 121.1 Protein: 3.4g Fat: 6.5g Carbohydrates: 15.7g

601.   Coriander and Walnut Pesto

Preparation time: 5 minutes
Cooking time: 0 minutes
Servings: 2
Ingredients:
- 1 coriander bundle
- 2 cloves of garlic
- 1 handful of walnuts
- Oil to taste

Direction:
1.   Blend coriander, garlic, salt and walnuts with a little oil to form a paste.
2.   Add oil little by little. Store in glass jars and refrigerate in the refrigerator.
Nutrition: Calorie: 35 Protein: 0g Fat: 4g Carbohydrates: 0g

602.   Tofu Cream: Spreadable Tofu Cheese

Preparation time: 5 minutes
Cooking time: 0 minutes
Servings: 2
Ingredients:
- ¼ lb. tofu
- 1 tbsp titanium nutritional yeast
- 1 tbsp of lemon juice
- Neutral oil
- Neutral vegan milk or water

Direction:
1.   Mix everything well. add oil little by little until it becomes consistent.
2.   Add, if necessary, vegan milk or water to lighten.
3.   Store in a plate in the refrigerator.
Nutrition: Calorie: 159.3 Protein: 5g Fat: 4.5g Carbohydrates: 23.7g

603.   Almond Milk

Preparation time: 8 hours
Cooking time: 0 minutes
Servings: 2
Ingredients:
- 100g raw almonds
- 1 liter of water

Direction:
1.   Put the liter of water in the transparent glass, put the previously soaked almonds for about 8 hours in the filter and crush with a hand mixer for one minute at maximum power.
2.   Drain well and store the milk in the fridge, which lasts about 3 days.
Nutritional Information: Calorie: 39 Protein: 1g Fat: 3g Carbohydrates: 3.5g

604.   Ginger Milk

Preparation time: 5 minutes
Cooking time: 5-10 minutes
Servings: 2
Ingredients:
- 1 ½ cup of vegetable milk
- Grated or powdered ginger
- Pinch of salt
- Muscovy sugar

Direction:
1.   Heat all ingredients in a saucepan over medium low heat. Stir well until it boils.
2.   Serve and enjoy!
Nutrition: Calorie: 200 Protein: 8g Fat: 10g Carbohydrates: 20g

605.   Fresh Mint and Basil Ice Cream

Preparation time: 5 minutes
Cooking time: 0 minutes
Servings: 4
Ingredients:
- ½ lb. raw cashews
- 1 lb. peeled and diced pears
- 1 ¾ oz. white raisins
- 3 ½ oz. fresh basil leaves
- 3 ½ oz. fresh mint leaves

- 1 ½ oz. of water (enough to mix)

Direction:
1.   Soak the cashews in water for about 12 hours and then remove the water.
2.   Put all the ingredients in a blender and blend until you get a uniform and homogeneous cream.
3.   If you have an ice cream maker, you can put the mix in it to finish the ice cream. If you don't have this machine, just put the mix in the freezer until it has a harder consistency.
Nutrition: Calorie: 247 Protein: 5g Fat: 16g Carbohydrates: 23g

606.   Watermelon Smoothie

Preparation time: 5 minutes
Cooking time: 0 minutes
Servings: 4
Ingredients:
- 1 lb. of watermelon
- 1 soy yogurt
- 2 glasses of crushed ice
Direction:
1.   The preparation of this watermelon smoothie is very simple; you just have to put the glass of the blender the watermelon cut into pieces and the soy yogurt. Whisk until well mixed and watermelon completely melts. A fairly liquid and homogeneous mixture will remain.
2.   To finish the smoothie, you just have to add the ice and beat again so that it melts.
3.   Let's enjoy it!
Nutrition: Calorie: 113.5 Protein: 4.3g Fat: 1.7g Carbohydrates: 22.1g

607.   Tart Apple Granita

Preparation time: 15 minutes, plus 4 hours freezing time
Cooking time: 0 minutes
Servings: 4
Ingredients:
- ½ cup granulated sugar
- ½ cup of water
- 2 cups unsweetened apple juice
- ¼ cup freshly squeezed lemon juice

Directions:
1.   In a small saucepan over medium-high heat, heat the sugar and water.
2.   Bring the mixture to a boil and then reduce the heat to low. Let it simmer for about 15 minutes or until the liquid has reduced by half.
3.   Remove the pan from the heat and pour the liquid into a large shallow metal pan.
4.   Let the liquid cool for about 30 minutes and then stir in the apple juice and lemon juice.
5.   Place the pan in the freezer.
6.   After 1 hour, run a fork through the liquid to break up any ice crystals that have formed. Scrape down the sides as well.
7.   Place the pan back in the freezer and repeat the stirring and scraping every 20 minutes, creating slush.
8.   Serve when the mixture is completely frozen and looks like crushed ice, after about 3 hours.
Nutrition: Calories: 157 Fat: 0g Carbohydrates: 0g Phosphorus: 10mg Potassium: 141mg Sodium: 5mg Protein: 0g

608.   Lemon-Lime Sherbet

Preparation time: 5 minutes, plus 3 hours chilling time
Cooking time: 15 minutes
Servings: 2
Ingredients:
- 2 cups of water
- 1 cup granulated sugar
- 3 tablespoons lemon zest, divided
- ½ cup freshly squeezed lemon juice
- Zest of 1 lime
- Juice of 1 lime
- ½ cup heavy (whipping) cream
Directions:
1.   Place a large saucepan over medium-high heat and add the water, sugar, and 2 tablespoons of the lemon zest.
2.   Bring the mixture to a boil and then reduce the heat and simmer for 15 minutes.
3.   Transfer the mixture to a large bowl and add the remaining 1 tablespoon lemon zest, the lemon juice, lime zest, and lime juice.
4.   Chill the mixture in the fridge until completely cold, about 3 hours.

5. Whisk in the heavy cream and transfer the mixture to an ice cream maker.
6. Freeze according to the manufacturer's instructions.
Nutrition: Calories: 151 Fat: 6g Carbohydrates: 26g Phosphorus: 10mg Potassium: 27mg Sodium: 6mg Protein: 0g

609. Tropical Vanilla Snow Cone

Preparation time: 15 minutes, plus freezing time
Cooking time: 0 minutes
Servings: 2
Ingredients:
• 1 cup pineapple
• 1 cup of frozen strawberries
• 6 tablespoons water
• 2 tablespoons granulated sugar
• 1 tablespoon vanilla extract
• 2 Peaches
Directions:
1. In a large saucepan, mix together the peaches, pineapple, strawberries, water, and sugar over medium-high heat and bring to a boil.
2. Reduce the heat to low and simmer the mixture, occasionally stirring for 15 minutes.
3. Remove from the heat and let the mixture cool completely, for about 1 hour.
4. Stir in the vanilla and transfer the fruit mixture to a food processor or blender.
5. Purée until smooth and pour the purée into a 9-by-13-inch glass baking dish.
6. Cover and place the dish in the freezer overnight.
7. When the fruit mixture is completely frozen, use a fork to scrape the sorbet until you have flaked flavored ice.
8. Scoop the ice flakes into four serving dishes.
Nutrition: Calories: 92 Fat: 0g Carbohydrates: 22g Phosphorus: 17mg Potassium: 145mg Sodium: 4mg Protein: 1g

610. Peanut Butter, Nut, and Fruit Cookies

Preparation time: 30 minutes

Cooking time: 0 minutes
Servings: 25
Ingredients:
• ¾ cup rolled oats
• ¼ cup chopped peanuts
• ½ cup coconut flakes, unsweetened
• ¼ cup and 2 tablespoons chopped cranberries, dried
• ¼ cup sliced almonds
• ¼ cup and 2 tablespoons raisins
• ¼ cup maple syrup
• ¾ cup peanut butter
Directions:
1. Take a baking sheet, line it with wax paper, and then set it aside until required.
2. Take a large bowl, place oats, almonds, and coconut flakes in it, add ¼ cup each of cranberries and raisins, and then stir until combined.
3. Add maple syrup and peanut butter, stir until well combined, and then scoop the mixture on the prepared baking sheet with some distance between them.
4. Flatten each scoop of cookie mixture slightly, press the remaining cranberries and raisins into each cookie, and then let it chill for 20 minutes until firm.
5. Serve straight away.
Nutrition: Calories: 140 Fat: 7g Protein: 3g Carbs: 18g Fiber: 5g

611. Stone Fruit Compote

Preparation time: 5 minutes
Cooking time: 10 minutes
Serving: 2½ cups
Ingredients:
• 1½ pounds (680 g) ripe peaches, plums, apricots, or cherries
• ½ cup freshly squeezed orange juice or filtered water
• Tiny pinch of fine sea salt (optional)
• 1 teaspoon arrowroot powder
• 2 teaspoons filtered water
• ½ teaspoon vanilla extract
Direction:
1. If using peaches, plums, or apricots, halve and pit them. Cut each half into ½-inch wedges and slice the wedges in half crosswise. If using cherries, pit them.

Put the fruit in a medium pot, add the orange juice and salt, and bring to a simmer over high heat. Cover the pot, reduce the heat to low, and simmer for 8 to 10 minutes, until the fruit is soft. Dissolve the arrowroot in the water in a small cup, then drizzle it into the pot, stirring constantly. Once the compote has returned to a simmer and thickened, remove from the heat and stir in the vanilla.

2. Serve warm or at room temperature. Store the cooled compote in a sealed jar in the fridge for up to 5 days.

Nutrition: Calories: 77 | fat: 0g | protein: 1g | carbs: 19g | fiber: 2g

612.   Apple-Oat Crisp

Preparation time: 10 minutes
Cooking time: 25 minutes
Serving: 4 to 6
Ingredients:
* 4 medium Granny Smith apples, cored and cut into ½-inch-thick slices
* ¾ cup pure maple syrup, divided
* 1 tablespoon lemon juice
* ½ teaspoon ground cinnamon
* 1/8 teaspoon ground nutmeg
* ¼ teaspoon tapioca starch
* 2/3 cup rolled oats
* 2/3 cup oat flour
* 1/3 cup unsweetened applesauce
Direction:
1. Preheat the oven to 350ºF (180ºC).
2. In a medium bowl, mix together the apples, ½ cup of maple syrup, the lemon juice, cinnamon, nutmeg, and tapioca starch until the apples are well coated.
3. Spread the apples out in a single layer in an 8-by-8-inch glass baking dish or a 9-inch pie plate.
4. In a medium bowl, mix together the oats, oat flour, remaining ¼ cup of maple syrup, and the applesauce until well combined. Scoop the oat mixture in dollops onto the apples, and spread gently, trying to cover all the apples.
5. Transfer the baking dish to the oven, and bake for 20 to 25 minutes, or until the oat mixture is golden brown. Remove from the oven.
Nutrition: Calories: 344 | fat: 3g | protein: 5g | carbs: 80g | fiber: 9g

613.   Sweet Potato Pie Nice Cream

Preparation time: 5 minutes
Cooking time: 0 minutes
Serving: 2
Ingredients:
* 2 medium cooked sweet potatoes
* ½ cup plant-based milk
* 1 tablespoon maple syrup (optional)
* 1 teaspoon vanilla extract
* ½ teaspoon ground cinnamon
Direction:
1. Line a baking sheet with parchment paper.
2. Remove the skin from the cooked sweet potatoes, and cut the flesh into 1-inch cubes. Place on the baking sheet in an even layer, then place in the freezer overnight, or for a minimum of 4 hours.
3. In a food processor, combine the frozen sweet potato, milk, maple syrup (if desired), vanilla, and cinnamon.
4. Process on medium speed for 1 to 2 minutes, or until the mixture has been blended into a smooth soft-serve consistency, and serve. (If you notice any sweet potato pieces stuck toward the top and sides of the food processor, you may need to stop and scrape them down with a spatula, then pulse until smooth.)
Nutrition: Calories: 155 | fat: 1g | protein: 2g | carbs: 34g | fiber:5 g

614.   Pumpkin Bread Pudding

Preparation time: 10 minutes
Cooking time: 25 minutes
Serving: 8
Ingredients:
* 1¼ cups pumpkin purée (a little over ½ of a 15-ounce / 425-g can)
* 1 cup unsweetened plant-based milk
* ½ cup 100% maple syrup (optional)
* 2 teaspoons pure vanilla extract
* 2 tablespoons cornstarch
* ½ teaspoon salt (optional)
* ½ teaspoon ground cinnamon

- ¾ teaspoon ground ginger
- ¼ teaspoon ground nutmeg
- ¼ teaspoon ground allspice
- 1/8 teaspoon ground cloves
- 8 slices stale whole wheat bread, cut into 1-inch cubes (about 6 cups)
- ½ cup golden raisins

Direction:

1. Preheat the oven to 350ºF (180ºC). Have ready an 8 × 8-inch nonstick or silicone baking pan.

2. In a large bowl, whisk together the pumpkin purée, plant-based milk, maple syrup (if using), and vanilla. Add the cornstarch, salt (if using), cinnamon, ginger, nutmeg, allspice, and cloves and whisk well. Stir in the bread cubes and raisins, and toss to coat completely.

3. Transfer the mixture to the prepared pan. Bake for 25 minutes, or until the top is golden brown and firm to the touch. Serve warm.

Nutrition: Calories: 192 | fat: 1g | protein: 4g | carbs: 31g | fiber: 2g

615. Vanilla Corn Cake with Roasted Strawberries

Preparation time: 20 minutes
Cooking time: 50 minutes
Serving: 1 cake
Ingredients:

- ¾ cup full-fat coconut milk
- 1 teaspoon fresh lemon juice
- 1 cup cornmeal
- 1 cup whole spelt flour
- 1 teaspoon lemon zest
- 1 tablespoon aluminum-free baking powder
- ¼ teaspoon baking soda
- 1 teaspoon fine sea salt (optional)
- ½ teaspoon ground turmeric (optional)
- ½ cup plus 2 tablespoons pure maple syrup (optional)
- ½ cup coconut oil, plus extra to grease pan
- 1 teaspoon vanilla bean paste or pure vanilla extract
- 4 cups whole strawberries

Direction:

1. Preheat the oven to 350ºF (180ºC). Lightly grease a 9-inch round cake pan with coconut oil. Cut a circle of parchment paper to fit in the bottom of the pan

and press it in. Lightly grease the parchment, and set aside.

2. In a medium bowl, whisk together the coconut milk and lemon juice. Let this mixture sit for 5 minutes so that the milk can curdle slightly.

3. In a large bowl, whisk together the cornmeal, spelt flour, lemon zest, baking powder, baking soda, sea salt, and turmeric, if using.

4. Make a well in the center of the cornmeal mixture. Add the maple syrup, oil, if using, vanilla, and coconut milk mixture. With a spatula, gently mix until you have a smooth and unified batter. Avoid overmixing.

5. Scrape the batter into the prepared cake pan and slide the pan into the oven. Bake the cake for 25 to 28 minutes or until the top is golden and a toothpick inserted into the center comes out clean. Let the cake cool completely. Raise the oven temperature to 400ºF (205ºC).

6. Cut the strawberries into halves or quarters (depending on size), and place them on a parchment-lined baking sheet. Slide the baking sheet into the oven and roast the strawberries until they become juicy and jammy, about 20 minutes.

7. Serve slices of the corn cake with a few roasted strawberries.

Nutrition: Calories: 394 | fat: 20g | protein: 6g | carbs: 52g | fiber: 5g

616. Pumpkin Pie Oatmeal Parfaits

Preparation time: 20 minutes
Cooking time: 7 hours
Serving: 6 parfaits
Ingredients:

- Nonstick cooking spray (optional)
- 2 cups steel-cut oats
- 4 cups water
- 2 teaspoons ground cinnamon, divided
- 1 teaspoon ground nutmeg, divided
- ½ teaspoon ground cloves
- ½ teaspoon ground ginger
- 1½ cups rolled oats
- ¾ cup chopped pecans (optional)

Direction:

1. Coat the inside of the slow cooker with cooking spray (if using) or line it with a slow cooker liner.

Place the unopened can of coconut cream into the refrigerator to chill.

2. Add the steel-cut oats, water, pumpkin purée, 1 teaspoon of cinnamon, ½ teaspoon of nutmeg, the cloves, ginger, and maple syrup (if using). Stir to combine. Cover and cook on Low for 7 hours. After cooking, stir well.

3. Just before serving, pour the cold coconut cream into a medium bowl. Using an electric beater, whip the cream for about 1 minute, until it becomes thick.

5. For each parfait, layer 3 tablespoons of the crumble, about ½ teaspoon of the maple syrup (if using), 2 to 3 tablespoons of the warm pumpkin oatmeal, and about 2 tablespoons of the whipped cream. Continue layering in this order until your glass is full, finishing with the whipped cream on top, a sprinkle of the crumble, and a tiny drizzle more of maple syrup.

Nutrition: Calories: 497 | fat: 18g | protein: 11g | carbs: 76g | fiber: 10g

617.   Berry Chia Pudding

Preparation time: 5 minutes
Cooking time: 5 minutes
Serving: 3 cups
Ingredients:
- 4 cups fresh or frozen berries
- 1½ cups freshly squeezed orange juice
- Pinch of fine sea salt (optional)
- ½ cup raw cashews or macadamia nuts
- 2 tablespoons coconut butter
- 2 teaspoons vanilla extract
- 6 tablespoons chia seeds

Direction:
1. Combine the berries, orange juice, and salt, if using, in a medium pot and bring to a boil over high heat. Cover, reduce the heat to low, and simmer for 5 minutes, or until the berries have softened and released their juices. Remove from the heat and allow to cool slightly.

2. Transfer the mixture to an upright blender, add the cashews, coconut butter, and vanilla, and blend until completely smooth. Pour into a widemouthed quart jar or a medium bowl, add the chia seeds, and whisk thoroughly, making sure there are no clumps of seeds hiding anywhere. Allow to sit for a few minutes and then whisk again. Leave the whisk in place and refrigerate for at least 1 hour, or until completely

chilled, whisking every now and then to distribute the chia seeds evenly and to help cool the pudding quickly. The pudding will thicken further overnight; if it gets too thick, stir in a splash of water or nut milk. Store the pudding in an airtight glass jar or other container in the fridge for up to 5 days.

Nutrition: Calories: 211 | fat: 14g | protein: 2g | carbs: 21g | fiber: 5g

618.   Vanilla Bean Whip

Preparation time: 5 minutes
Cooking time: 0 minutes
Serving: 2 cups
Ingredients:
- ½ cup cashews, soaked overnight and drained
- ½ cup 100% pure maple syrup (optional)
- 2 tablespoons fresh lemon juice
- Pinch salt (optional)
- 1 vanilla bean

Direction:
1. Combine the tofu, cashews, maple syrup (if using), lemon juice, and salt (if using) in a blender. Purée until smooth. Scrape down the sides of the blender to incorporate all the ingredients.

2. Slice the vanilla bean in half lengthwise with a sharp knife and scrape the seeds into the blender. Blend the mixture until very smooth.

3. Transfer the mixture to a bowl and cover with plastic wrap. Chill for several hours in the refrigerator, or until firm.

Nutrition: Calories: 143 | fat: 6g | protein: 5g | carbs: 17g | fiber: 0g

619.   Pistachio Protein
Ice Cream

Preparation time: 25 minutes
Cooking time: 0 minutes
Serving: 8
Ingredients:
- 1 can low-fat coconut milk
- 2 scoops organic pea protein
- 1 tablespoon vanilla extract
- ½ cup shelled pistachios

Optional Toppings:

- Pomegranate seeds
- Fresh mint
- Chopped dark chocolate

Direction:

1. Add all ingredients to a blender and blend into a smooth mixture.
2. Alternatively, add all ingredients to a medium bowl, cover it, and process using a handheld blender.
3. Add any desired toppings and freeze for at least 2 hours.
5. Store the ice cream in the freezer for a maximum of 90 days and thaw for 5 minutes at room temperature before serving.

Nutrition: Calories: 115 | fat: 4g | protein: 9g | carbs: 10g | fiber: 2g

620. Blackberry Lemon Muffins

Preparation Time: 11 minutes
Cooking Time: 31 minutes
Serving: 6
Ingredients

- 1 cup All-purpose flour
- ¾ cup Whole Wheat flour
- ½ cup granulated sugar
- 2 tablespoons baking powder
- ½ tablespoon baking soda
- 1 tablespoon Grated lemon or orange peel
- 1 and a ½ cups Coffee Rich
- ½ cup Margarine (Melted)
- 2 egg whites
- 1 cup Fresh or frozen unsweetened blackberries

Direction

1. Preheat oven to 375 F.
2. Incorporate flours with sugar, baking powder, baking soda, and lemon peel.
3. In a medium bowl, whisk Coffee Rich® with margarine and egg whites until blended. Stir Coffee Rich® mixture into flour mixture just until combined.
4. Fold in blackberries.
5. Scoop batter into lightly greased, paper lined muffin tins.
6. Bake for 21 minutes.

Nutrition: 564 calories 13g protein 40mg potassium 161mg sodium

621. Quick Canned Pear Dessert

Preparation Time: 9 minutes
Cooking Time: 15 minutes
Serving: 4
Ingredients

- cup unsifted flour
- ¼ cup Sugar
- ¼ cup unsalted Butter or Margarine
- 3 cups canned pears
- 2 tablespoons Lemon juice
- ¼ cup Sherry
- ¼ tsp. Nutmeg

Direction

1. Preheat oven to 350 0F
2. In a medium bowl, mix flour and sugar together.
3. Using two knives or pastry blender, slice margarine or butter and flour until mixture is crumbly.
4. Set aside. Drain canned pears.
5. Place sliced pears into a well-greased 9-inch pie plate.
6. Drizzle fruit with lemon juice, sherry and nutmeg; dust flour mixture over top.
7. Bake for 15 minutes

Nutrition: 399 calories 16g protein 31mg potassium 144mg sodium

622.   Basic Vanilla Chia Pudding

Preparation time: 5 minutes
Cooking time: 0 minutes
Serving: 4
Ingredients:

- 1 cup almond milk
- 1 tablespoon coconut sugar (optional)
- 1 teaspoon vanilla bean powder
- Pinch of salt (optional)

Direction:
1. Whisk all the ingredients together in a medium bowl. Stir every few minutes until thickened, about 15 minutes. Serve, or refrigerate for up to 48 hours.
Nutrition: Calories: 153 | fat: 14g | protein: 5g | carbs: 14g | fiber: 6g

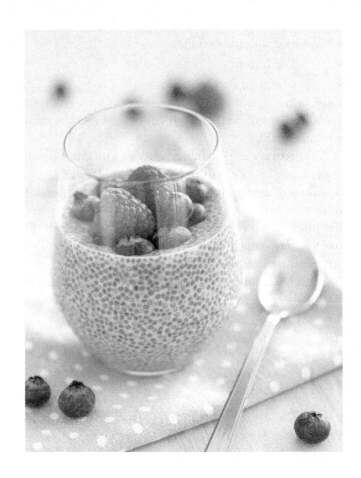

Chapter 15. Four-Week Meal Plan

First Week

Day	Breakfast	Lunch	Dinner
Day-1	Frankenstein Avocado Toast	Savory Collard Chips	Tofu Greek Salad
Day-2	Showy Avocado Toast	Roasted Red Pepper Hummus	Eggplant Arugula Salad
Day-3	Almond Butter Toast with Sweet Potatoes and Blueberries	Thai-Style Eggplant Dip	Cauliflower Salad
Day-4	Oatmeal Seasoned with Vegetables	Collard Salad Rolls with Peanut Dipping Sauce	Kale Sprouts Salad
Day-5	Pumpkin and Spice Oatmeal	Simple Roasted Broccoli	Broccoli Salad
Day-6	Fruit and Nut Oatmeal	Roasted Mint Carrots	Tempeh Caprese Salad
Day-7	Flaxseed Pancakes	Vegetable Couscous	Apple & Spinach Salad

Second Week

Day	Breakfast	Lunch	Dinner
Day-8	Savory Zucchini Pancakes	Veggie Kabobs	Mixed Berries Salad
Day-9	Beginnings with Sweet Potato	Nutty Brussels Sprout	Beet & Spinach Salad
Day-10	Oatmeal Breakfast Muffins	Vegetable Kebab	Cucumber & Tomato Salad
Day-11	Cherry and Poppy Seed Muffins	Golden Eggplant Fries	Zucchini & Tomato Salad
Day-12	Brown Rice Breakfast Pudding with Dates	Very Wild Mushroom Pilaf	Quinoa, Bean, & Mango Salad
Day-13	Quinoa With Berries	Sporty Baby Carrots	Quinoa & Veggie Salad
Day-14	Breakfast Scramble	Saucy Garlic Greens	Red Beans & Corn Salad

Third Week

Day	Breakfast	Lunch	Dinner
Day-15	Parmesan Zucchini Frittata	Garden Salad	Quinoa & Veggie Salad
Day-16	Apple Cinnamon Rings	Spicy Cabbage Dish	Red Beans & Corn Salad
Day-17	Yogurt Bulgur	Quinoa with Mushrooms	Chickpeas & Veggie Salad
Day-18	Deviled Eggs	Couscous Stuffed Bell Peppers	Peaches, Peas, and Beans Summer Salad
Day-19	Goat Cheese Omelet	Tantalizing Cauliflower and Dill Mash	Shaved Root Salad with Crispy Lentils
Day-20	Breakfast Potato Latkes With Spinach	Peas Soup	Lentil, Lemon and Mushroom Salad
Day-21	Easy Turnip Puree	Enjoyable Green Lettuce and Bean medley	Bulgur Lettuce Cups

Fourth Week

Day	Breakfast	Lunch	Dinner
Day-22	Gentle Apple Porridge	Kale and Garlic Platter	Pineapple Meringues
Day-23	Simple Granola Platter	Blistered Beans and Almond	Baked Custard
Day-24	Delicious Apple and Cinnamon Oatmeal	Cucumber Soup	Strawberry Pie
Day-25	Avocado Toast	Eggplant Salad	Apple Crisp
Day-26	Vegan Pancakes	Cajun Crab	Almond Cookies
Day-27	Oatmeal Soaks with Goji Berries	Mushroom Pork Chops	Lime Pie
Day-28	Cheesy Scrambled Eggs with Fresh Herbs	Caramelized Pork Chops	Buttery Lemon Squares

Conclusion

A renal diet is an eating regimen that helps to prevent and control kidney disease while also protecting the kidneys from additional harm. Maintaining a healthy renal diet is essential because it helps our body manage waste and clear the buildup of toxins in the kidneys. With good maintenance, we can live much longer and happier lives with less pain. I hope this article has helped to understand better renal diet and how it works so you can be proactive about your health now or in the future!

It is best to maintain a healthy, balanced diet to keep your kidneys healthy rather than significantly changing your diet unless your healthcare expert suggests it. This can help you avoid any adverse health complications. Your food options should be based on various foods, including vegetables, fruits, whole grains, and protein sources such as lean meats and eggs. Reducing sodium intake through minimizing salt and salting foods at the table can also prevent kidney complications.

Certain fruits and vegetables like beets and cranberries that contain high amounts of oxalates have increased calcium crystals within the kidneys. Doctors recommend that patients with acute or chronic kidney failure avoid these foods as much as possible. At this time, there isn't enough data to suggest avoiding other vegetables and fruits that don't contain oxalates.

Doctors recommend having a diet that includes a variety of food choices, such as drinking plenty of water and eating five or more servings of fruits and vegetables each day. Reducing sodium intake through minimizing salt and salting foods at the table can also help prevent kidney complications. It is also essential to eat only one or two servings of high-protein foods each day, including lean meats, poultry, fish, eggs, beans, nuts, seeds, soy products, etc. These foods are best consumed in moderation rather than being wholly avoided to maintain kidney health.

The best way to preserve kidney health, according to the National Institute of Diabetes and Digestive and Kidney Diseases, is to consume a nutritious diet that includes a variety of foods. However, undergoing dialysis or a kidney transplant may be recommended if this is not feasible. Depending on your specific health needs, using a special diet for kidney health may be an option.

Made in United States
Orlando, FL
06 April 2022

16576075R00128